AF616162

Medical Intelligence Unit

Pancreatic Islet Transplantation Volume II:

Immunomodulation of Pancreatic Islets

Editors:

Robert P. Lanza, M.D.

William L. Chick, M.D.

BioHybrid Technologies Inc.
Shrewsbury, Massachusetts
U.S.A.

R.G. Landes Company
Austin

Medical Intelligence Unit

PANCREATIC ISLET TRANSPLANTATION VOLUME II:
IMMUNOMODULATION OF PANCREATIC ISLETS

R.G. LANDES COMPANY
Austin

CRC Press is the exclusive worldwide distributor of publications of the Medical Intelligence Unit.
CRC Press, 2000 Corporate Blvd., NW, Boca Raton, FL 33431. Phone: 407/994-0555.

Submitted: May 1994
Published: July 1994

Please address all inquiries to the Publisher:
R.G. Landes Company, 909 Pine Street, Georgetown, TX 78626
or
P.O. Box 4858, Austin, TX 78765
Phone: 512/ 863 7762; FAX: 512/ 863 0081

ISBN 1-57059-134-2
Series ISBN 1-57059-179-2
CATALOG # LN9134

While the authors, editors and publisher believe that drug selection and dosage and the specifications and usage of equipment and devices, as set forth in this book, are in accord with current recommendations and practice at the time of publication, they make no warranty, expressed or implied, with respect to material described in this book. In view of the ongoing research, equipment development, changes in governmental regulations and the rapid accumulation of information relating to the biomedical sciences, the reader is urged to carefully review and evaluate the information provided herein.

Library of Congress Cataloging-in-Publication Data

Pancreatic islet transplantation series / editors, Robert P. Lanza, William L. Chick.
p. cm.—(Medical intelligence unit)
Includes bibliographical references and index.
Contents: v. 1. Procurement of pancreatic islets—v. 2. Immunomodulation of pancreatic islets—v. 3. Immunoisolation of pancreatic islets.
ISBN 1–57059–133–4 (v. 1).—ISBN 1–57059–134–2 (v. 2).—ISBN 1–57059–135–0 (v. 3)
1. Islands of Langerhans—Transplantation. 2. Diabetes—Surgery.
I. Lanza, R.P. (Robert Paul), 1956– . II. Chick, William L. (William Louis), 1938– . III. Series.
[DNLM: 1. Islets of Langerhans Transplantaiton. 2. Pancreas—immunology. 3. Islets of Langerhans—immunology. 4. Organ Procurement. 5. Tissue Culture. WK 800 P188 1994]
RD599.5. I84P36 1994
617.5'570592—dc20
DNLM/DLC 94-25951
for Library of Congress CIP

To Our Readers

R.G. Landes Company publishes four book series: *Medical Intelligence Unit, Molecular Biology Intelligence Unit, Neuroscience Intelligence Unit,* and *Biotechnology Intelligence Unit.* Our goal is to publish the most recent information in biomedical science for sophisticated researchers and physicians.

To achieve this goal we have accelerated our publishing program to conform to the fast pace in which information grows in biomedical science. The book you have in hand, like all titles in our series, was published *90 to 120 days within receipt of the manuscript.*

As you might expect, this causes a few problems for us; sometimes it makes our office more like a big city newspaper than a scholarly publisher. So as you look through this book you may see something that isn't just right. Please let us know. Or if you have an idea for improving our books, we'd like very much to hear from you. If the problem you describe hasn't already been discovered or if your idea is provocative enough to promote a discussion here, we'll give you a free book of your choice. Just list three titles in order of preference and we'll send you one, based on availability—with our thanks. Our address is printed on the copyright page of each of our books.

Elinda McKenna
Director of Operations
R.G. Landes Company

Dedicated to the memory of Elinor Sara Chick DeLuca,

beloved sister and special friend

and to

Eugene O'Donnell,

for his inspiration and example.

CONTENTS

CONTENTS

CONTENTS

EDITORS

Robert P. Lanza, M.D.
Director, Transplantation Biology
BioHybrid Technologies Inc., Shrewsbury, Massachusetts, USA
and
Clinical Associate Professor of Surgery, Tufts University
North Grafton, Massachusetts USA

William L. Chick, M.D.
President and Scientific Director
BioHybrid Technologies Inc., Shrewsbury, Massachusetts USA

CONTRIBUTORS

Eleni S. Athan, Ph.D.
Department of Surgery
Columbia University College of Physicians and Surgeons
New York, New York, USA
Chapter 10

Clyde F. Barker, M.D.
Professor and Chairman
Department of Surgery
University of Pennsylvania School of Medicine
Philadelphia, Pennsylvania, USA
Chapter 8

Pierre Y. Benhamou, M.D., Ph.D.
Research Fellow
UCLA Islet Transplant Program
Diabetes Research Center
UCLA School of Medicine
Los Angeles, California, USA
Chapter 9

Louis Campos, M.D.
Post-Doctoral Fellow
Harrison Department of Surgical Research
University of Pennsylvania School of Medicine
Philadelphia, Pennsylvania, USA
Chapter 8

Charles B. Carpenter, M.D.
Professor of Medicine
Harvard Medical School
Director of Immunogenetics and Transplantation
Brigham and Women's Hospital
Boston, Massachusetts, USA
Chapter 13

Margaret J. Dallman, D.Phil.
University of Oxford
Nuffield Department of Surgery
John Radcliffe Hospital
Oxford, United Kingdom
Chapter 4

CONTRIBUTORS

Barbara C. Deli, B.A.
University of Pennsylvania School of Medicine
Philadelphia, Pennsylvania, USA
Chapter 8

Denise Faustman, M.D., Ph.D.
Director, Immunobiology Laboratories
Massachusetts General Hospital
Assistant Professor of Medicine
Harvard Medical School
Boston, Massachusetts, USA
Chapter 11

Carl G. Figdor, M.D.
Professor
Tumor Immunology
University Hospital Nijmegen St. Radboud
Nijmegen, The Netherlands
Chapter 5

Elliot R. Goodman, M.D.
Department of Surgery
Columbia University College of Physicians and Surgeons
New York, New York, USA
Chapter 10

Paul F. Gores, M.D.
Associate Professor of Surgery
University of Minnesota Medical School
Minneapolis, Minnesota, USA
Chapter 6

Mark A. Hardy, M.D.
Auchincloss Professor of Surgery
Director of Organ Transplantation
Department of Surgery
Columbia University College of Physicians and Surgeons
New York, New York, USA
Chapter 10

David M. Harlan, M.D.
Immune Cell Biology Program
Naval Medical Research Institute
Department of Medicine
Uniformed Services University of the Health Sciences
Bethesda, Maryland, USA
Chapter 12

Carl H. June, M.D.
Director, Immunobiology
Naval Medical Research Institute
Department of Medicine
Uniformed Services University of the Health Sciences
Bethesda, Maryland, USA
Chapter 12

Y. van Kooyk, Ph.D.
Tumor Immunology
University Hospital Nijmegen
Nijmegen, The Netherlands
Chapter 5

CONTRIBUTORS

Andrew I. Lazarovits, M.D., F.R.C.P.C.
Director, Renal Transplantation
University Hospital
John P. Robarts Research Institute
and Associate Professor of Medicine
Microbiology and Immunology
University of Western Ontario
London, Ontario, Canada
Chapter 2

George L. Mayo, M.D., Ph.D.
University of Pennsylvania School of Medicine
Philadelphia, Pennsylvania, USA
Chapter 8

Yoko Mullen, M.D., Ph. D.
Director, UCLA Islet Transplant Program, Department of Surgery
UCLA School of Medicine
Los Angeles, California, USA
Chapter 9

Ali Naji, M.D., Ph.D.
J. William White Professor of Surgery
University of Pennsylvania School of Medicine
Philadelphia, Pennsylvania, USA
Chapter 8

Soji F. Oluwole, M.D.
Associate Professor of Surgery
Department of Surgery
Columbia University College of Physicians and Surgeons
New York, New York, USA
Chapter 10

Leendert C. Paul, M.D., Ph.D., F.R.C.P.
Keenan Professor of Medicine
University of Toronto
Director, Renal Division
St. Michael's Hospital
30 Bond Street
Toronto, Ontario, Canada
Chapter 3

Andrew M. Posselt, M.D., Ph.D.
Instructor, Department of Medicine
University of California
San Francisco, California, USA
Chapter 8

Mohamed H. Sayegh, M.D.
Assistant Professor of Medicine
Harvard Medical School
Brigham and Women's Hospital
Boston, Massachusetts, USA
Chapter 13

Helena P. Selawry, M.D., Ph.D.
Professor of Medicine
Department of Veterans Affairs Medical Center
Memphis, Tennessee, USA
Chapter 7

David E. R. Sutherland, M.D., Ph.D.
Professor of Surgery
University of Minnesota Medical School
Minneapolis, Minnesota, USA
Chapter 6

CONTRIBUTORS

Francis T. Thomas, M.D.
Professor of Surgery
Division of Transplantation
Department of Surgery
East Carolina University School of Medicine
Greenville, North Carolina, USA
Chapter 14

Lee Anne Tibbles, M.D., F.R.C.P.C.
Nephrology Subspecialty Resident
John P. Robarts Research Institute
University Hospital
The University of Western Ontario
London, Ontario, Canada
Chapter 2

Howard L. Weiner, M.D.
Robert L. Kroz Chair in Neurologic Disease
Director, Multiple Sclerosis Program and
Co-Director, Center for Neurologic Diseases,
Brigham and Women's Hospital and
Harvard Medical School
Boston, Massachusetts, USA
Chapter 13

Kathryn J. Wood, D. Phil.
Lecturer in Immunology
University of Oxford
Nuffield Department of Surgery
John Radcliffe Hospital
Oxford, United Kingdom
Chapter 1

FOREWORD

In 1949, Jacobsen and colleagues reported that mice could survive otherwise lethal irradiation if the spleen were protected by a lead shield. Shortly thereafter, Lorenz and co-workers showed that the same irradiation-protection could be achieved by an infusion of marrow cells. In 1955, Ford et al used cytogenetics to demonstrate that the marrow of an irradiated mouse protected by an infusion of marrow cells contained cells of donor, not host, origin. These experiments marked the beginning of the field of cell transplantation.

The field of solid organ transplantation had its beginning at almost the same time. In 1959, Schwartz and Damasek reported that 6–mercaptopurine was an immunosuppressive agent that could confer a form of tolerance. Following this demonstration, Hitchings and Ilion developed imuran and Murray and Starzl and colleagues used these immunosuppressive agents along with superb surgical skills to open up the field of transplantation of kidney, heart and liver.

During the following two decades marrow grafting was applied with increasing success to diseases such as aplastic anemia, leukemia and a series of genetic diseases. The increasing knowledge of human histocompatibility typing, additional immunosuppressive agents and improved supportive care made possible the progress.

Yet, until quite recently transplantation of hematopoietic progenitor cells was the only form of cell transplantation being actively pursued. It had been known for more than 15 years that marrow grafting also involved grafting of donor pulmonary macrophages and Kupffer cells. Recently, Starzl and colleagues demonstrated that solid organ transplants also involved systemic "microchimerism" of donor cells, presumably dendritic cells. Clearly, transplantation of cells other than marrow stem cells can be achieved. Why not transplant other cells needed because of disease — liver cells, pancreatic islet cells, glial cells?

This series of presentations focuses on the transplantation of pancreatic islet cells. Despite the wealth of knowledge about diabetes and the availability of recombinant insulin, diabetes remains a major scourge of mankind. The present series demonstrates the wealth of scientific technology being brought to bear on the possibility of therapy by islet cell transplantation. Although the problem is formidable, progress in science often occurs with great rapidity. The investigators reporting here are to be congratulated on their vision and resourcefulness to insure continued progress in developing improved treatment for diabetics.

E. Donnall Thomas, M.D.

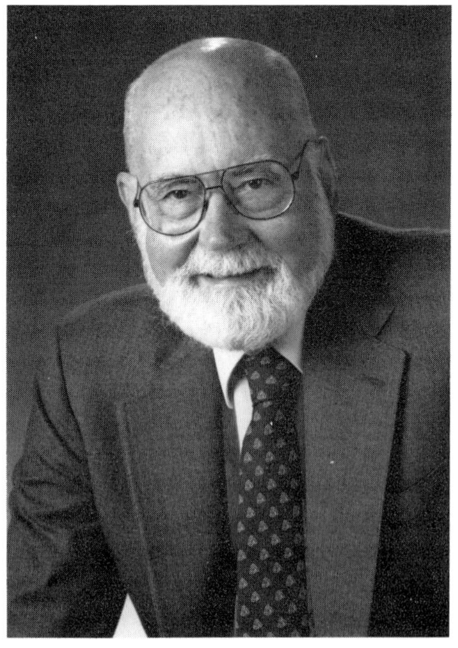

E. Donnall Thomas, M.D.
Nobel Laureate 1990

Dr. Thomas is one of the pioneers who ushered in the modern era of cell transplantation. In 1956, he performed the first human marrow transplant and was the first to treat acute leukemia by bone marrow transplantation while working at the Mary Imogene Bassett Hospital in Cooperstown, New York.

PREFACE

The modern era of clinical cell transplantation was ushered in approximately 40 years ago when E. Donnall Thomas performed his pioneering work using bone marrow transplantation as a therapy for leukemia. At approximately the same time, Joseph Murray and colleagues performed the first successful long-term renal transplant between identical twins at the Peter Bent Brigham Hospital in Boston. This technology was subsequently extended to transplantation between more distantly related and unrelated kidney donors through the use of immunosuppressive drugs such as imuran and glucocorticoids and more recently cyclosporin A. To date, almost 400,000 patients worldwide have received life sustaining renal transplants.

Medical applications of transplantation technology have grown significantly during the past decade to include pancreas, heart and liver. In addition to transplanting whole organs, isolation and transplantation of cells and tissues with specific differentiated functions (e.g., beta cells which secrete insulin) represents an important conceptual and technological advance. It is readily apparent that transplantation of organs, tissues and cells into patients with a wide variety of serious disorders will constitute a major segment of the health care industry over the next several decades. The potential economic impacts of transplantation as a treatment for human disease are enormous given the fact that the cost of a renal transplant is presently $35,000, while heart and liver transplants fall in the $100,000 to $200,000 range.

Further advancement and wider application of tissue and cell transplantation will require solving several problems including development of new strategies to overcome present formidable obstacles and to simplify implantation procedures. These problems include: (1) requirements for immunosuppressive drugs which expose patients to a wide variety of serious complications including cancer, infection, renal failure and osteoporosis; (2) lack of sufficient human donor tissue, which is so severe that patients may die while awaiting procurement of a matched donor organ; (3) requirements for extensive surgery such as transplantation of the whole pancreas with vascular anastomoses in diabetics when only 1-2% of the tissue produces insulin.

Solution of these problems would open the door to widespread practical applications of cell and tissue transplantation. Diabetes mellitus is likely to be the initial major disease to which these advances will be applied for several reasons: (1) pancreatic islet transplantation is an area of current intense investigation, and would demonstrate improved treatment of a disorder currently affecting 80 million diabetics worldwide, at an estimated $92 billion annual cost for health care and lost wages in the U.S. alone; (2) pancreatic islets can be isolated from a wide variety of animal sources; animal insulins are fully active in man and have been used to treat diabetics for 70 years; and, (3) the quantity of differentiated islet tissue to be transplanted is within a reasonable range (<1 g).

The last several years of research and technology development have produced a dramatic advancement in islet isolation techniques, and in our knowledge of the human immune system, autoimmune disease, and immune rejection processes. This has resulted in a reliable source of human and animal islets, and in the development of procedures for immune modulation and immune isolation of donor islets that have the potential for preventing rejection of islet allografts and islet xenografts in patients without need for a life long regimen of generalized immunosuppression. This remarkable progress has furnished the stimulus for this series.

It appears increasingly likely that as we approach the 21st century islet transplantation will assume increasing importance as a treatment for diabetes. The resultant improvements in glycemic control will serve to prevent or to greatly retard the development of the dreaded complications of this disease which have claimed the health and life of millions.

We wish to express our indebtedness and gratitude to all our coauthors, who generously contributed their time and knowledge in the preparation of this series.We also thank Ms. Kathy Vairo for her valuable secretarial assistance.

March 1994
Robert P. Lanza, M.D.
William L. Chick, M.D.

CHAPTER 1

Approaches to Achieving Tolerance

Kathryn J. Wood

When T cells encounter any foreign antigen they make a choice as to how they will respond. One of three possible courses of action are available to the cell, activation, indifference or inactivation irrespective of the nature of the antigen to which the cells are responding (Fig. 1.1). Nominal, allo- and xeno-antigens will all cause a T cell or cells capable of recognizing the antigen to choose one of these three options.

Activation is arguably the most frequent outcome following the interaction of a T cell with its antigen presented by an APC following transplantation, unless active steps, such as the administration of immunosuppressive drugs, are taken to prevent it (for a detailed discussion of T cell activation see a general immunology text such as[1] and chapter 2 of this volume). If the interaction between the antigen and its TCR is of sufficient affinity and the other essential molecular interactions between the APC and the T cell occur (Fig. 1.2), the T cell will be activated as a result of the encounter. A T cell requires at least two signals for full activation.[2] The first, signal 1, is delivered as a result of the interaction between the antigen and TCR and is transmitted by the CD3 molecule. This signal may be reinforced by the interaction of a number of different accessory molecules with the appropriate ligand expressed by the APC. For example if the T cell recognizes antigen in association with a major histocompatibility complex (MHC) class II molecule, in other words is class II restricted, the CD4 molecule will bind to the β_2 domain of the MHC class II molecule expressed by the APC[3] and a signal will be delivered to the T cell via $p56^{lck}$, a tyrosine kinase associated with the cytoplasmic domain of CD4.[4] CD8 fulfils a similar role for MHC class I restricted T cells. However, none of these interactions can deliver the critical second signal, signal 2, to the cell. This can only be transmitted following the interaction of the T cell surface molecule, CD28 with one of its ligands, e.g. B7, on the APC.[5,6] T cell activation then ensues and results in (i) the induction of genes not expressed by the cell in its resting state, for example CD25 the α chain of the interleukin-2 receptor (IL-2R) as well as the cytokine it binds, IL-2; (ii) transformation of the cell into a T cell blast and eventually (iii) clonal expansion of the cell by cell division. Activation of T cells is clearly the most effective course of action when the immune

Pancreatic Islet Transplantation Volume II: Immunomodulation of Pancreatic Islets, edited by Robert P. Lanza, MD, William L. Chick, MD; ©1994 R.G. Landes Company.

system is dealing with an invading pathogen. However, in the context of transplantation T cell activation will lead to the destruction of the transplanted tissue and is therefore highly undesirable.

The second possible outcome is that the T cell feigns indifference following the antigen encounter. This scenario can result if, for example, the affinity of the interaction between T cell receptor (TCR)/CD3 complex expressed by the responding cell and antigen is too low to trigger signal transduction. Indifference may also occur when the overall avidity of the interaction between the T cell and antigen presenting cell (APC) is too low. This situation can arise when the appropriate interactions between T cell accessory molecules and their ligands expressed by the APC, including for example the interaction between LFA-1 (CD58) and ICAM-1 (CD11a/18), do not occur. Indifference to one antigen encounter does not necessarily mean that subsequent encounters will be treated in the same way, as we will see below.

The third possible result of a T cell encountering its antigen is inactivation of the cell. Inactivation of the responding cell can take more than one guise, the most final of which is elimination or deletion of the cell from the repertoire. T cell deletion occurs most commonly during the induction of tolerance to self antigens during ontogeny.[7] Less final, but nevertheless effective, is the functional inactivation of the responding cell, such that when it encounters the same antigen for a second time it is no longer capable of responding.[8] For the induction of tolerance to an organ graft of any type, this is clearly the most desirable outcome any encounter between a recipient's T cells and donor antigen. Functional inactivation of a T cell results from a suboptimal encounter between the T cell and the APC such that a negative rather than a positive signal is delivered to the T cell causing it to be switched off rather than on. Suboptimal encounters can occur in a number of different ways but probably the best documented is when a T cell receives the correct signal following engagement of TCR, signal 1, but subsequently fails to receive signal 2.[9,10] Thus if the APC fails to express a ligand for CD28 it will not be able to deliver the second signal and therefore the T cell will be inactivated.[11] Alternatively, deliberate intervention to inhibit the interaction of CD28 and its ligands can pre-

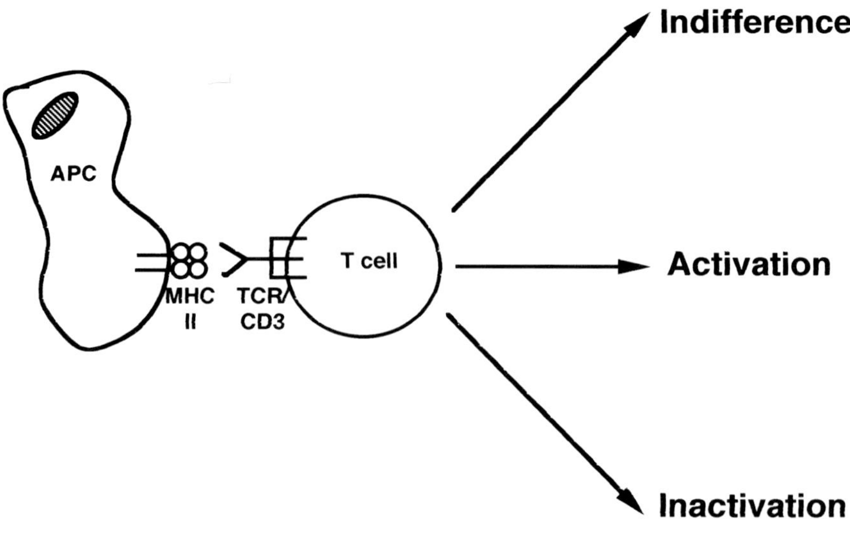

Fig. 1.1. Possible T cell responses following antigen recognition.

vent the delivery of the second signal and turn the responding T cell off. This is not the only strategy to prevent T cell activation. Inhibiting other molecular interactions, such as that between CD4 and the class II molecule or LFA-1 and ICAM-1, can result in the T cell failing to receive all of the signals it requires resulting in its inactivation. A further mechanism for inactivating the responding T cell is to deliver a suboptimal version of signal 1 through the TCR itself. This can occur if the T cell interacts with a modified version of its antigen it is capable of recognizing. This situation has been demonstrated in vitro for T cells that recognize nominal antigens as peptides in association with an MHC molecule, where a single amino acid change in the peptide presented has been shown to render the T cell incapable of responding to the correct peptide in a subsequent encounter.[12] However, to date this has not been shown for allo- or xeno-antigens, but these data suggest an intriguing strategy that may be applicable for the inactivation of T cells capable of responding to allo- or xeno-antigens.

Increasing the immunological specificity of the immunosuppressive therapy that is used to prevent the rejection of transplanted tissues is one of the fundamental aims of research designed to develop new approaches for the prevention of graft rejection. The final objective of work in this area is to identify a strategy for the induction of transplantation tolerance in vivo which would result in the immune system of a transplant recipient becoming specifically unresponsive to the foreign histocompatibility antigens of the organ or tissue donor. This can only be achieved if immunosuppressive therapy targets the leukocytes capable of responding to the foreign histocompatibility antigens expressed by the transplanted tissue and not those capable of responding to other antigens. As T cells are essential for the rejection response (see chapter 2, this volume), it is the T cell and its interaction with the APC that holds the key to the induction of transplantation tolerance. If the T cell can either be prevented from recognizing the stimulating antigen or switched off as a result of the antigen encounter, unresponsiveness will dominate.

A strategy that allowed the immune system to be manipulated or reprogrammed in such a way as to induce specific immunological unresponsiveness or tolerance to the allo-, or in the future, xeno-antigens of the tissue donor would offer many advantages over the immunosuppressive drug therapy currently used in clinical transplantation. Strategies targeting only leukocytes reactive with donor antigens would be affected by the therapy leaving those capable of responding to other antigens unaffected. Transplant recipients would therefore be able to respond effectively to other immunological stimuli they encounter after transplantation as the remainder of the T cell repertoire would be unaffected. Furthermore, if it proved possible to reprogram the immune system permanently, once tolerance was established immunosuppressive therapy would no longer be required to maintain the survival of the transplanted tissue. The non-immunological side effects associated with the long-term administration of immunosuppressive drug therapy would therefore also be eliminated.

This all sounds wonderful in theory, but is there any information to suggest that it is possible to induce tolerance to donor antigens in vivo? The first indication that exposing the immune system to foreign antigens could lead to a state of immunological tolerance, came from observation of twins born from a common placenta, so-called Freemartin cattle. Such cattle were able to accept skin grafts donated by the other twin permanently. Tolerance was thought to arise as a result of mixing of 'blood cells' between the twins in utero.[13,14] Medawar and his colleagues then showed that this same phenomenon could be induced deliberately if mice were treated with semi-allogeneic lymphocytes within 24 hours of birth.[15] The immaturity of the recipient's immune system was key to the establishment of tolerance in both of these situations. The induction of tolerance in an adult where the immune system is already fully developed and the T cell repertoire established represents a much more challenging, although not impossible task.

One of many lessons that have been learned from these pioneering experiments is that if it were possible to revert the immune system to a more immature state, it may be relatively more straightforward to induce tolerance to donor antigens. Many approaches for tolerance induction have attempted to exploit this observation (see below). However, complete ablation of the immune system would result in the recipient becoming severely immunocompromised. As understanding of the immune response to transplanted tissues has developed, experimental data have shown that it may not be necessary to ablate the immune system in adult recipients before introducing donor antigens completely to facilitate the induction of tolerance. It may be possible to target strategically certain components of the response to promote the induction of tolerance.

Much experimental work is currently in progress exploring new approaches for the induction of specific unresponsiveness to, for the most part alloantigens in adult recipients, although work exploring strategies for tolerance induction to xenoantigens is also underway.[16] The approaches under investigation can be divided into two broad categories. The first including strategies designed to induce unresponsiveness in the long-term after transplantation and the second those aiming to achieve what is often described as 'the ultimate goal', by attempting to make recipients unresponsive to the donor from the time the tissue is transplanted. Strategies that fit into the former category accept that the immunosuppressive therapy selected will lack immunological specificity in the early post-transplantation period, but that it will create an environment that will allow immunological unresponsiveness to the transplanted tissue to emerge in the long-term. If this could be achieved clinically it would represent a major step forward over conventional immunosuppressive strategies currently in clinical use. Not least, it should allow the dose of each of the non-specific immunosuppressive drugs to be reduced and ultimately withdrawn without compromising the survival of the transplanted tissue thereby eliminating the nonimmunological side effects associated with the long-term administration of non-specific immunosuppressive drug therapy. Strategies that fall into the second category are clearly aiming higher, as the induction of unresponsiveness to donor antigens before transplantation will require the reprogramming of an immune system that is already fully developed in adult recipients awaiting transplantation.

Those who think that the induction of specific unresponsiveness even in the long-term after transplantation is ambitious in the clinical setting should remember that there are a small number of cases reported in the clinical literature where unresponsiveness, and in some cases tolerance, to an organ graft has developed. In some of these cases patients simply stopped taking their immunosuppressive drugs, non-compliance, but in others the drug dose has been reduced in a controlled way under the supervision of the transplant team, without the patient losing their graft. One of the best documented series being in patients who received total lymphoid irradiation (TLI) before kidney transplantation.[17] These cases highlight the fact that it is possible to induce tolerance to a graft in the clinical setting. The critical question that remains to be answered is whether the adult immune system can be manipulated to facilitate the reliable induction of a state of unresponsive to the alloantigens presented by the tissue donor?

Islets of Langerhans may offer a unique opportunity for developing a strategy for the induction of tolerance in clinical transplantation as they can be manipulated more easily than whole organ grafts before transplantation. This may allow several approaches for the induction of tolerance to be linked together resulting in a more effective approach for this to be investigated in the clinical setting. Furthermore, the opportunities for encapsulation of the islet tissue to protect it from the hostile immunological environment within the recipient (discussed in volume 3 of this series) may allow tolerance to islet grafts to be more easily achieved.

In this chapter I will simply outline some of the approaches for tolerance induction that are currently being explored in experimental models of transplantation. Detailed discussions of many of the approaches I will mention will be provided by other chapters in this volume.

STRATEGIES FOR TOLERANCE INDUCTION

Reduction of Tissue Immunogenicity Before Transplantation

Presentation of the same antigen by different cell types has a different outcome depending on the activation state of the responding T cell. In a primary immune response activation of a resting T cell can most efficiently be accomplished by a dendritic cell.[18] Activated B cells can also trigger T cell activation, but higher numbers of cells are required to achieve an equivalent response. Both dendritic cells and activated B cells express molecules capable of interacting with CD28.[5,6] In contrast, in secondary responses, previously activated T cells can be restimulated by a variety of APCs providing they express the appropriate antigen molecule. APCs for secondary responses include resting B cells, macrophages and epithelial cells. Thus different populations of leukocytes resident within a graft may have a different capacity of activating a rejection response, depending on the status of the recipient. Some leukocytes, such as resting B cells, may also be able to turn T cells off;[19] an observation that merits further examination.

Removal or inactivation of resident leukocytes, most commonly referred to as passenger leukocytes, before transplantation should therefore reduce the immunogenicity of the transplanted tissue; a theory that has been in the literature for some time.[20,21] Different strategies for pretreating isolated islet tissue before transplantation have been reported in the literature. These include, culturing the islets in 95% oxygen[22] or at low temperatures,[23] treating the islets with antibodies to remove the dendritic cells[24] or exposing the islets to UVB irradiation[25] before transplantation. In experimental systems, pretreatment of islets using these approaches has proved successful in facilitating acceptance of the graft.

Interestingly, although pretreatment of the islets using these strategies alters the immunogenicity of the graft, the antigenicity of the tissue is unaffected. Thus passenger depleted islet grafts will not initiate a rejection response, but if the immune system of the recipient is activated deliberately by challenging with leukocytes or a skin graft from the same strain of animal as the islet donor, rejection of both recently transplanted and established islet grafts will occur.[26,27] Thus, this approach appears to result in antigen reactive T cells becoming indifferent to the transplanted islet tissue, rather than inactivated and may therefore not provide the permanent state of unresponsiveness that would be desirable.

Manipulation of the Antigen Presenting Cells

Approaches designed to prevent effective presentation of donor antigens after transplantation are currently being explored in experimental models of islet transplantation. These approaches utilize either monoclonal antibodies (mabs) or genetically engineered recombinant molecules to prevent adhesion or, probably more effectively, signalling between the APC and the responding T cell.

Mabs provide an effective means of targeting cell surface molecules specifically in vivo. As the name suggests, a monoclonal antibody is produced by a single clone of B cells that has been immortalized in vitro and that will theoretically produce antibodies with a single defined antigen specificity forever. Mabs can be used as therapeutic agents to manipulate immune responses, including graft rejection, in vivo.[28] A large body of work also suggests that they may be an effective way of manipulating the immune system to promote the induction of tolerance to donor antigens.

As the characterisation of molecules expressed by both APC and T cells proceeds, potential candidate molecules that may allow the initiation of an immune response to be prevented have been highlighted. With respect to the APC, probably highest on the list at present, with the exception of B7 and other related ligands for CD28 or CTLA-4, are the adhesion molecules (for review see[29,30]). Experimental work using mabs specific for adhesion molecules in vivo is still in its infancy and will be reviewed in depth later in this volume (see Figdor and van Kooyk, chapter 5). However, preliminary data using strategies targeting ICAM-1 (CD54) and VLA-4 (CD49d/29) either alone or in combination with other cell surface molecules do look promising.[31,32]

Recombinant DNA technology can be used to produce biologically active molecules with potential for the manipulation of immune responses in vivo. The application of these techniques to this area is very attractive as large quantities of molecules with potent biological activity, that would normally be present in very low amounts or as cell surface molecules in vivo, can be produced and purified for administration in vivo.

As mentioned above, 2 signals are required for effective T cell activation. If the delivery of signal 2 via the CD28 molecule to T cells capable of responding to donor antigens could be blocked, this might provide an effective way of both preventing activation and result in the responding T cells being switched off, thereby inducing unresponsiveness to the donor antigens. Interestingly, signalling through CD28 cannot be inhibited by cyclosporine. This pathway may therefore be relatively unaffected by conventional immunosuppressive drug therapy. Their are potentially two ways to block the delivery of the second signal (i) by using mabs specific for either CD28 or its ligands which would prevent effective interaction between the responding T cell and the antigen presenting cell[33] or (ii) by using a soluble form of one of the naturally occurring ligands for B7. CTLA-4 is a second receptor that can interact with B7 and other related molecules with a higher avidity than CD28 that is expressed by activated T cells.[34] A soluble form of CTLA-4 has been engineered by fusing the extracellular domains of the gene to the constant domains of IgG. This soluble recombinant molecule, known as CTLA-4Ig, has been shown to block T cell dependent immune responses in vitro and suppress humoral responses in vivo. CTLA-4Ig has also been used to modify the rejection response to cardiac allografts and islet xenografts in vivo.[35,36] This strategy will be discussed in detail by Harland and June in chapter 12 of this volume. Suffice to say at this point, that this approach also looks very promising.

Manipulation of T Cells

As T cells are central to nearly every immune response, not least allograft rejection (see chapter 2), and are therefore the most logical target for any form of therapy designed to control responses made by the immune system. Polyclonal preparations of antilymphocyte (ALG/ALS) or antithymocyte globulins (ATG) have been used as immunosuppressive agents for many years. Indeed, there are reports in the literature of ALS inducing specific unresponsiveness to islet allografts.[37] However, it is difficult to produce polyclonal reagents that have consistent reactivity and potency. Furthermore, as more knowledge of the cell surface molecules expressed by leukocytes is acquired it has become clear that there may be advantages to targeting distinct subpopulations of T cells through the cell surface molecules they express, eg. those that act as subset markers, such as CD4 or CD8 or molecules that are known to be critical for T cell activation such as CD28 (see above).

Which leukocyte cell surface molecule to target remains a major matter for debate (Fig. 1.2). In the past decade our understanding of the molecular interactions that occur when T cells recognize antigen has increased exponentially. To block an immune response in vivo, it may be sufficient to simply inhibit the interaction between T cells and APCs to prevent T cell activation, for example by using mabs to target and bind to cell surface molecules, thereby preventing their interaction with a ligand on the other cell. Alternatively, rather than just blocking a critical interaction, it may be more effective to deliver negative or tolerogenic signals to cells by binding mabs or soluble ligands to cell surface molecules with signal transduction activity, in other words molecules with the potential to transmit a signal to the cell. At present, strategies designed to influence or prevent T cell activation by targeting single cell surface molecules are under investigation, but it may also be possible to reinforce a negative signal by targeting more than one cell surface molecule at once. For example, it has been shown that TCR and CD28 signal T cells by distinct signalling pathways. The pathway triggered by the binding of antigen to T cell receptor (TCR) is inhibitable by the immunosuppressive drug cyclosporine, but the CD28 pathway is insensitive to this drug. As more information on the molecules and signal transduction pathways involved in T cell activation becomes available, strategies that target more than one cell surface molecule, each interacting with a different intracellular signalling pathway, may ultimately prove more effective.

Anti-CD4

The $CD4^+$ subset of T cells has been shown to play a central role in the initiation and amplification of the immune response against an allograft (chapter 2). Targeting this subset of T cells using mabs specific for the CD4 molecule has resulted in effective immunosuppression in a number of different immunological situations, including transplantation and autoimmune disease in rodent and primate models (for reviews see[38, 39] and chapter 7). The question to be addressed in relation to this discussion is does specific unresponsiveness to the organ graft develop following anti-CD4 mab therapy?

In the early phase after anti-CD4 mab treatment, the immunosuppression induced is not immunologically specific. This can be clearly demonstrated in vivo, as a recipient treated with anti-CD4 mab will accept grafts from a number of different donors. The lack of immunological specificity at this stage is not surprising as the mab therapy targets all $CD4^+$ T cells irrespective of their antigen specificity. However, importantly as the length of time the primary transplant survives increases, immunological specificity begins to emerge. This can be demonstrated experimentally in vivo by transplanting a second graft from either the same strain as the original organ donor or a third party allogeneic strain. Anti-CD4 mab therapy has been shown to prolong the survival of islet

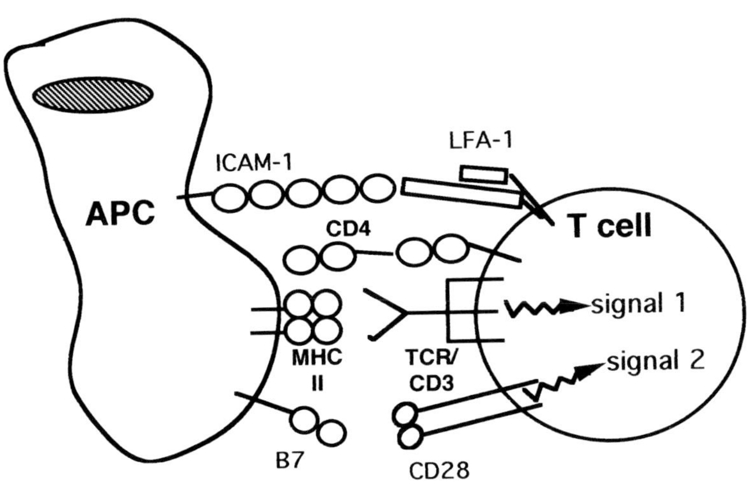

Fig. 1.2. Some of the molecular interactions that occur between T cells and APC capable of triggering primary responses.

allografts in a mouse model, ultimately leading to the induction of tolerance to the donor antigens.[40] The ability of anti-CD4 mab therapy to induce tolerance may depend on the type of tissue transplanted and the antigenic disparity between the donor and recipient,[41] but nevertheless, anti-CD4 mabs may be able to create an environment for the induction of tolerance to donor antigens in the long-term.

Anti-LFA-1 (CD18/CD11a)

Lymphocyte function antigen-1 (LFA-1) (CD18/CD11a) may be another leukocyte cell surface molecule that can be targeted using mab therapy to induce tolerance to alloantigen in vivo (Fig. 1.1). LFA-1 is a member of the integrin family, an $\alpha_L\beta_2$ integrin to be precise, and is involved in leukocyte adhesion by binding to members of the ICAM family of molecules, ICAM-1, 2 or 3.[30] LFA-1 is involved in the antigen independent adherence of leukocytes to endothelial cells, an important event when recipient leukocytes infiltrate the graft after transplantation. This interaction occurs in addition to the antigen dependent interaction of leukocytes with APCs. In addition to its role in cell adhesion, LFA-1 may also be involved in the signalling events that occur during T cell activation. Treatment with anti-LFA-1 mabs may therefore intervene in the response to an allograft at a number of points, leukocyte adhesion to graft endothelium, leukocyte adhesion in response to alloantigen stimulation and T cell activation.

Mabs specific for LFA-1 have been used in the context of transplantation and have been shown to both prolong graft survival and promote tolerance induction in rodents.[31,32,42,43] They have also been shown to have potential in the blockade of effector T cell activity during allograft rejection in primates.[44] A clinical trial assessing the effects of administering an anti-LFA-1 mab during the first 10 days after renal transplantation is currently in progress in France (Soulillou and colleagues, unpublished). However, data from a randomized trial using anti-LFA-1 mab treatment conducted in Boston did not show any significant beneficial effects of the anti-LFA-1 therapy.

Anti-IL-2 Receptor (CD25)

IL-2 plays a critical role in the expansion of antigen specific T cells following antigen recognition. It is secreted by activated T cells and interacts with IL-2 receptors (IL-2Rs) in an autocrine and paracrine fashion. IL-2Rs are composed of three polypeptide chains, the γ chain is expressed constitutively by T cells, the β or p75 chain is expressed constitutively by $CD8^+$ cytotoxic T cells but not by $CD4^+$ helper T cells and can be further induced on T cell activation, whereas expression of the α chain (CD25) is induced during T cell activation. Together the three chains form a high affinity receptor for IL-2.[45]

It has been suggested that the IL-2R, particularly the inducible CD25 chain, may provide a route for targeting only those T cells actively involved in graft rejection. T cells not involved in the rejection process would be unaffected by this therapy, as they would remain in the resting state and not express IL-2R α chain. (This argument assumes that the transplant recipients are not experiencing any form of infection). Immunological specificity might therefore be achieved in the early stages after transplantation as well as in the longer term using this approach.

Kirkman and his colleagues were the first to demonstrate that anti-CD25 mabs could be used as immunosuppressive agents.[46] Subsequently a large number of experimental studies have been reported in the rat, where panels of mabs specific for different epitopes present on the CD25 chain have been used. Efficacy in prolonging graft survival was found to correlate with the ability of the mab to block the functional interaction of IL-2 with its receptor. In the rat, anti-IL2R (CD25) mabs were found to induce tolerance to the organ donor in the long-term after transplantation. Tolerance induction was demonstrated in recipients bearing long-term surviving renal or cardiac allografts resulting from anti-IL2R mab therapy by the survival of donor specific but not third party skin grafts.[47]

Clinical trials of anti-CD25 mab therapy in renal transplantation have been carried out.

The data from the study undertaken by Soulillou and his colleagues in Nantes using the anti-IL-2 receptor mab 33B3.1 as a prophylactic treatment for rejection showed that the mab was as effective as ATG in preventing rejection and resulted in fewer infections and side effects.[48,49] This trial did not set out to determine if this mab could be used to create an environment for the induction of tolerance to the donor antigens. However, this information may be forthcoming when the long-term follow-up of the group of patients treated with the anti-CD25 mab is completed.

An alternative, but related approach to the use of anti-CD25 mabs is to use the cytokine molecule itself conjugated to a toxin, such as diphtheria toxin, to target and eliminate cells expressing the cytokine receptor. Cells that express the appropriate cytokine receptor and bind the toxin conjugated recombinant molecule would be destroyed and therefore nolonger able to participate in the response. This approach is currently being explored using IL-2-toxin conjugates.[50,51]

Anti-cytokine Mabs or Soluble Cytokine Receptors

Cytokines are soluble molecules produced by APCs and T cells that participate in the immune response to a transplant (see chapter 4 this volume). It may be possible to modify the course of an immune response by eliminating active cytokines from the environment of the graft, a related approach to that described above using mabs to block the binding site for IL-2 on the IL-2R thereby preventing amplification of the response. Two strategies exist for the implementation of this approach. The use of mabs specific for individual cytokines or alternatively soluble forms of cytokine receptors some of which are produced naturally, eg. the IL-1R antagonist.[52] Soluble cytokine receptors have been shown to compete for their cytokine with the cell surface receptor molecule of the same specificity. Soluble forms of cytokine receptors can be genetically engineered by manipulating the cytokine receptor gene or genes, (many are composed of more than one polypeptide chain), to remove the transmembrane region thereby ensuring that it is secreted from the cell rather than inserted into the cell membrane. Soluble forms of the receptor molecules for some of the cytokines known to be important in the rejection process (see chapter 4) may be an effective way of removing unwanted cytokines and redirecting the progress of the rejection response. The use of soluble cytokine receptors in transplant models is currently under investigation. It is, as yet, unclear whether it will be possible to achieve a sufficient concentration of the soluble molecule in vivo to block the interaction of the natural ligand with the membrane bound receptor effectively.

Antigen Pretreatment

The strategies outlined above may prove effective for the induction of specific unresponsiveness to alloantigen, and perhaps xenoantigens, in the long-term after transplantation. However, none of these approaches selectively target T cells capable of reacting with donor allo- or xeno-antigens. All of the approaches described above target molecules expressed by T cells, resting and/ or activated, irrespective of their antigen specificity. To achieve specific unresponsiveness at the time of transplantation, T cells expressing TCR molecules capable of reacting with donor antigens must be targeted selectively to ensure that only cells capable of interacting with the donor antigens are switched off. To target the TCR itself donor antigen in some form, it may be possible to use peptides for this purpose, must be incorporated into the immunosuppressive strategy.

Medawar and his colleagues were the first to achieve long-term survival of skin allografts in adult mice without the need for any other immunosuppressive therapy at the time of transplantation, by administering semi-allogeneic bone marrow and spleen cells to the mice within 24 hours of birth.[15] As mentioned above, this strategy took advantage of the immaturity of the immune system in new-born recipient mice. In primates the immune system develops in utero. As the majority of patients in need of an islet transplant are not identified until after birth when the immune system is already mature; a more challenging state from the point of view of reprogramming the response and tolerance induction presents itself. Even so, the administration of donor antigen, most frequently in the form of blood transfusion, before transplantation has been shown to result in the improved survival of vascularized organ allografts.[53]

A more successful approach may be to combine antigen administration with another strategy, such as those described above. Monaco and his colleagues first investigated this approach in the 1960s by using donor bone marrow, as the source of donor antigen, in combination with ALS and found that this strategy resulted in the prolonged survival of skin allografts in mice.[54] This strategy relied on the properties of ALS to create a suitable environment for the administration of donor bone marrow cells after transplantation allowing them to engraft and promote the induction of specific unresponsiveness to the graft. It has been suggested that lymphocytes newly emerging from the thymus may be tolerized more easily than those already resident in the periphery. Thus the use of ALS may promote this process by depleting lymphocytes from the periphery. This system has been used successfully to induce tolerance to renal allografts in primates[55] and is currently being explored in the clinical setting (see below).

The use of mabs or soluble recombinant molecules, such as CTLA-4Ig, that specifically target subsets of T cells in combination with donor antigen may provide a more subtle approach[56, 57] (chapter 12). The persistence of donor antigen may be important for the induction of unresponsiveness, to this end some groups have been investigating whether it is possible to create mixed allogeneic or xenogeneic chimeras, i.e. of donor and recipient leukocytes, before transplantation, thereby inducing tolerance to a subsequent allo- or xeno-geneic organ graft.[58, 59]

MECHANISMS OF TOLERANCE INDUCTION

Above I have described just a few of the strategies that are currently being explored for the induction of tolerance to donor antigens in adult recipients. The mechanisms responsible for the induction of unresponsiveness after antigen pretreatment and the induction and maintenance phases of the response after transplantation are still being investigated, particularly at the molecular level. Below is a brief description of the mechanisms that have been shown to operate in different situations. It is not intended to be a comprehensive discussion but to act as an introduction to the mechanisms responsible for the induction of tolerance to islet grafts; these will be dealt with for the specific situations described in the chapters that follow.

Four or five, according to how you define each state, non-mutually exclusive hypotheses have been proposed to explain the induction of peripheral tolerance to donor antigens in vivo. These are in broad terms, deletion, anergy, ignorance or indifference, helplessness or exhaustion and suppression. The immune status of the recipient before tolerance induction may influence which of these mechanisms operates in any one particular situation. What is apparent from all studies is that tolerance induction is a dynamic process and any or all of these mechanisms may be operating at different stages of the induction and maintenance process.[8] What is also clear is the confusion generated by different definitions for the terms are used to describe what may be the same phenomena!

DELETION

Deletion of antigen reactive T cells has been shown to be an important mechanism for the induction of tolerance to self antigens during development of the immune system.[7] As a mechanism for the induction of peripheral tolerance it may be less important, but nevertheless it has been identified as the mechanism responsible for the induction of tolerance to a superantigen, Mls1a, in thymectomised adult mice.[60] A similar series of experiments examining the mechanism of tolerance induction to the same superantigen did not identify deletion as a mechanism.[61] However, in this case, mice were not thymectomised. These two studies highlight the importance of the status of the recipient in determining which mechanism is operating.

Ignorance

If T cells remain ignorant or incapable of responding to antigen that is present in vivo they are by definition unresponsive. The phenomenon was first described in an experimental system in mice made transgenic for a glycoprotein from the lymphocytic choriomeningitis virus (LCMV).[62] The transgene, which was expressed by pancreatic β cells was ignored by the immune system. The LCMV antigen was only recognized when mice which were also transgenic for the LCMV-specific TCR were immunised with LCMV glycoprotein. Following immunisation the LCMV specific T cells destroyed the pancreatic β cells and the mice became diabetic.

Ignorance may be a feature of low affinity T cells. Work from Miller and his colleagues has shown that in transgenic mice where H-$2K^b$ is expressed predominantly by pancreatic β cells, high affinity T cells were deleted in the thymus as a result of low level expression of K^b in the thymus.[63] T cells that escape deletion, were able to cause the rejection of skin grafts expressing Kb, but were seemingly unaware of K^b expressed by β cells in the same mouse. Only when high levels of IL-2 were present are the β cells destroyed. These data suggest that the site of antigen expression may also play a role in determining how T cells respond to an antigen. This is an important observation, as islet cells can be transplanted to a number of different sites in vivo. It may be that some sites are more suitable for the induction of tolerance to the graft than others.

Anergy

The induction of anergy or the functional inactivation of alloreactive T cells is the mechanism that currently receives most support in the transplantation tolerance literature. However, the molecular mechanisms responsible for the induction of this state of T cell inactivity remain unclear.

Anergic T cells are usually identified because although they are present in a tolerant animal they are unable to respond when stimulated through their antigen receptor with either antigen or a mab specific for the TCR they express.[61,64-68] In some models anergy has also been shown to be associated with a down regulation of cell surface expression of TCR and accessory molecules such as CD8.[8,69]

In a transplantation model, where tolerance was induced by pretreatment with donor alloantigen, we have shown although donor reactive cytotoxic cells are present within the grafts of tolerant recipients,[70] the graft infiltrating cells are unable to respond to or produce functional IL-2 in vitro.[67] These data suggest that the donor reactive cells present within these grafts are anergic. Interestingly, mRNA for IL-2 is still detectable in the graft infiltrating population, implying that the defect in the IL-2 pathway is not at the level of gene transcription. This finding is in contrast to those reported recently using in vitro systems, where transcription of the IL-2 gene in anergic cells was down regulated because of the absence of transcription factors such as AP-1.[71]

The cytokine environment may also play a role in influencing the outcome when T cells encounter antigen (see chapter 4 this volume). It has been suggested that the cytokines, IL-4 and IL-10 that are produced by Th2 cells, may be associated with the development of unresponsiveness[72,73] or alternatively that a low or defective production of the T_H1 cytokines, IL-2 and interferon-γ (IFNγ) might be responsible.[67,74,75] Clearly the two situations may be related. However, convincing evidence that the development of a Th2-like environment is the critical factor for the induction of tolerance to alloantigen is still awaited, so far only casual associations have been implied. Clear evidence supporting these ideas will likely only be obtained from studies which attempt to manipulate the cytokine environment in vivo. So far little has been done in this area, but studies using for example antibodies to IFN-γ, an important Th1 cytokine, have proved ineffective to date at both inhibiting graft rejection and inducing tolerance.[76]

Suppression

In many transplant models, it is possible to adoptively transfer cells from animals bearing long-term surviving allografts to a fresh syngeneic recipient and show that these are able to modify the rejection response to a fresh graft.[77] It is important to note that suppressor cells are most frequently described in the maintenance phase of graft survival, usually 50 or more days after transplantation in rodent models. Thus it may be that the mechanisms responsible for tolerance induction converge and become unified in the longer term after transplantation. It is important to note however that cells that can adoptively transfer unresponsiveness have also been described during the induction phase after antigen pretreatment alone,[78] thus the situation is undoubtedly complex. Although it remains possible to demonstrate the phenomenon of suppression, the idea that suppressor cells control unresponsiveness has largely fallen into disrepute because even with advances in technology, it has proved very difficult to isolate and characterize cells with suppressor activity. In addition, the experimental systems used to demonstrate suppression often, but not always, required manipulation of the secondary recipient before the putative suppressor cells were transferred, eg. using low doses of irradiation.[77] It may be interesting to re-evaluate these studies in the light of recent observations in experimental models of autoimmune disease where irradiation has been shown to abolish the activity of naturally occurring regulatory cells.[79] In the recent literature suppressor or regulatory cells seem to be enjoying a revival of interest and it may not be too long before speculation regarding their existence is finally put to rest.

Another phenomenon which can be considered as fitting into the same category as suppression is that of infectious tolerance. Again demonstrable in recipient bearing long-term surviving allografts, where the transfer of naive syngeneic lymphocytes to the recipient will not induce graft rejection.[40,80] Waldmann and his colleagues have shown that in mice rendered tolerant to skin grafts by treatment with anti-CD4 and anti-CD8 mabs, a $CD4^+$ population of cells in the tolerant host is responsible for switching off the naive cells.[81] Interestingly, the naive cells must be resident in the tolerant host for 14 days before they lose the capacity to reject a fresh graft. Experiments of this type may help elucidate the molecular properties of the cells responsible for maintaining tolerance to alloantigen in the long-term.

References

1. Austyn J, Wood K, Principles of cellular and molecular immunology. 1993, Oxford University Press.
2. Bretscher P, Cohn M, A theory of self-nonself discrimination. Science 1970; 169:1042.
3. Konig R, Huang L-Y, Germain RN, MHC class II interaction with CD4 mediated by a region analogous to the MHC class 1 binding site for CD8. Nature 1992; 356:796.
4. Rudd CE, CD4, CD8 and the TcR-CD3 complex: a novel class of protein-tyrosine kinase receptor. Immunol. Today 1990; 11:400.
5. Linsley PS, Clark EA, Ledbetter JA, T cell antigen CD28 mediates adhesion with B cells by interacting with activation antigen B7/BB1. Proc. Natl. Acad. Sci. 1990; 87:5031.
6. Larsen CP, Ritchie SC, Pearson TC, et al., Functional expression of the costimulatory molecule, B7/BB1, on murine dendritic cell populations. J Exp Med 1992; 176:1215.
7. Marrack P, Kappler J, The T cell repertoire for antigen. Immunol. Today 1988; 9:308.
8. Arnold B, Schonrich G, Hammerling GJ, Multiple levels of peripheral tolerance. Immunol. Today 1993; 14:12.

9. Schwartz RH, A cell culture model for T lymphocyte clonal anergy. Science 1990; 248:1349.
10. Jenkins MK, The role of cell division in the induction of clonal anergy. Immunol. Today 1992; 13:69.
11. Schwartz RH, Costimulation of T lymphocytes: the role of CD28, CTLA-4, and B7/BB1 in interleukin-2 production and immunotherapy. Cell 1992; 71:1065.
12. Sloan-Lancaster J, Evavold BD, Allen PM, Induction of T cell anergy by altered T cell receptor ligand on live antigen presenting cells. Nature 1993; 363:156.
13. Owen RD, Immunogenetic consequences of vascular anastomoses between bovine twins. Science 1945; 102:400.
14. Billingham RE, Lampkin GH, Medawar PB, et al., Tolerance to homografts, twin diagnosis, and the freemarting condition in cattle. Heredity 1952; 6:201.
15. Billingham RE, Brent L, Medawar PB, Actively acquired tolerance of foreign cells. Nature 1953; 172:603.
16. Sykes M, Aksentijevich I, Sharabi Y, et al., Xenotolerance through bone marrow transplantation, in Xenotransplantation, D. Cooper, et al., Editors. 1991, Springer-Verlag: Berlin. 121.
17. Strober S, Dhillon M, Schubert M, et al., Acquired immune tolerance to cadaveric renal allografts: A study of three patients treated with total lymphoid irradiation. New Engl. J. Med. 1989; 321:28.
18. Inaba K, Steinman RM, Resting and sensitized T lymphocytes exihibit distinct stimulatory requirements for growth and lymphokine release. J. Exp. Med. 1984; 160:1711.
19. Fuchs E, Matzinger P, B cells turn off virgin but not memory T cells. Science 1992; 258:1156.
20. Snell G, The homograft reaction. Annual Review of Microbiology 1957; 11:439.
21. Lafferty K, Prowse S, Simeonovic C, Immunology of tissue transplantation: a return to the passenger leukocyte concept. Ann. Rev. Immunol. 1983; 1:143.
22. Huag C, Gill R, Babcock S, et al., Cyclosporine-induced tolerance requires antigens capable of initiating an immune response. J. Immunol. 1987; 139:2947.
23. Lacy P, Davie J, Finke E, Prolongation of islet allograft survival following in vitro culture (24°C) and a single injection of ALS. Science 1979; 204:312.
24. Faustman DL, Steinman RM, Gebel HM, et al., Prevention of rejection of murine islet allografts by pretreatment with anti-dendritic cell antibody. Proceedings of the National Academy of Sciences 1984; 81:3864.
25. Lau H, Reemtsma K, Hardy M, Prolongation of rat islet allograft survival by direct ultraviolet irradiation of the graft. Science 1984; 223:607.
26. Bowen K, Prowse S, Lafferty K, Reversal of diabetes by islet transplantation: vulnerability of the established allograft. Science 1981; 213:1261.
27. Morrow C, Sutherland D, Steffes M, et al., Lack of donor specific tolerance in mice with established anti-IA treated islet allografts. Transplantation 1983; 36:691.
28. Ortho Multi Centre Study Group, A randomised trial of OKT3 monoclonal antibody for acute rejection of cadaveric renal transplantation. New Engl. J. Med. 1985; 313:337.
29. Springer TA, Adhesion receptors of the immune system. Nature 1990; 346:425.
30. Hynes RO, Integrins: versatility, modulation, and signalling in cell adhesion. Cell 1992; 69:11.
31. Isobe M, Yagita H, Okumura K, et al., Specific acceptance of cardiac allografts after treatment with antibodies to ICAM-1 and LFA-1. Science 1992; 255:1125.
32. Paul LC, Davidoff A, Benediktsson H, et al., The efficacy of LFA-1 and VLA-4 antibody treatment in rat vascularized cardiac allograft rejection. Transplantation 1993; 55:1196.
33. Harding FA, McArthur JG, Gross JA, et al., CD28-mediated signalling co-stimualtes murine T cells and prevents induction of anergy in T-cell clones. Nature 1992; 356:607.
34. Linsley PS, Wallace PM, Johnson J, et al., Immunosuppression in vivo by a soluble form of the CTLA-4 T cell activation molecule. Science 1992; 257:792.

35. Turka LA, Linsley PS, Lin H, et al., T cell activation by the CD28 ligand B7 is required for cardiac allograft rejection in vivo. Proc. Natl. Acad. Sci. 1992; 89:11102.
36. Lenschow DJ, Zeng Y, Thistlethwaite JR, et al., Long-term survival of xenogeneic pancreatic islet grafts induced by CTLA4Ig [see comments]. Science 1992; 257:789.
37. Gotoh M, Porter J, Monaco A, et al., Induction of antigen-specific unresponsiveness to islet allografts by antilymphocyte serum. Transplantation 1988; 45:429.
38. Waldmann H, Manipulation of T-cell responses with monoclonal antibodies. Ann. Rev. Immunol. 1989; 7:407.
39. Wood KJ, Pearson TC, Darby C, et al., CD4: A potential target molecule for immunosuppressive therapy and tolerance induction. Transplant. Rev. 1991; 5:150.
40. Shizuru JA, Gregory AK, Chao CT-B, et al., Islet allograft survival after a single course of treatment of recipient with antibody to L3T4. Science 1987; 237:278.
41. Hao L, Wang Y, Gill R, et al., Role of the L3T4+ T cell in allograft rejection. J. Immunol. 1987; 139:4022.
42. Benjamin RJ, Qin S, Wise MP, et al., Mechanisms of monoclonal antibody-facilitated tolerance induction: a possible role for the CD4 (L3T4) and CD11a (LFA-1) molecules in self-non-self discrimination. Eur. J. Immunol. 1988; 18:1079.
43. Talento A, Nguyen M, Blake T, et al., A single administration of LFA-1 antibody confers prolonged allograft survival. Transplantation 1993; 55:418.
44. Berlin PJ, Bacher JD, Sharrow SO, et al., Monoclonal antibodies against human T cell adhesion molecules—modulation of immune function in nonhuman primates. Transplantation 1992; 53:840.
45. Taniguchi T, Minami Y, The IL-2/IL-2 receptor system: A current overview. Cell 1993; 73:5.
46. Kirkman RL, Barret LV, Gaulton GN, et al., Administration of an anti-interleukin-2 monoclonal antibody prolongs cardiac allograft survival in mice. J. Exp. Med. 1985; 162:358.
47. Tellides G, Immunosuppression with monoclonal antibodies to rat lymphocyte activation antigens. 1988, University of Oxford:
48. Soulillou JP, Peyronnet P, Le Mauff B, et al., Prevention of rejection of kidney transplants by monclonal antibody directed against interleukin-2 receptor. Lancet 1987; 1:1339.
49. Soulillou J-P, Cantarovich D, Le Mauff B, et al., Randomised controlled trial of a monoclonal antibody against the interleukin-2 receptor (33B3.1) as compared with rabbit antithymocyte globulin for prophylaxis against rejection of renal allografts. New Engl. J. Med. 1990; 322:1175.
50. Kirkman RL, Bacha P, Barrett LV, et al., Prolongation of cardiac allograft survival in murine recipients treated with a diphtheria toxin-related interleukin-2 fusion protein. Transplantation 1989; 47:327.
51. Lorberboum GH, Barrett LV, Kirkman RL, et al., Cardiac allograft survival in mice treated with IL-2-PE40. Proc Natl Acad Sci U S A 1989; 86:1008.
52. Arend WP, Interleukin-1 receptor antagonist. Adv Immunol 1993; 54:167.
53. Wood K, Morris P, The blood transfusion effect, in Transplantation Immunology, F. Bach and Auchincloss, Editors. 1994, Wiley and sons: in press.
54. Monaco AP, Wood ML, Russel PS, Studies on heterologous anti-lymphocyte serum in mice: III. Immunologic tolerance and chimerism produced across the H-2 locus with adult thymectomy and anti-lymphocyte serum. Annals of the New York Academy of Sciences 1966; 129:190.
55. Thomas JM, Carver M, Cunningham P, Promotion of incompatible allograft acceptance in rhesus monkeys given posttransplant anti-thymocyte globulin and donor bone marrow. I. In vivo parameters and immunohistologic evidence suggesting microchimerism. Transplantation 1987; 43:332.
56. Posselt AM, Barker CF, Tomaszewski JE, et al., Induction of donor-specific unresponsiveness by intrathymic islet transplantation. Science 1990; 249:1293.

57. Pearson TC, Madsen JC, Larsen C, et al., Induction of transplantation tolerance in the adult using donor antigen and anti-CD4 monoclonal antibody. Transplantation 1992; 54:475.
58. Sykes M, Sachs DH, Mixed allogeneic chimerism as an approach to transplantation tolerance. Immunol. Today 1988; 9:23.
59. Jin M, Englestad K, Oluwole S, Induction of stable chimerism and transplantation tolerance to rat islet and heart allografts by ultraviolet-B modulation of bone marrow cells. Transplantation 1992; 54:113.
60. Webb S, Morris C, Sprent J, Extrathymic tolerance of mature T cells: clonal elimination as a consequence of immunity. Cell 1990; 63:1249.
61. Rammensee H-G, Kroschewski R, Frangoulis B, Clonal anergy induced in mature Vβ6$^+$ T lymphocytes on immunising Mls-1^b mice with Mls-1^a expressing cells. Nature 1989; 339:541.
62. Ohashi PS, Oehen S, Buerki K, et al., Ablation of "tolerance" and induction of diabetes by virus infection in viral antigen transgenic mice. Cell 1991; 65:305.
63. Heath WR, Allison J, Hoffmann MW, et al., Autoimmune diabetes as a consequence of locally produced interleukin-2. Nature 1992; 359:547.
64. Lo D, Burkly LC, Widera G, et al., Diabetes and tolerance in transgenic mice expressing Class II MHC molecules in pancreatic β bells. Cell 1988; 53:159.
65. Burkley LC, Lo D, Kanegawa O, et al., T-cell tolerance by clonal anergy in transgenic mice with nonlymphoid expression of MHC class II I-E. Nature 1989; 342:564.
66. Qin S, Cobbold S, Benjamin R, et al., Induction of classical transplantation tolerance in the adult. J. Exp. Med. 1989; 169:779.
67. Dallman MJ, Shiho O, Page TH, et al., Peripheral tolerance to alloantigen results from altered regulation of the interleukin-2 pathway. J. Exp. Med. 1991; 173:79.
68. Alters SE, Shizuru JA, Ackerman J, et al., Anti-CD4 mediates clonal anergy during transplantation tolerance induction. J Exp Med 1991; 173:491.
69. Kisielow P, Bluthmann H, Staerz UD, et al., Tolerance in T-cell-receptor transgenic mice involves deletion of nonmature CD4$^+$8$^+$ thymocytes. Nature 1988; 333:742.
70. Dallman MJ, Wood KJ, Morris PJ, Specific cytotoxic T cells are not found in the nonrejected kidneys of blood transfused rats. J. Exp. Med. 1987; 165:566.
71. Kang S-M, Beverly B, Tran A-C, et al., Transactivation by AP-1 is a molecular target of T cell clonal anergy. Science 1992; 257:1134.
72. Takeuchi T, Lowry RP, Konieczny B, Heart allografts in murine systems - The differential activation of TH2-like effector cells in peripheral tolerance. Transplantation 1992; 53:1281.
73. Papp I, Wieder KJ, Sablinski T, et al., Evidence for functional heterogeneity of rat CD4+ T cells in vivo. Differential expression of IL-2 and IL-4 mRNA in recipients of cardiac allografts. J Immunol 1992; 148:1308.
74. Mohler KM, Streilein JW, Lymphokine production by MLR-reactive reaction lymphocytes obtained from normal mice and mice rendered tolerant of Class II MHC antigens. Transplantation 1989; 47:625.
75. Bugeon L, Cuturi M-C, Hallet J, et al., Peripheral tolerance of an allograft in adult rats - characterisation by low interleukin-2 and interferon-γ mRNA levels and by strong accumulation of major histocompatibility complex transcripts within the graft. Transplantation 1992; 54:219.
76. Paineau J, Priestley C, Fabre J, et al., Effects of gamma interferon and interleukin-2 and of gamm-interferon antibodies on the rat response against allografts. Transplant. Proc. 1989; 21:999.
77. Hutchinson IV, Suppressor T cells in allogeneic models. Transplantation 1986; 41:547.
78. Quigley RL, Wood KJ, Morris PJ, Mediation of the induction of immunologic unresponsiveness following antigen pretreatment by a CD4 (W3/25$^+$) T cell appearing transiently in the splenic compartment and subsequently in the TDL. Transplantation 1989; 47:689.

79. Fowell D, Mason D, Evidence that the T cell repertoire of normal rats contains cells with the potential to cause diabetes. Characterisation of the CD4+ T cell subset that inhibits this autoimmune potential. J. Exp. Med. 1993; 177:627.
80. Billingham RE, Brent L, Medawar PB, Quantitative studies on tissue transplantation immunity. III. Actively acquired tolerance. Philosophical transactions of the Royal Society (London). Series B 1956; 239:357.
81. Qin S, Cobbold SP, Pope H, et al., Infectious transplantation tolerance. Science 1993; 259:974.

CHAPTER 2

THE ROLE OF T CELLS IN TRANSPLANT REJECTION

Lee Anne Tibbles

Andrew I. Lazarovits

The primary role of the immune system is to recognize "self" and to destroy anything that is not "self," i.e. viruses, bacteria, and tumor cells. To accomplish this goal, a huge array of various cell types interact by means of chemical messengers and direct contact to recognize invaders, alert the immune system, and activate the cells responsible for effecting their destruction. A transplanted organ is recognized as foreign by the immune system and becomes a target. A better understanding of how the immune system "sees" foreign antigens and how it becomes activated to attack will allow us to develop improved immunosuppressive drugs to subvert this process.

THE MHC GENE PRODUCTS AS A TARGET FOR ALLORECOGNITION

The immune system recognizes "self" via cell surface molecules called human leukocyte antigens (HLA), the genes for which reside in the major histocompatibility complex (MHC) on the short arm of the 6th chromosome. The function of these molecules is to present foreign antigen, in the form of short peptides, to the T cells. These T cells recognize the HLA antigens in association with the peptides via their T cell receptors (TCR). There are two structural types of HLA antigen, which perform related but distinct roles.

Class I antigens (HLA A, B, C) are present on all nucleated cells. They consist of two polypeptide chains. The α chain (45kD) has three extracellular, one transmembrane, and one intracellular domain (see Fig. 2.1A). It is bound non-covalently to β-2 microglobulin (12kD). This chain and the $\alpha3$ domain of the α chain are structurally homologous to certain immunoglobulin domains. Class I antigens have a peptide binding groove located between the α helices of the $\alpha1$ and $\alpha2$ domains of the heavy chain. In the HLA A-2, for example, there are six pockets within the groove to accommodate the side-chains of the various amino acids in the nonapeptide bound.[1] Mutations using amino acid substitutions in any of these six pockets alter the peptide binding affinity of the HLA molecule, which may cause changes

Pancreatic Islet Transplantation Volume II: Immunomodulation of Pancreatic Islets, edited by Robert P. Lanza, MD, William L. Chick, MD; ©1994 R.G. Landes Company.

in the peptide repertoire bound within the groove. This results in changes in its recognition by effector cytotoxic T cells.[1] However, other mutations to the HLA structure which affect amino acid residues outside of the peptide binding groove and do not alter the peptides bound, also affect T cell recognition of the complex.[2] Therefore it seems that parts of the HLA molecule itself, in addition to the bound peptide, are recognized by the T cell receptor. Also, X-ray crystallographic[3] and other studies[4] suggest that subtle conformational changes induced by the peptides themselves can alter T cell recognition of the MHC/peptide complex.

The Class I HLA system is responsible for presenting endogenously produced peptides to the immune system. Therefore "self" peptides as well as viral peptides translated in infected cells are acquired during the post-translational processing of the HLA molecule. As it traverses from rough endoplasmic reticulum through the Golgi apparatus and to the cell surface, peptides are bound within the groove. This intracellular trafficking of the molecule also depends on the presence of the β-2 microglobulin chain. The class I molecules are present on the cell surface as tetramers.[5] Class I molecules only associate with the TCR in the presence of a CD8 molecule.

The HLA class II molecule is a heterodimer consisting of an α and β chain (see Fig. 2.1B). It is expressed on the cell surface of B cells, macrophages, and dendritic cells. In addition it can be induced on the surface of renal tubular epithelial cells and endothelium.[6]

The class II molecule has a binding groove for peptides located between the α_1 and β_1 domains. It is involved in presentation of endogenous and exogenous peptides to T cells of the CD4+ phenotype. Class II molecules can present processed peptides from self or (in the case of a transplanted organ) foreign class I and class II molecules.

During the formation of the class II molecule, the α and β chains are associated with another polypeptide called the invariant chain (Ii) which aids in assembly of the complex and protects the binding groove from being saturated with endogenously

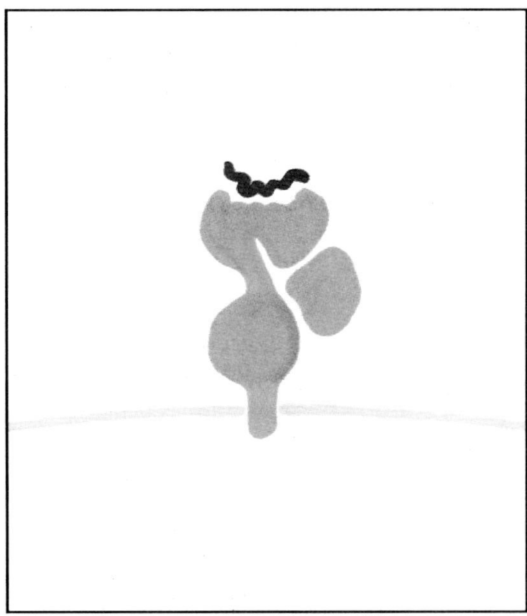

Fig. 2.1A. Class I HLA antigen consists of two polypeptide chains: a 45kD α chain and β-2 microglobulin.

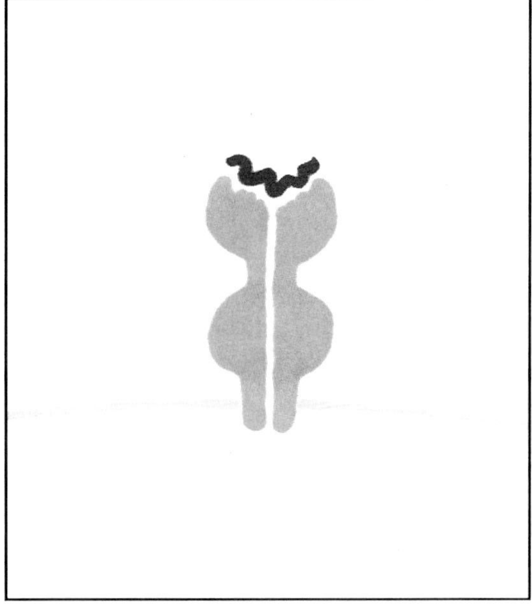

Fig. 2.1B. Class II HLA antigen consists of two polypeptide chains. Both class I and class II have a peptide binding groove shown here with black peptide bound.

produced peptides. The invariant chain also targets the αβ dimers to an endocytic compartment[7] where the invariant chain is proteolytically cleaved, and the binding groove becomes available to bind endocytosed and processed antigens.[8] The molecules undergo a conformational change after binding with peptide, and are transported to the cell surface.[9] The availability of peptide for binding has some influence on the amount of class II expressed on the cell surface,[9] although there are some "empty" molecules located on the surface as well.[9]

In addition to presenting antigens to T cells the MHC class II complex acts as a signal transduction system. When the class II molecule interacts with its corresponding T cell receptor, it transmits a signal to increase the cell surface expression of another molecule involved in immune activation, B7[10] (vide infra).

class I HLA molecules are present on all nucleated cells and therefore on all transplanted cells. They present antigen only to CD8+ T cells (formerly called T suppressor or cytotoxic T cells, based on their phenotype). Presentation of foreign antigen in this manner does not induce an acute rejection response; in fact it can lead to specific tolerance of the graft. Various experimental approaches to induce donor-specific class I antigens into the host prior to transplantation have resulted in long-term graft survival.[11]

Class II HLA molecules present foreign antigen, including degraded HLA molecules, to CD4+ (formerly termed T helper cells) and induce T cell activation and rejection of the organ. Since class II HLA are present on hematopoetic cells, the presence of "passenger" leukocytes in a transplanted organ facilitates the presentation of foreign antigen to helper T cells and the escalation of an immune response.

STRUCTURE OF THE TCR

The T cell "sees" antigen with a complex organization of cell surface glycoproteins (Fig. 2.2). This multimer is composed of the TCR, the CD3 family of proteins and the CD4 or CD8 associated molecules.

The TCR is a heterodimer of α and β (or less often γ and δ) chains. Each chain is assembled by recombination of variable, (± diversity), joining and constant regions of

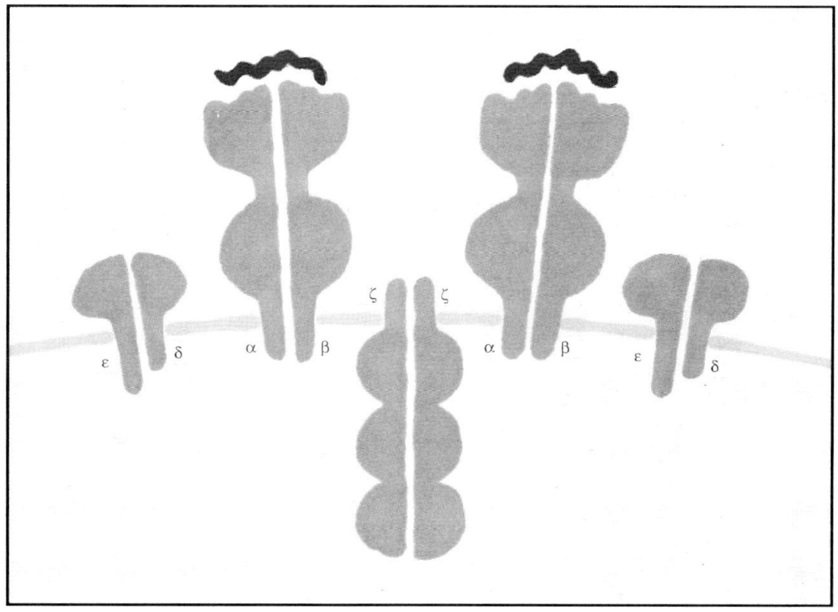

Fig. 2.2. The T cell receptor complex consists of two αβ T cell receptor dimers, and associated CD3 polypeptides arranged as either two εδ or two εγ dimers. Also associated is a ζζ dimer. The N-terminal regions of the TCR bind processed peptides.

the gene in a manner analogous to the generation of antibody diversity in B cells. Within each T cell precursor, the genes rearrange under the control of recombinase genes and the proteins derived from transcription of these genes therefore each have unique antigen binding regions. The hypervariable regions of the TCR α or β proteins are located at their amino termini, and face the cell exterior for interaction with peptides bound to HLA molecules on opposing cells.

The TCR chains have very short intracytoplasmic domains which are incapable of signalling to the cell interior when ligand is bound to them. They are associated, however, with multiple accessory chains termed the CD3 polypeptides which act as signal transducers. These are 20-28 kD molecules arranged as $^{TM}\gamma$ or $^{TM}\delta$ heterodimers; as well as ζζ or ζγ dimers. Each of these chains has recognition motifs for cytoplasmic proteins involved in signal transduction.[12] The stoichiometry is for example: 2 αβ TCR dimers associated with either 2 $^{TM}\delta$, or 2 $^{TM}\gamma$ dimers and a zz dimer (Fig. 2.2).[12] Various other combinations also occur. The CD3 chains are the target of the anti-T cell drug OKT3 used in transplant rejection, and the side effects of this drug are probably due to signalling through the CD3 molecules.

Associated with the TCR/CD3 complex in mature T cells is either a CD4 or CD8 co-receptor. These are cell surface structures which belong to the immunoglobulin gene superfamily. CD4 is a single chain which binds to a nonpolymorphic region of the HLA class II molecule on the opposing cell. CD8 is a dimer (αα or αβ) which binds to a similar nonpolymorphic region of HLA class I. CD4+ T cells bind only to HLA class II cells. CD8+ T cells bind to cells expressing HLA class I. Both CD4 and CD8 are thought to function as co-receptors with the TCR/CD3 receptor, and are responsible for signal transduction (vide infra).

THYMIC SELECTION OF THE T CELL REPERTOIRE

The multiple rearrangements of the TCR lead to proteins which can bind an enormous number of different peptides. To avoid having T cells reactive to self proteins, and the induction of autoimmune disease, self-reactive clones of T cells must be controlled. The initial check point is within the thymus. The stages of thymocyte (pre T cell) differentiation are classified by the cell surface characteristics which the cells express. Initial T cells have the CD4- CD8- TCR- phenotype. At this stage, the β chain of the TCR undergoes recombination. Once one β chain rearranges successfully, the other allele is prevented from doing so (allelic exclusion). β chain dimers in association with the CD3 polypeptides are expressed on the cell surface, and CD4 and CD8 also appear (double positive stage). β chain rearrangements appear necessary for this step to occur.[13]

The TCR α chain undergoes recombination under the action of the recombinase activation genes (RAG-1 and RAG-2). αβ TCR receptors are expressed on the cell surface. At this stage, cells strongly reactive to self HLA or self peptides are deleted or clonally inactivated - a process called negative selection. In elegant experiments using transgenic mice it has been shown that the co-receptor CD8 is required in some,[14] but not all negative selection events.[15] Other cell surface molecules also participate in this process.[16]

While destruction of autoreactive clones is necessary, it is also important to select T cells which have some affinity for their own HLA antigens and peptides so they can recognize self vs. non-self antigen in the periphery. This process is called positive selection and it is dependant on the CD8 co-receptor[15,17] binding to the same HLA molecule as the TCR.[15] CD4 may be similarly required for positive selection in T cells.[18] Although the CD8 molecule is necessary, it does not require association with the intracellular protein lck[19] which is thought to be important in the activation of mature T cells.

After positive selection, the T cells mature into CD4+ CD8- or CD4- CD8+ cells. The commitment to develop along one of these mutually exclusive pathways may depend on the affinity of the TCR, and whether it preferentially binds MHC class I or class II molecules on the antigen presenting cells.[20]

THE BIOCHEMISTRY OF SIGNAL TRANSDUCTION

In many receptor mediated processes binding of the ligand to the extracellular domain of a receptor initiates a cascade of activation signals. Many receptors have intracellular domains which have enzymatic activity — specifically they are kinases which phosphorylate protein substrates on tyrosine residues. This activates the substrates which diffuse away from the receptor and interact with other proteins. The end result of these biochemical pathways is a change in gene transcription, leading to a change in the cell's activation state and the initiation of proliferation.

In T cells the cytoplasmic domains of the αβ TCR chains are very short and have no kinase domains. The CD3 γδ and $^{TM}\gamma$ and the ζζ or ζη chains also lack enzymatic activity. These polypeptides, however, do have conserved amino acid motifs called antigen receptor homology-1 (ARH-1) regions[12,21] which mediate attachment of cytoplasmic proteins to the receptor complex. Each of these motifs has a tyrosine residue which can become phosphorylated on TCR binding. These motifs bind to SH2 (Src-homology-2)

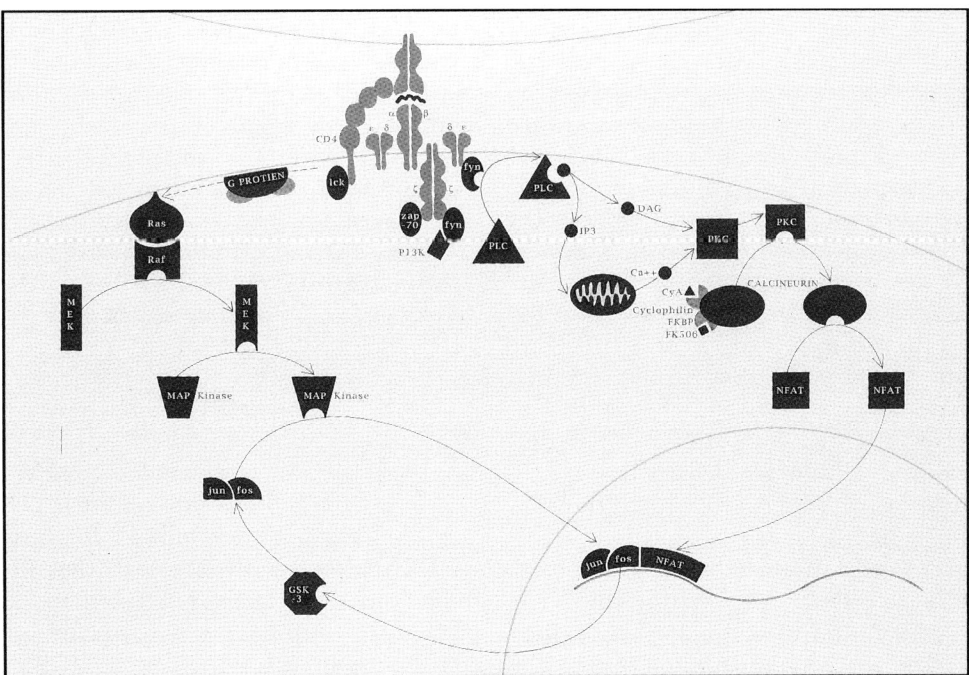

Fig. 2.3. The T cell signal transduction pathway. Enzymes and proteins are represented by geometric shapes. Activated enzymes have cut out active sites. Protein tyrosine kinases lck, fyn and zap-70 bind to elements of the TCR. Phospholipase Cγ1 (PLC) is phosphorylated by fyn (±lck) and translocates to the plasma membrane, releasing inositol triphosphate (IP3) and diacylglycerol (DAG) IP3 releases Ca++ from mitochondia. DAG and Ca++ activate protein kinase C which translocates to the plasma membrane and phosphorylates and activates calcineurin, a protein phosphatase. Calcineurin dephosphorylates nuclear factor of activated T cells (NFAT) which traverses the nuclear membrane and binds to the DNA in association with jun and fos nuclear binding proteins to promote IL2 and IL2 receptor gene activation.
The TCR may also activate pathways dependant on G proteins, leading to the activation of ras, raf, mek (map kinase kinase) and MAP kinase. Certain MAP kinases phosphorylate jun and fos which translocate to their nuclear binding sites. Jun and fos are phosphorylated at other sites by GSK-3 to inactivate them.
The TCR-protein tyrosine kinase pathway may intersect with the mitogen activated kinase pathway at the level of the IL2 regulatory genes. Cyclosporine A (CYA) and FK506 are shown with their respective cellular binding proteins, binding to calcineurin.

domains on interacting tyrosine kinases. The CD3 chains bind $p59^{fyn}$, a tyrosine kinase thought to be important in early post receptor signalling (see Fig. 2.3). Genetic overexpression of fyn produces T cells hyper-responsive to stimulation, whereas transgenic mice with a mutant kinase-negative fyn have diminished responsiveness.[22] The ζ chain of the TCR binds to fyn as well. In experimental systems in nonhemopoetic cells, cross-linking of transfected ζ and fyn can produce signalling similar to TCR engagement.[23]

The ζ chains also bind a protein tyrosine kinase called ZAP-70 (for zeta associated protein). This is a member of the Syk family of kinases. Co-clustering of ZAP-70 and fyn at the cell surface, by clustering of fusion proteins constructed of CD16 extracellular domains and ZAP-70 and fyn intracellular domains can mimic the secondary events of TCR stimulation.[24]

The associated molecules CD4 and CD8 bind noncovalently to a tyrosine kinase $p56^{lck}$. Lck appears to be important in signal transduction, as expression of a constitutively active mutant lck can induce T cell activation after TCR cross-linking even in the absence of CD4 or CD8.[25]

T cell receptor activation by binding to peptide/HLA therefore induces the action of at least three protein tyrosine kinases - fyn, ZAP-70 and lck. These and possibly other kinases are responsible for initiating the activation cascade in T cells.

How does an increase in protein tyrosine kinase activity translate into a T cell response to antigen binding? One of the earliest changes in the T cell after ligand binding is an increase in calcium mobilization within the cell. Activation of the T cell and subsequent tyrosine kinase activity leads to the phosphorylation of phospholipase Cγ-1,[26] an enzyme which releases diacylglycerol and inositol triphosphate from membrane phospholipids. Lck and fyn have been shown to bind to and activate PLCγ-1.[27-30] and fyn may be the more physiologic transducer.[30] Inositol triphosphate mediates the release of calcium from intracellular stores, such as mitochondria.

The increased intracellular calcium, along with the diacylglycerol, causes protein kinase C (PKC) to translocate to the inside of the plasma membrane and activate this serine/threonine kinase. Protein kinase C is an important member of the signal transduction pathway, as stimulation of PKC directly with phorbol esters such as phorbol myristate acetate (PMA) will produce T cell activation, bypassing the initial TCR mediated steps. Protein kinase C activates many substrates by phosphorylating them. One of these substrates is calcineurin, a protein phosphatase, which becomes activated when it is phosphorylated.[31-33] Calcineurin is a pivotal step in T cell activation.[34,35] Cyclosporine A, bound to cyclophilin (its cellular binding protein), interacts with calcineurin to inhibit its activity and dampen the T cell activation sequence. A new immunosuppressive drug FK506 binds to its cytosolic binding protein (FKBP) and also interacts with calcineurin, again inhibiting its activity.[34,35] Both cyclophilin and FKBP are rotamase enzymes, although interference with this activity does not seem to mediate the action of cyclosporine A and FK506.

The usual substrates for calcineurin include proteins like NFAT[36] (nuclear factor of activated T cells) which, when dephosphorylated, bind to regulatory areas of DNA and induce the transcription of IL-2 and the IL-2 receptor genes. Thus, activation of NFAT and possibly other nuclear binding proteins can alter the expression of cytokine and other genes culminating in the change from naive T cell to the activated effector T cell phenotype.

The T cell may be stimulated by other signal transduction systems as well as the tyrosine kinase pathway just described. A role for G proteins in T cell activation has been sought for many years, and recently a new family of G proteins with slower kinetics than those previously known may provide a link to the cyclic nucleotide system.[37] $p21^{ras}$, an oncogene product in the GTP-mediated cascade of mitogenic signal transduction is activated after TCR binding.[38] $p21^{ras}$ interacts directly with raf,[39] another proto-oncogene product to form an activation cascade which leads to the phosphorylation of MEK (MAP kinase kinase), then MAP kinase (mitogen activated protein kinase).[40] MAP kinases phosphorylate and activate the ubiquitous nuclear transcription factors c-jun and c-fos to promote DNA transcription at a DNA binding site termed AP-1.[41,42] Recently it has been shown that c-jun and c-fos interact with NFAT to form multimeric complexes that bind to DNA at the NFAT site, an upstream regulator of IL-2 and IL-2 receptor transcription.[36] This provides a link between the tyrosine kinase pathway of T cell signal transduction, and that mediated by mitogen-activated kinases; interacting at the gene transcription level.

There are presumably many other pathways involved in the transition of T cells from the naive to the effector phenotype. Some of these may involve alternate lipid kinase systems such as PI3 kinase which initiates a lipid kinase cascade distinct from that of PLCγ-1.[43] Indeed, PI3 kinase has been shown to interact with the SH3 (src-homology-3) domain of fyn.[44]

Despite this array of signalling pathways, it has been shown that binding of the TCR to its ligand, without co-stimulatory signals provided by other cell surface molecules, leads to T cell inactivation or anergy.[45] The role of these accessory molecules will be the focus of the following section.

ACCESSORY MOLECULES IN T CELL ACTIVATION

The presentation of co-stimulatory signals by antigen presenting cells may increase the appropriate response of T cells to foreign antigens, while limiting the potential of autoimmune reactions. In fact, the requirement for costimulation may be a mechanism of induction of peripheral tolerance to hidden self antigens, which, when presented without costimulation, promote T cell unresponsiveness.[46]

Many cell surface molecules have been shown to play a role in T cell activation subsequent to TCR/MHC engagement (see Fig. 2.4). Of greatest importance are the co-receptors CD4 or CD8, which have been discussed in the previous section on signal

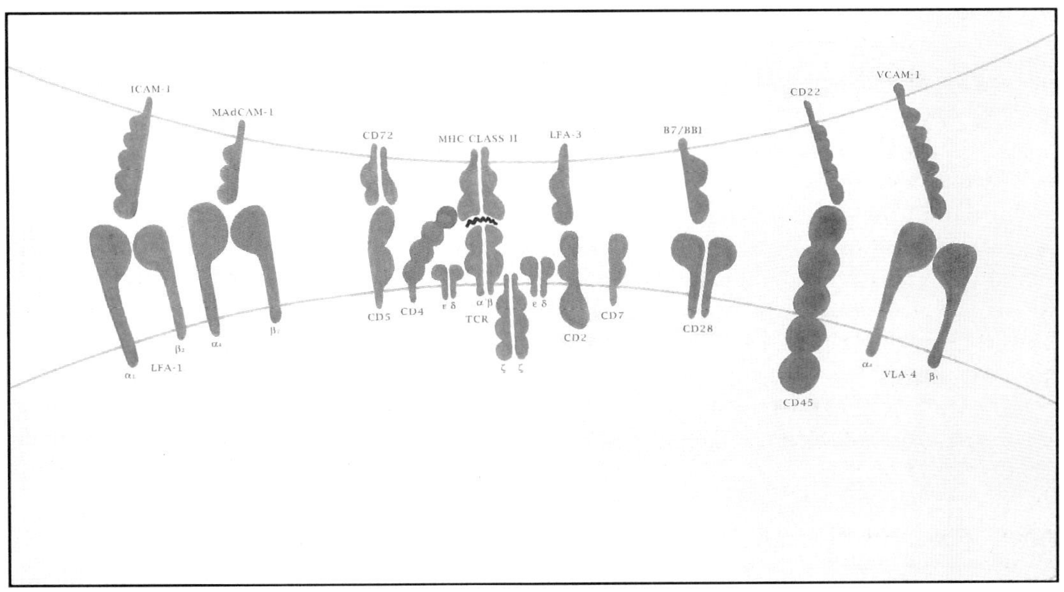

Fig. 2.4. Accessory cell surface molecules. The T cell surface is depicted at the bottom; an opposing cell at the top. The TCR is shown interacting with an MHC class II molecule and associated peptide. CD4 binds to a non-polymorphic region of MHC class II. CD2 and CD5 have been shown to be associated with the TCR. Other ligand/receptor pairs are shown: ICAM-1/LFA-1; MAdCAM-1/integrin α4β7; CD5/CD72; CD2/LFA-3; CD28/B7/BB1; CD45/CD22; VLA-4/VCAM-1. The ligand for CD7 is unknown at this time. See text for further details.

transduction. These molecules restrict the T cell to either MHC class I or class II specificity; they increase cell-cell adhesion by binding to the HLA molecule, and their associated p56^{lck} protein tyrosine kinase is required for TCR signalling.

The leukocyte common antigen, CD45, is a receptor protein tyrosine phosphatase found on all hematopoetic cells except mature erythrocytes. It binds to the CD22 antigen on B cells.[47] CD45 has been shown to be necessary for signal transduction in T cells, as CD45 deficient cell lines are unable to signal via their T cell receptors.[48] Reconstitution of CD45 in these cell lines by transfection of CD45 cDNA restores their signalling ability.[49] In vivo, CD45 exon 6 deficient mice have been prepared which are unable to transduce signals through their T cell receptors.[50]

The mechanism of action of CD45 is thought to be through its phosphatase activity. Monoclonal antibodies to CD45 have been shown to increase this activity.[51] Proposed targets of the dephosphorylation are the negative regulatory tyrosines of fyn and lck tyrosine kinases, and these have been shown to be substrates for CD45 in vitro.[51-54] If this mechanism occurs in vivo it would lead to increased signals via the T cell receptor initiated pathways.

CD45 exists as multiple isoforms, produced by differential splicing of exons 4-7, leading to different epitopes near the N-terminal of the proteins.[50,54,55] The roles of these various isoforms are not well characterized, but they seem to have a role in T cell ontogeny[50] and they may relate to previous antigen exposure[56] or to different requirements for activation.[52] The various isoforms may also associate preferentially with other cell surface molecules.[52]

In clinical transplantation, the CD45 antigen is a major target of antilymphocyte globulin used in the therapy of transplant rejection. We have shown that monoclonal antibodies to certain isoforms of CD45 inhibit the mixed lymphocyte reaction and inhibit the generation of cytotoxic T cells in vitro.[57] CD45 therefore may be an appropriate target for in vivo immunotherapy.

An essential co-stimulatory signal for T cell activation is provided through the CD28 cell surface antigen. CD28 and the related CTLA-4 bind to B cell activation antigen B7 (also known as BB1)[58] and B7-2.[59] CD28 does not need to be co-associated with the T cell receptor to provide synergism to TCR activation.[60] Stimulation through CD28 causes an increase in tyrosine phosphorylation similar to that seen with TCR binding. In addition however, CD28 stimulation causes an increase in the production of D-3 phosphoinositides by phosphatidyl inositol 3 kinase,[43] an increase in the stability of mRNA for cytokines[59] and a change in IL-2 gene transcription via a CD28 dependant nuclear DNA binding protein.[61] At least some of these pathways are cyclosporine A resistant.[59] Lenschow and Bluestone[59] have suggested a time and activation dependent binding cascade, where naive T cells with their constitutive CD28 interact with B7-2 on activated B cells initially, then the T cell expresses CTLA-4 which binds to B7 on the B cell. In fact, binding of the T cell receptor to MHC class II receptor can induce the expression of B7 on B cells.[10] In transgenic mice deficient in CD28, T cell responses to mitogenic lectins are inhibited, and B cell help is not adequately provided, demonstrating a role of CD28 in mediating T cell dependant immune responses.[62]

In experimental systems, the B7/CD28 pathway has been shown to play an important role in cardiac allograft rejection in vivo,[60] as blocking this pathway with a soluble CTLA-immunoglobulin fusion protein (CTLA-Ig) leads to prolonged graft survival. In xenogeneic islet cell transplants, treatment of recipients with CTLA-Ig leads to specific tolerance to the graft.[59] This may occur when other accessory signals are prevented from working due to cross-species differences in binding.[59] The B7/CD28 pathway may therefore have potential as a target of immunosuppressive strategies.

Several T cell surface antigens augment the signals initiated with T cell receptor binding to ligand and are candidates for costimulation in vivo. CD5 is a 67 kd glycoprotein which binds to the B-cell CD72 antigen. It has been shown that CD5 signalling can provide an accessory signal[63] and it is physically associated with the TCR.[64,65] Since CD5 is phosphorylated on tyrosine after CD3 stimulation[66] it may be involved in the tyrosine kinase pathway of T cell activation.

CD2 stimulation leads to phosphorylation of identical substrates as does the T cell receptor[67] and is therefore thought to stimulate the same tyrosine kinase pathway, perhaps via physical interaction.

Monoclonal antibodies against cell surface receptors have been used to prevent and treat transplant rejection. For example, OKT3 is the most effective therapy for the rapid reversal of acute rejection.[68] We have shown that a chimeric human/mouse monoclonal antibody against the T cell surface molecule CD7 can delay transplant rejection in renal transplants to the same degree as prophylactic OKT3, without the generalized cytokine release that accompanies OKT3 therapy.[69] Anti-CD7 therapy shows promise for the prevention of transplant rejection.

A number of other cell surface molecules have been shown to augment T cell receptor mediated signals. Several of these molecules belong to the integrin family of proteins. Integrins are heterodimeric glycoproteins composed of α and β subunits which combine in various ways to produce an array of cell adhesion molecules. Certain integrins bind to members of the immunoglobulin gene superfamily (ICAM, VCAM, MAdCAM) as well as to matrix proteins like fibronectin and laminin. They are responsible for some cell-substratum, and cell-cell interactions, as well as lymphocyte homing to tissue specific compartments.[70-74] These molecules can be activated to bind their ligands with greater affinity, therefore transmitting signals from the inside of the cell to influence the interactions at the cell exterior.[70] Of greater interest in T cell activation, however, is their ability to signal from the outside in to provide synergism to T cell receptor events.[75] VLA integrins have been shown to co-stimulate T cell activation by inducing the AP-1 transcription factor which controls IL-2 production in an independent fashion from CD3/TCR.[76] VLA-4 ($\alpha4\beta1$) initiates this process via a tyrosine kinase pathway distinct from that triggered by the T cell receptor.[75] Integrin LFA-1 ($\alpha L\beta2$) binding to ICAM-1 has been shown to potentiate T cell receptor tyrosine kinase pathways and to prolong the tyrosine phosphorylation of phospholipase Cγ-1.[77] We have prepared a monoclonal antibody Act I which binds to a late lymphocyte activation antigen,[78] $\alpha4\beta7$ integrin. This integrin has been shown to bind to MAdCAM, the Peyer's patch addressin[71] and is involved in homing of T memory cells to mucosal sites.[72,73]

Integrins mediate both lymphocyte adhesion, and therefore their invasion of the transplant, and their activation state. With their multiple combinations, and their specific regulation on different subsets of lymphocytes[79] they are uniquely suited as targets for immunosuppressives.

In experimental systems, anti-LFA-1 ($\alpha L\beta2$) and anti-VLA-4 ($\alpha4\beta1$) monoclonal antibodies prolong vascularized cardiac graft survival in rats.[80] A phase 1 clinical trial using monoclonal antibodies to ICAM-1, the cognate receptor for LFA-1 has shown a decrease in primary non-function and an increased graft survival in high risk renal transplants.[81] Further clinical trials are underway.

The T cell receptor confers the specificity of lymphocyte activation on binding to ligands, but the varied and diverse second signals provided by the accessory cell surface molecules amplify and modify these signals to control T cell responses. Further understanding and ultimately therapy directed at these secondary activation pathways shows promise in control of transplant rejection.

The generation of and interactions of cytokines obviously also play a role in T cell activation, but will not be further discussed here as they are dealt with in another chapter in this text book. Likewise the role of antibody mediated events will be covered by Dr. Paul.

CYTOTOXIC T CELLS

The mechanism by which recipients of allogeneic grafts reject the foreign tissue depends on presentation of the foreign MHC gene products to the host cells. Their recognition as "non-self" by the host T cell receptor mediated activation sequences and the second signal delivered to augment the T cell response. These comprise the afferent arm of the immune response – alerting the host to invasion. The efferent arm involves destruction of the graft by activated lymphocytes. Killing of target cells can occur by membrane lysis, similar to the final components of the complement cascade. Cytotoxic cells produce granules which contain enzymes to lyse membranes (granzymes and perforin).[82] Distribution of these granules to the cell surface and exocytosis depend on activation events and calcium fluxes.[82] Other lymphocytes mediate killing by initiating apoptosis or programmed cell death in their targets.[82]

Several phenotypically different cell populations have been implicated in graft rejection. Natural killer cells are devoid of T cell receptors, but may "see" antigen via multiple isoforms of the cell surface molecule CD56. Monoclonal antibodies to CD56 can inhibit NK cell cytotoxicity in vitro.[83] T cells with the $\gamma\delta$ T cell receptor also have a cytotoxic capacity, and constitutively express granules filled with perforin.[84]

The most widely studied cytotoxic cells, however, are the CD8 positive T cells. The CD8 antigen is not invariably associated with a killer phenotype, though, since CD8 cells also comprise the majority of suppressor T cells, and some CD4 positive cells are effective killers. A transgenic mouse strain has been developed which has the β-2 microglobulin gene knocked out, and therefore cannot express class I MHC gene products.[85] This leads to a deficiency of CD8+ cells as MHC class I is necessary for the maturation of thymocytes to a CD8+ lineage. In these CD8 deficient mice, pancreatic islet allografts have a prolonged survival, but are eventually rejected in most animals[85] suggesting that although CD8 cells are primarily involved in rejection of these grafts, other cells can also mediate target cell destruction.

CONCLUSION

In organ transplantation, the T cell orchestrates the recognition of the graft and the response to the graft including its destruction by rejection. T cells do this by a highly involved cascade of biochemical events — the foundation of the immune response. The more knowledge we gain about the discrete events involved in T cell activation and effector function, the more we will be able to modify the rejection response. The ultimate goal, of course, is to modulate the immune response to accept the graft as "self" and to become "tolerant". We are currently at the beginning of such a process and we are developing the tools to do so. Monoclonal antibodies are ideal for modifying cell surface events like HLA/TCR interactions, and the interference with accessory molecular signals. Pharmacologic immunosuppressives impact on the intracellular activation cascade, and new drugs are being developed that will alter other signal transduction pathways. Eventually, therapy aimed at controlling certain gene transcription events may be possible.

In this way, further developments in transplant immunology will also allow us to selectively immunosuppress the host to the transplant, without affecting their ability to combat viruses and neoplasms. One hopes that this will lead to permanent graft acceptance without undue toxicity.

ACKNOWLEDGEMENTS

The authors' experiments have been supported by the Kidney Foundation of Canada. We gratefully acknowledge Mr. Ralph Tibbles of Ralph Tibbles Design Inc., who kindly provided the illustrations, and the excellent secretarial support of Ms. K. McCormick.

References

1. Matsui M, Hioe CE, Frelinger JA. Roles of the six peptide-binding pockets of the HLA-A2 molecule in allorecognition by human cytotoxic T cell clones. Proc Natl Acad Sci USA 1993;90:674-678.
2. Grandea AG, Bevan MJ. Single-residue changes in class I major histocompatibility complex molecules stimulate responses to self peptides. Proc Natl Acad Sci USA 1992;89:2794-2798.
3. Fremont DH, Matsumura M, Stura EA, et al. Crystal structures of two viral peptides in complex with murine MHC class I H-2Kb. Science 1992;257:919-927.
4. Chen W, McCluskey J, Rodda S, et al. Changes at peptide residues buried in the major histocompatibility complex (MHC) class I binding cleft influence T cell recognition: a possible role for indirect conformational alterations in the MHC class I or bound peptide in determining T cell recognition. J Exp Med 1993;177:869-873.
5. Krishna S, Benaroch P, Pillai S. Tetrameric cell-surface MHC class I molecules. Nature 1992;357:164-167.
6. Benson EM, Colvin RB, Russell PS. Induction of IA antigens in murine renal transplants. J Immunol 1985;134:7-9.
7. Romagnoli P, Layet C, Yewdell J, et al. Relationship between invariant chain expression and major histocompatibility complex class II transport into early and late endocytic compartments. J Exp Med 1993;177:583-596.
8. Kelley WL, Georgopoulos C. Chaperones and protein folding. Curr Opin Cell Biol 1992;4:984-991.
9. Germain RN, Hendrix LR. MHC class II structure, occupancy and surface expression determined by post-endoplasmic reticulum antigen binding. Nature 1991;353:134-139.
10. Nabavi N, Freeman GJ, Gault A, et al. Signalling through the MHC class II cytoplasmic domain is required for antigen presentation and induces B7 expression. Nature 1992;360:266-268.
11. Wood KJ. The induction of tolerance to alloantigens using MHC class I molecules. Curr Opin Immunol 1993;5:759-762.
12. Chan AC, Irving BA, Weiss A. New insights into T-cell antigen receptor structure and signal transduction. Curr Opin Immunol 1992;4:246-251.
13. von Boehmer H. Thymic selection: a matter of life and death. Immunol Today 1992;13:454-458.
14. Ingold AL, Landel C, Knall C, et al. Co-engagement of CD8 with the T cell receptor is required for negative selection. Nature 1991;352:721-723.
15. Fung-Leung WP, Wallace VA, Gray D, et al. CD8 is needed for positive selection but differentially required for negative selection of T cells during thymic ontogeny. Eur J Immunol 1993;23:212-216.
16. Carlow DA, van Oers NSC, Teh SJ, et al. Deletion of antigen-specific immature thymocytes by dendritic cells requires LFA-1/ICAM interactions. J Immunol 1992;148:1595-1603.
17. Wallace VA, Penninger J, Mak TW. CD4, CD8 and tyrosine kinases in thymic selection. Curr Opin Immunol 1993;5:235-240.
18. Takeuchi Y, Horiuchi T, Hamamura K, et al. Role of CD4 molecule in intrathymic T cell development. Immunology 1991;74:183-190.
19. Chan IT, Limmer A, Louie MC, et al. Thymic selection of cytotoxic T cells independent of CD8α-Lck association. Science 1993;261:1581-1584.
20. Robey EA, Fowlkes BJ, Gordon JW, et al. Thymic selection in CD8 transgenic mice supports an instructive model for commitment to a CD4 or CD8 lineage. Cell 1991;64:99-107.
21. Cambier JC. Signal transduction by T- and B-cell antigen receptors: converging structures and concepts. Curr Opin Immunol 1992;4:257-264.
22. Cooke MP, Abraham KM, Forbush KA, et al. Regulation of T cell receptor signaling by a src family protein-tyrosine kinase (p59fyn). Cell 1991;65:281-291.
23. Hall CG, Sancho J, Terhorst C. Reconstitution of T cell receptor ζ-mediated calcium mobilization in nonlymphoid cells. Science 1993;261:915-921.

24. Kolanus W, Romeo C, Seed B. T cell activation by clustered tyrosine kinases. Cell 1993;74:171-183.
25. Abraham N, Miceli MC, Parnes JR, et al. Enhancement of T-cell responsiveness by the lymphocyte-specific tyrosine protein kinase p56lck. Nature 1991;350:62-66.
26. Weiss A, Koretzky G, Schatzman RC, et al. Functional activation of the T-cell antigen receptor induces tyrosine phosphorylation of phospholipase C-γ1. Proc Natl Acad Sci USA 1991;88:5484-5488.
27. Weber JR, Bell GM, Han MY, et al. Association of the tyrosine kinase lck with phospholipase C-γ1 after stimulation of the T cell antigen receptor. J Exp Med 1992;176:373-379.
28. Shiroo M, Goff L, Biffen M, et al. CD45 tyrosine phosphatase-activated p59fyn couples the T cell antigen receptor to pathways of diacylglycerol production, protein kinase C activation and calcium influx. EMBO J 1992;11:4887-4897.
29. Liao F, Shin HS, Rhee SG. In vitro tyrosine phosphorylation of PLC-γ1 and PLC-γ2 by SRC-family protein tyrosine kinases. Biochem Biophys Res Comm 1993;191:1028-1033.
30. Archuleta MM, Schieven GL, Ledbetter JA, et al. 7,12-dimethylbenz[α]anthracene activates protein-tyrosine kinases fyn and lck in the HPB-ALL human T cell line and increases tyrosine phosphorylation of phospholipase C-γ1, formation of inositol 1,4,5-trisphosphate, and mobilization of intracellular calcium. Proc Natl Acad Sci USA 1993;90:6105-6109.
31. Strom TB. Molecular immunology and immunopharmacology of allograft rejection. Kidney Int 1992;42:182-187.
32. Hashimoto Y, King MM, Soderling TR. Regulatory interactions of calmodulin-binding proteins: phosphorylation of calcineurin by autophosphorylated Ca2+/calmodulin-dependent protein kinase II. Proc Natl Acad Sci USA 1988;85:7001-7005.
33. Cyert MS, Kunisawa R, Kaim D, et al. Yeast has homologs (CNA1 and CNA2 gene products) of mammalian calcineurin, a calmodulin-regulated phosphoprotein phosphatase. Proc Natl Acad Sci USA 1991;88:7376-7380.
34. Clipstone NA, Crabtree GR. Identification of calcineurin as a key signalling enzyme in T-lymphocyte activation. Nature 1992;357:695-697.
35. O'Keefe SJ, Tamura J, Kincaid RL, et al. FK-506- and CsA-sensitive activation of the interleukin-2 promoter by calcineurin. Nature 1992;357:692-694.
36. Jain J, McCaffrey PG, Miner Z, et al. The T-cell transcription factor NFATp is a substrate for calcineurin and interacts with Fos and Jun. Nature 1993;365:352-355.
37. Harnett M, Rigley K. The role of G-proteins versus protein tyrosine kinases in the regulation of lymphocyte activation. Immunol Today 1992;13:482-486.
38. Downward J, Graves JD, Warne PH, et al. Stimulation of p21ras upon T-cell activation. Nature 1990;346:719-723.
39. Vojtek AB, Hollenberg SM, Cooper JA. Mammalian ras interacts directly with the serine/threonine kinase raf. Cell 1993;74:205-214.
40. Crews CM, Erikson RL. Extracellular signals and reversible protein phosphorylation: what to mek of it all. Cell 1993;74: 215-217.
41. Pulverer BJ, Hughes K, Franklin CC, et al. Co-purification of mitogen-activated protein kinases with phorbol ester-induced c-jun kinase activity in U937 leukaemic cells. Oncogene 1993;8:407-415.
42. Pulverer BJ, Kyriakis JM, Avruch J, et al. Phosphorylation of c-jun mediated by MAP kinases. Nature 1991;353:670-674.
43. Ward SG, Westwick J, Hall ND, et al. Ligation of CD28 receptor by B7 induces formation of D-3 phosphoinositides in T lymphocytes independently of T cell receptor/CD3 activation. Eur J Immunol 1993;23:2572-2577.
44. Prasad KVS, Janssen O, Kapeller R, et al. Src-homology 3 domain of protein kinase p59fyn mediates binding to phosphatidylinositol 3-kinase in T cells. Proc Natl Acad Sci USA 1993;90:7366-7370.
45. Johnson JG, Jenkins MK. Accessory cell-derived signals required for T cell activation. Immunol Res 1993;12:48-64.

46. Waldmann H, Cobbold S. Monoclonal antibodies for the induction of transplantation tolerance. Curr Opin Immunol 1993;5:753-758.
47. Aruffo A, Kanner SB, Sgroi,D, Ledbetter JA, Stamenkovic I. CD22-mediated stimulation of T cells regulates T-cell receptor/CD3-induced signaling. Proc Natl Acad Sci USA 1992;89:10242-10246.
48. Koretzky GA, Picus J, Schultz T, et al. Tyrosine phosphatase CD45 is required for T-cell antigen receptor and CD2-mediated activation of a protein tyrosine kinase and interleukin 2 production. Proc Natl Acad Sci USA 1991;88:2037-2041.
49. Koretzky GA, Kohmetscher MA, Kadleck T, et al. Restoration of T cell receptor-mediated signal transduction by transfection of CD45 cDNA into a CD45-deficient variant of the jurkat T cell line. J Immunol 1992;149:1138-1142.
50. Kishihara K, Penninger J, Wallace VA, et al. Normal B lymphocyte development but impaired T cell maturation in CD45-exon6 protein tyrosine phosphatase-deficient mice. Cell 1993;74:143-156.
51. Goldman SJ, Uniyal S, Ferguson LM, et al. Differential activation of phosphotyrosine protein phosphatase activity in a murine T cell hybridoma by monoclonal antibodies to CD45. J Biol Chem 1992;267:6197-6204.
52. Donovan JA, Koretzky GA. CD45 and the immune response. J Am Soc Nephrol 1993;4:976-985.
53. Ledbetter JA, Deans JP, Aruffo A, et al. CD4, CD8 and the role of CD45 in T-cell activation. Curr Opin Immunol 1993;5:334-340.
54. Thomas ML. The leukocyte common antigen family. Ann Rev Immunol 1989;7:339-369.
55. Merkenschlager M. Confusion over CD45 isoform. Nature 1991;352:28.
56. Trowbridge IS. CD45: A prototype for transmembrane protein tyrosine phosphatases. J Biol Chem 1991;266:23517-23520.
57. Lazarovits AI, Poppema S, White MJ, et al. Inhibition of alloreactivity in vitro by monoclonal antibodies directed against restricted isoforms of the leukocyte-common antigen (CD45). Transplantation 1992;54:724-729.
58. Linsley PS, Clark EA, Ledbetter JA. T-cell antigen CD28 mediates adhesion with B cells by interacting with activation antigen B7/BB-1. Proc Natl Acad Sci USA 1990;87:5031-5035.
59. Lenschow DJ, Bluestone JA. T cell costimulation and in vivo tolerance. Curr Opin Immunol 1993;5:747-752.
60. Turka LA, Linsley PS, Lin H, et al. T-cell activation by the CD28 ligand B7 is required for cardiac allograft rejection in vivo. Proc Natl Acad Sci USA 1992;89:11102-11105.
61. Fraser JD, Irving BA, Crabtree GR, et al. Regulation of interleukin-2 gene enhancer activity by the T cell accessory molecule CD28. Science 1991;251:313-316.
62. Shahinian A, Pfeffer K, Lee KP, et al. Differential T cell costimulatory requirements in CD28-deficient mice. Science 1993;261:609-612.
63. Geppert TD, Davis LS, Gur H, et al. Accessory cell signals involved in T-cell activation. Immunol Reviews 1990;117:5-66.
64. Osman N, Ley SC, Crumpton MJ. Evidence for an association between the T cell receptor/CD3 antigen complex and the CD5 antigen in human T lymphocytes. Eur J Immunol 1992;22:2995-3000.
65. Osman N, Lazarovits AI, Crumpton MJ. Physical association of CD5 and the T cell receptor/CD3 antigen complex on the surface of human T lymphocytes. Eur J Immunol 1993;23:1173-1176.
66. Davies AA, Ley SC, Crumpton MJ. CD5 is phosphorylated on tyrosine after stimulation of the T-cell antigen receptor complex. Proc Natl Acad Sci USA 1992;89:6368-6372.
67. Ley SC, Davies AA, Druker B, et al. The T cell receptor/CD3 complex and CD2 stimulate the tyrosine phosphorylation of indistinguishable patterns of polypeptides in the human T leukemic cell line Jurkat. Eur J Immunol 1991;21:2203-2209.
68. Ortho Multicenter Transplant Study Group. A randomized clinical trial of OKT3 monoclonal antibody for acute rejection of cadaveric renal transplants. N Engl J Med 1985;313:337-342.

69. Lazarovits AI, Rochon J, Banks L, et al. Human mouse chimeric CD7 monoclonal antibody (SDZCHH380) for the prophylaxis of kidney transplant rejection. J Immunol 1993;150:5163-5174.
70. Hynes RO. Integrins: versatility, modulation, and signaling in cell adhesion. Cell 1992;69:11-25.
71. Berlin C, Berg EL, Briskin MJ, et al. α4β7 integrin mediates lymphocyte binding to the mucosal vascular addressin MAdCAM-1. Cell 1993;74:1-20.
72. Schweighoffer T, Tanaka Y, Tidswell M, et al. Selective expression of integrin α4β7 on a subset of human CD4+ memory T cells with hallmarks of gut-trophism. J Immunol 1993;151:717-729.
73. Hu MCT, Crowe DT, Weissman IL, et al. Cloning and expression of mouse integrin βp(β7): A functional role in Peyer's patch-specific lymphocyte homing. Proc Natl Acad Sci USA 1992;89:8254-8258.
74. Lazarovits AI, Karsh J. Differential expression in rheumatoid synovium and synovial fluid of α4β7 integrin. J Immunol 1993;151:6482-6489.
75. Nojima Y, Rothstein DM, Sugita K, et al. Ligation of VLA-4 on T cells stimulates tyrosine phosphorylation of a 105-kD protein. J Exp Med 1992;175:1045-1053.
76. Yamada A, Nikaido T, Nojima Y, et al. Activation of human CD4 T lymphocytes. J Immunol 1991;146:53-56.
77. Kanner SB, Grosmaire LS, Ledbetter JA, et al. β2-integrin LFA-1 signaling through phospholipase C-γ1 activation. Proc Natl Acad Sci USA 1993;90:7099-7103.
78. Lazarovits AI, Moscicki RA, Kurnick JT, et al. Lymphocyte activation antigens: I. A monoclonal antibody anti-Act I, defines a new late lymphocyte activation antigen. J Immunol 1984;133:1857-1862.
79. Horgan KJ, Ginther Luce GE, Tanaka Y, et al. Differential expression of VLA-α4 and VLA-β1 discriminates multiple subsets of CD4+CD45RO+ "memory" T cells. J Immunol 1992;149:4082-4087.
80. Paul LC, Davidoff A, Benediktsson H, et al. The efficacy of LFA-1 and VLA-4 antibody treatment in rat vascularized cardiac allograft rejection. Transplantation 1993;55:1196-1199.
81. Haug CE, Colvin RB, Delmonico FL, et al. A phase I trial of immunosuppression with anti-ICAM-1 (CD54) mab in renal allograft recipients. Transplantation 1993;55:766-773.
82. Taylor MK, Cohen JJ. Cell-mediated cytotoxicity. Curr Opin Immunol 1992;4:338-343.
83. Suzuki N, Suzuki T, Engleman EG. Evidence for the involvement of CD56 molecules in alloantigen-specific recognition by human natural killer cells. J Exp Med 1991;173:1451-1461.
84. Nakata M, Smyth MJ, Norihisa Y, et al. Constitutive expression of pore-forming protein in peripheral blood γ/δ T cells: implication for their cytotoxic role in vivo. J Exp Med 1990;172:1877-1880.
85. Desai NM, Bassiri H, Kim J, et al. Islet allograft, islet xenograft, and skin allograft survival in CD8+ T lymphocyte-deficient mice. Transplantation 1993;55:718-722.

CHAPTER 3

ALLO- AND XENO- ANTIBODY MEDIATED EVENTS OF PANCREATIC ISLET GRAFTS

Leendert C. Paul

Antibodies, along with major histocompatibility complex molecules and T cell antigen receptors, comprise the three classes of molecules used by the immune system to specifically recognize antigens. Of these three, antibodies are distinguished by the widest range of antigenic structures they can recognize, by the greatest ability to distinguish between different antigens, and by the greatest strength of binding to antigens. The biological properties of antibodies are determined by their antigenic specificity and their ability to activate a variety of biological effector mechanisms. They bind to their antigens through the antigen-binding site in the hypervariable regions located on the F(ab)2 region of the molecule. Once the antibody is bound, different consequences may ensue, depending on the structure, anatomic localization, and isotype of the antibody.

The interest in antibodies as mediators of graft rejection or acceptance has fluctuated over the years. The first clinical observation in the 1960s that suggested that antibodies are able to mediate immediate graft rejection of a vascularized organ transplant[1] stimulated a wide interest in antibody-mediated graft damage. Experimental studies from the 1970s suggested that antibodies may also play a major role in the early rejection of non-vascularized islet grafts.[2-4] The recent interest in xenotransplantation[5] and the potential role of naturally-occurring xenoantibodies in the rapid destruction of transplants exchanged between distantly related donor-recipient combinations has led to a revived curiosity in the mechanisms of antibody mediated graft destruction. Kaliss's work on the role of antibodies in the protection of tumor transplants in the 1960s had established that antigen-specific antibodies can protect allogeneic transplants from rejection and "enhance" their growth.[6] Several experimental studies have tried to induce long-term graft acceptance of islet allografts by treatment of the grafts with antibodies against donor-specific antigens. I will review in this chapter the mechanisms of antibody mediated tissue damage and potential for graft protection by donor specific antibodies.

Pancreatic Islet Transplantation Volume II: Immunomodulation of Pancreatic Islets, edited by Robert P. Lanza, MD, William L. Chick, MD;

TISSUE DAMAGE BY ANTIBODIES

Passive transfer of alloantisera containing high titers of antibodies against donor antigens into recipient rats that are tolerant to donor antigens after neonatal injections of bone marrow cells results in destruction of well-functioning allogeneic islet grafts within one to six days.[2-4] This susceptibility to antibody mediated graft destruction seems specific to islets as vascularized pancreas grafts or fetal pancreata placed under the renal capsule seemed resistant to the damaging effects of antibodies.[3] The specificity of the antibodies responsible for graft rejection have not been established but as islets express normally mostly class I MHC antigens and no or very little class II antigens,[7,8] it would seem most likely that high titers of class I antibodies were responsible for the induction of graft damage. Anti-class II antibodies may, however, at least at some point, contribute to further damage since combinations of cytokines like interferon-γ in combination with tumour necrosis factor-α may induce expression of class II MHC antigens on fraction of the islet β cells.[8] Antibody-mediated damage of β cells may be mediated through complement-dependent and/or complement independent pathways such as antibody-dependent cell-mediated cytotoxicity.

COMPLEMENT ACTIVATION BY ANTIBODIES

The complement system consists of a family of serum proteins that are activated by a proteolytic cascade to generate the effector molecules that mediate many of the cytolytic and inflammatory effects of humoral immunity.[9] The complement system can be activated through the so-called "classical" or the "alternative" activation routes.

The classical activation pathway is triggered when one of the complement proteins, C1q, binds to the C_H3 domain of IgM or C_H2 domain of complement binding IgG molecules. A single C1q molecule must bind simultaneously to at least two immunoglobulin Fc portions; therefore a minimum of one pentameric IgM or two IgG molecules bound closely together at a cell surface are required for activation. Soluble IgM does not bind the C1 because the Fc regions are inaccessible for the C1 protein in solution but binding of the antibody molecule to a cell surface induces a conformational change that exposes the Fc regions, allowing the C1q molecule of the C1 complex to bind. Binding of two or more of the C1q subunits of the C1 molecule leads to enzymatic activation of the molecule which can now act on the C4 and C2 molecules of the classical activation pathway, leading to the formation of a C4b2a complex, which functions as the classical pathway C3 convertase.

In the alternative pathway, C3b is generated spontaneously at low levels or by IgA antibodies[10] and binds to a protein called Bb generated by proteolytic cleavage of a protein called Factor B. The C3bBb complex is the alternative pathway C3 convertase, functioning, like the classical pathway convertase, to further breakdown and generate more C3b.

The next step in both pathways is the binding of C3b to the C3 convertase enzymes, changing them to C5 convertases, which catalyze the proteolytic cleavage of the C5 protein. Although the C5 convertases of the two pathways are molecularly distinct, they catalyze identical reactions and act on identical substrates. Once C5 is cleaved, both pathways share the same terminal step. These terminal events do not involve proteolysis, but rather the sequential binding of several soluble complement proteins called C6, C7, C8, and C9, to the activating surface. This leads to the formation of a lipid soluble pore structure, called the membrane attack complex, which causes osmotic lysis of cells.

Different effector functions are mediated by different complement proteins produced during complement activation. Inflammation, consisting of the recruitment and activation of leukocytes, is mediated by cleavage products of C3, C4, and C5, called C3a, C4a, and C5a, respectively. Granulocytes and monocytes are attracted to sites of complement activation by the chemotactic factor C5a and the trimolecular C5,6,7 complex; C5a also stimulates the release of leukocyte lysosomal enzymes and may play a role in the granulocyte-dependent induction of inflammatory edema.[11]

When C3b is bound to cells of a transplant, circulating recipient cells with C3b receptors can adhere to graft cells and be activated. C3b acts in this way as an opsonin for monocytes and polymorphonuclear granulocytes. Likewise, C3b can cause immune adherence of erythrocytes. In addition, in experimental animals but not in man, C3b can cause immune adherence of platelets which may lead to the release of vasoactive amines and nucleotides from platelets. C3a and C5a furthermore stimulate mast cells to release histamine, contract smooth muscle cells, and increase capillary permeability, while a fragment of C2 has kinin activity.

Cytolysis is mediated by the membrane attack complex. Although one membrane attack complex, which consists ultrastructurally of a doughnut-like structure with a 200 Å diameter electron lucent rim and a 100 Å electron-opaque centre, is sufficient to cause lysis of an erythrocyte, metabolically more active nucleated cells are more resistant to lysis due to their ability to rapidly eliminate the C5b-9 complex, to repair the plasma membrane, and the osmoregulatory properties of nucleated cells. Therefore, although prompt leakage of ions can be demonstrated at low doses of complement, cytolysis occurs only after the formation of several transmembrane channels and an appreciable time delay.[12] Even if the membrane attack complex does not cause lysis it may contribute to the development of tissue damage through the stimulation of the production of potent mediators of inflammation such as reactive oxygen metabolites, prostaglandins, and interleukin-1 like cytokines.[13,14]

Uncontrolled complement activation leads to formation of the membrane attack complex on tissues and excessive generation of inflammatory mediators. This does not normally happen because both the classical and alternative activation cascades are tightly regulated by several fluid-phase and membrane proteins that interact in specific ways with the various complement components. The proteolytic activity of C1 is inhibited by C1 inhibitor while the formation of the classical pathway C3 convertase is inhibited by the C4 binding protein (C4bp) and the membrane bound type 1 complement receptor (CR1). Both proteins bind to C4b and competively inhibit the binding of C2b, thus preventing the assembly and accelerating the dissociation of the classical pathway C3 convertase. C4bp and CR1 as well as another protein called membrane cofactor protein (MCP) act as cofactors that promote the proteolysis of C4b by a protein called Factor I. The formation of the classical pathway C3 convertase is also inhibited by decay accelerating factor (DAF), a 70 kD phosphatidylinositol-linked or transmembrane glycoprotein found on all peripheral blood cells, endothelium, and various mucosal epithelial cells. Like C4bp and CR1, DAF binds to C4b, in competition with C2, thereby inhibiting classical pathway convertase formation and promoting dissociation of C3 convertase after it is formed.

Factor H, a soluble serum protein, inhibits the alternative pathway C3 convertase. Factor H competes with Factor B and Bb for binding to C3b. In addition, the two membrane proteins, CR1 and DAF, bind to C3b and competitively inhibit the binding of Factor B, thus preventing the assembly of the alternative pathway C3 convertase. The formation of the alternative convertase, C3bBb is inhibited by Factor I-mediated proteolysis of C3b. Factor I cleavage of C3b is promoted by at least three different cofactors, including Factor H, CR1 and MCP.

Different cells express different amounts of the regulatory proteins, MCP and CR1, thus controlling the site at which C3b and the alternative pathway C3 convertase are formed. This is particularly important because the C3 tickover mechanism is capable of continuously generating C3b, with the potential to form more and more alternative pathway convertase. Most normal cells express high levels of MCP and/or CR1, which protect these cells from complement mediated injury. In contrast, many foreign particles and xenogeneic surfaces either lack or express MCP and CR1 in a form that does not interact with human C3b so that C3b deposited on these surfaces is not inactivated and binds Factor B with higher affinity than Factor H promoting the formation of the

C3bBb complex which leads to complement activation on these foreign surfaces.

Homologous restriction factor (HRF) and CD59, also called membrane inhibitor of reactive lysis or MIRL, inhibit the formation of the membrane attack complex. Both these membrane proteins show the property of homologous restriction; i.e., they efficiently inhibit MAC mediated lysis only when the terminal complement components are from the same species as the cells on which HRF and CD59 are expressed. The insertion of the terminal complement components into lipid membranes is inhibited by S protein, also called vitronectin. HRF may further protect tissues from complement-mediated damage.

Antibody-Dependent Cell-Mediated Cytotoxicity

Several different leukocyte populations such as neutrophils, eosinophils, mononuclear phagocytes and NK cells are capable of lysing various target cells that are precoated with specific IgG through a cytolytic process called antibody-dependent cell-mediated cytotoxicity (ADCC). Recognition of bound antibody occurs through low-affinity receptors for Fcγ on the leukocyte, called FcRIII or CD16. In the case of NK cells, the predominant cellular mediators of ADCC, it is now appreciated that IgG serves two distinct functions. Cell bound IgG provides a cognitive function in that those target cells that have IgG bound on their surface are preferentially killed compared with cells that are not coated with IgG. Occupancy of the FcRIII furthermore serves to activate the NK cell to synthesize and secrete cytokines such as tumour necrosis factor and interferon-γ as well as to discharge their granules. The released cytokines and granule proteins mediate very likely the cytolytic functions of this cell type and may upregulate the expression of various antigens and adhesion molecules involved in allogeneic cellular interactions.[8,15]

Since CD16 is a low affinity receptor that binds aggregated IgG more efficiently than monomeric IgG, monomeric plasma IgG does not activate NK cells nor does it compete effectively with cell-bound IgG for the Fc receptor. Only small amounts of cell-bound antibody are required to localize and trigger the effector cells in ADCC and this mechanism may increase the effectiveness of low concentrations of antibody. ADCC mechanisms are capable of killing histoincompatible target cells in vitro and the antibody concentrations involved are too low to initiate complement-mediated cytotoxicity. Xenogeneic skin graft rejection in the mouse initiated by noncomplement-fixing antibodies may be an example of graft rejection mediated by ADCC.[16]

Polymorphonuclear cells and monocytes express receptors for the Fc regions of IgA antibodies and may mediate antibody-dependent cell mediated cytotoxicity.[17]

Other Fc Receptor Dependent Antibody-Mediated Tissue Damage

A pharmacologically potent cell with Fc receptors is the platelet. Platelets may interact with graft bound antibodies through either their Fc receptors or via complement-dependent pathways. Platelets contain potent vasoconstrictive, proaggregatory, and proinfammatory substances including platelet-derived growth factor, epidermal growth factor, serotonins, thromboxanes, and platelet-activating factor. The release of these compounds from the platelets causes a wide variety of physiological changes including vasoconstriction and organ dysfunction. The importance of platelets in antibody-mediated damage of islet grafts remains to be investigated.

ANTIBODIES IN XENOGENEIC ISLET CELL GRAFTING

The succesfull clinical implementation of islet transplantation will certainly increase the demand for islet grafts and organ shortage may become the limiting factor. Therefore, the use of islets from xenogeneic donors might be considered. Porcine islets seem an attractive option as they can be obtained relatively easily with high yields and there is a close structural similarity between porcine and human insulin.

The role of preformed natural antibodies in the rapid rejection of xenogeneic grafts is presently not well defined but in vitro incubation of pancreatic islets with antibody containing xenogeneic antisera results in decreased insulin output, consistent with the hypothesis that antibodies cause cytolysis of β cells.[18] The higher primary non-function rate of islet xenografts between more distantly related large animals compared with more related species is also consistent with the hypothesis that xeno-reactive antibodies may play a role in the rapid islet graft destruction.[19] Transplantation of pancreatic microfragments from newborn Landrace pigs underneath the kidney capsule of normoglycemic LEW rats that had no antibodies against pig lymphocytes or pancreas fragments survived for up to 3 weeks in recipients treated with azathioprine and cyclosporine.[20] LEW rats contain, however, antibodies against LEWE minipig pancreatic islets and transplantation of LEWE islets underneath the kidney capsule resulted in rapid islet destruction,[21] consistent with the hypothesis that preformed antibodies are responsible for the early rejection.

Indirect immunofluoresence studies of normal human sera with tissue sections from Dutch Landrace pigs has shown that 70 to 80% of sera contain naturally occurring antibodies against pancreas vascular endothelium; 60% of the sera contained IgA antibodies against islet cells, 36% IgM antibodies and 26% IgG antibodies.[22] The presence of IgA antibodies is of special interest since human IgA antibodies can activate the alternative complement activation route, as discussed,[10] and seem to have highly inflammatory potential.[23] Other investigators investigated sera from IDDM patients for antibodies against pancreatic tissues from several different races of pigs and found that all sera contained either IgG and/or IgM antibodies against various pancreatic elements.[24] Athough this study found a much lower incidence of antibodies in normal sera than the study from Schaapherder et al,[22] they found that sera from diabetic patients contained significantly more often strong antibody reactivity against islet cells compared with normal control sera: 30% versus 4%. Of interest is the observation that up to 1/5 of sera from diabetic patients did not contain antibodies against porcine endocrine islet cells from seven different pig strains.[24] It has been suggested that many of these xenoreactive antibodies are directed against carbohydrate epitopes.[18]

Several studies have shown that membrane-bound inhibitors of C3 convertases on xenogeneic surfaces are incapable of inactivating the "normally" occuring recipient alternate pathway complement activation and formation of C3 convertase, leading to unantagonized complement activation and tissue destruction. Guinea pig red blood cells can be lysed by normal rat serum through alternative pathway activation and transplantation of a guinea pig heart into a normal LEW rat results in hyperacute rejection in association with normal levels of C2 and C4 but low levels of C3, consistent with alternative pathway activation.[25] It is presently unclear whether this tissue damaging pathway is used in xenogeneic islet rejection.

Preliminary clinical data on the transplantation of fetal porcine islet-like clusters into three human diabetic recipients have been reported.[26] All three patients had previously undergone renal transplantation and were on immunosuppressive drugs; one patient had evidence of engraftment, as indicated by the presence of porcine C-peptide in the serum and urine. All three patients had IgM and one had non-IgM cytotoxic antibodies against peripheral blood cells and pancreatic tissues prior to transplantation but these antibodies did not cause hyperacute rejection of the transplanted islets.

Thus, following xenogeneic transplantation of islets into a recipient with performed natural antibodies, the islets are exposed to several mediators that may be involved in β cell damage such as antibodies, complement, cytokines, macrophages, and natural killer cells but it is presently not clear under what conditions these mediators cause irreversible tissue damage. The development of microencapsulation methods that do not allow the passage of immunoglobulins should be able to overcome the detrimental effects of antibodies on pancreatic islet cell grafts.[27]

DIABETES-ASSOCIATED AUTOANTIBODIES

Screening of patients with type 1 diabetes have shown that many of these individuals have antibodies against both non-β-cell specific components like tubulin,[28] β cell specific compounds[29,30] and insulin.[31] The importance of these antibodies in the post-transpant islet cell destruction is not clear. However, implantation of an SV-40 transformed pancreatic β-cell line derived from an NOD mouse into a diabetic NOD mouse results in their destruction within 3 weeks as a result of β-cell directed autoimmunity. Implantation of the cells within an immunoisolation device that prevents the entry of cells but allows the passage of antibodies and complement did not result in tissue destruction, suggesting that antibodies alone do not cause β-cell destruction.[32]

ANTIBODY-MEDIATED PROTECTION OF ALLOGRAFTED TISSUES

Injection of antidonor antibodies into the recipient at about the time of transplantation can enhance the survival of a vascularized transplant and induce long-term graft survival.[33,34] The phenomenon of antibody induced prolongation of graft survival has been studied extensively in the late 1970s and early 1980s. In general, passive enhancement works best in low-responder donor-recipient combinations and is effective for kidney grafts, may be effective for heart grafts, and has very little influence on skin graft rejection. Some subclasses of IgG work better than others while IgM tends to accelerate rejection. Intact antibody, as opposed to Fab fragments, is required for suppression in most but not all experimental models of vascularized organ allografts.[35] Several mechanisms have been proposed to explain antibody-mediated prolongation of graft survival, including "masking" of donor antigens, removal or inactivation of passenger leukocytes, Fc-receptor mediated feed-back suppression of allogeneic immune reactions and anti-idiotypic antibody mediated suppression.

The concept of masking of donor antigens is that a layer of recipient "self" protein coats the antigens of the graft and prevents recognition. Although this concept has not received much support in vascularized organ grafts, several groups have presented evidence to support this possibility in islet allografts. As MHC class I molecules are the prominent antigens expressed on islets,[7,8] several investigators have targeted these molecules. The observation that in vitro treatment of islets with donor class I directed monoclonal antibody or its F(ab)2 fragments abolishes the generation of islet-directed cytotoxic cells in mixed allogeneic islet-splenocyte co-cultures is consistent with this hypothesis.[36] The survival of antibody-pretreated islets was in one study not different from that of non-treated islets[37] while the results from another study showed that preincubation with donor-specific F(ab)2 anti-class I antibody fragments but not the intact antibody molecule prolonged graft survival from 7 days to 200 days.[38] The MHC class I molecules seem of particular importance because F(ab)2 fragments from a polyclonal antiserum raised against human islets failed to produce prolonged graft survival after removal of the anti-class I antibodies.[38] It was furthermore shown that in vitro antibody treatment and graft acceptance was associated with the development of systemic tolerance which allowed the survival of unmodified cell grafts administered at a later time period.

Snell introduced in the 1950s the concept that organ allografts are immunogenic by virtue of their content of passenger leukocytes present in the graft at the time of transplantation;[39] such cells leave the graft after transplantation and stimulate the recipient immune system. This concept has been further expanded by Lafferty et al who showed that thyroid allografts depleted of bone-marrow derived passenger cells by prior in vitro culture enjoyed prolonged survival in non-immunosuppressed recipients.[40] The passenger leukocytes responsible for induction of graft immunity are cells with a striking dendritic morphology that express large quantities of class II MHC antigens and are potent stimulators of mixed leukocyte reactions. Pancreatic islet tissue, cultured in vitro under conditions believed to destroy passenger leukocytes and capillary endothelial cells can sometimes be transplanted successfully from allogeneic and even xenogeneic donors into recipient mice without chronic immunosuppression while uncultured grafts are rejected.[41]

Since β cells of normal islets do not express class II antigens,[7,8] antibodies against class II antigens may deplete class II positive cells, i.e. passenger cells, and, dependent on the species, the class II positive capillary endothelial cells within the islet, resulting in decreased immunogenicity.[24] Faustman et al eliminated class II-positive and dendritic cells from mouse islet allografts pretreated with antibody and complement which resulted in prolongation of graft survival times to more than 200 days.[42,43] Other investigators have failed, however, to induce prolonged survival using similar protocols in both mice and rats,[44,46] despite substantial reductions in numbers of class II positive cells per islet. Although it is conceivable that the lack of in vivo efficacy is quantitative rather than qualitative, i.e. incomplete depletion of class II positive non-endocrine cells, the available data do not support the hypothesis that antidonor class II antibodies cause prolongation of graft survival because of their ability to decrease the number of class II positive immunogenic cells from the graft.

Antidonor IgG antibodies may enhance graft acceptance through Fc receptor mediated mechanims.[47] The Fc portion of the antibody interacts with Fc receptors on B cells, crosslinking the Fc receptor and the surface immunoglobulin B-cell receptor which results in a rise in intracellular cyclic-AMP levels and unresponsiveness.[48] The Fc receptor and antigen-specific receptor could also be on different cells types such as macrophages and B cells.

T cell receptors capable of binding free antigenic determinants in immune complexes containing MHC antigens can become coated with antibody molecules and thereby be opsonized and phagocytosed by Fc receptor bearing macrophages.[49] The evidence in favor of this mechanism of antigen-reactive cell opsonization is that radiolabeled donor-specific T lymphocytes are opsonized by serum from long-surviving kidney graft recipients and that radiolabeled antidonor T cells, injected intravenously into long-term survivors, are selectively destroyed in the liver.[50]

Anti-idiotypic antibodies, antibodies specific for the antigen-binding site of other antibodies or the T cell receptor, can block the activation of the antigen-receptor bearing cell, tolerize the cell, mark it for destruction through blocking antigen recognition, cross-linking cell surface receptors to cause inactivation, complement-mediated lysis, or opsonization.

CONCLUSIONS

Available data suggest that antibodies against allogeneic or xenogeneic cell surface antigens of the β cells may cause damage and loss of functions of these cells although there are no data available to demonstrate this pathway in vivo. Several models of antibody-mediated prolongation of graft survival have been described but there is no consistent evidence to support the hypothesis that intact antibodies against graft alloantigens cause prolongation of islet allograft survival in vivo. More work needs to be done to define the specificity and pathogenicity of the various anti-β cell antibodies.

REFERENCES

1. Kissmeyer-Nielsen F, Olsen S, Petersen VP, et al. Hyperacute rejection of kidney allografts associated with pre-existing humoral antibodies against donor cells. Lancet 1: 662-5, 1966.
2. Naji A, Reckard CR, Ziegler MM, et al. Vulnerability of pancreatic islets to immune cells and serum. Surg Forum 26: 459-60,1975.
3. Frangipane LG, Poole TW, Barker CF, et al. Vulnerability of allogeneic and xenogeneic pancreatic islets to alloantisera. Tranplant Proc 9: 371-3,1977.
4. Perloff PJ, Naji A, Barker CF. Islet sensitivity to humoral antibody. Surg Forum 32: 390-1, 1981.
5. Cooper DKC, Kemp E, Reemtsma K, et al. (eds). Xenotransplantation. The transplantation of organs and tissues between species. Springer-Verlag, 1991.

6. Kaliss N. Immunological enhancement: conditions for its expression and its relevance for grafts of normal tissues. Ann N Y Acad Sci 129: 155-63, 1966.
7. Faustman D, Hauptfeld V, Davie JM, et al. Murine pancreatic β-cells express H-2K and H2-D but not Ia antigens. J Exp Med 151: 1563-8, 1980.
8. Campbell IL, Oxbrow L, West J, et al. Regulation of MHC protein expression in pancreatic β-cells by interferon-γ and tumor necrosis factor-α. Mol Endocrinol 2: 101-7, 1988.
9. Abbas A, Lichtman AH, Pober JS. Cellular and molecular immunology. WB Saunders Company. Harcourt Brace Jovanovich, Inc., Philadelphia, London, Toronto, Montreal, Sydney and Tokyo. 1991.
10. Hiemstra PS, Gorter A, Stuurman ME,et al. Activation of the alternative pathway of complement by human serum IgA. Eur J Immunol 17: 321-6, 1987.
11. Wedmore CV, Williams TJ. Control of vascular permeability by polymorphonuclear leukocytes in inflammation. Nature 289: 646-50, 1981.
12. Kim S-H, Carney DF, Hammer CH, et al. Nucleated cell killing by complement: effects of C5b-9 channel size and extracellular $Ca2^{+}$ on the lytic process. J Immunol 138: 1530-6, 1987.
13. Lovett D, Hansch G, Resch K, et al. Activation of glomerular mesangial cells by terminal complement components. Stimulation of prostanoid and interleukin-1 like factor release. Immunology 168: 34-5, 1984.
14. Adler S, Baker PJ, Johnson RJ, et al. Complement membrane attack complex stimulates production of reactive oxygen metabolites by cultured rat mesangial cells. J Clin Invest 77: 762-7, 1986.
15. Campbell IL, Cutri A, Wilkinson D, et al. Intercellular adhesion molecule I is induced on isolated islet cells by cytokines but not reovirus infection. Proc Natl Acad Sci USA 86: 4282-6, 1989.
16. Berden JH, Bogman MJ, Hageman GH, et al. Complement-dependent and independent mechanisms in acute antibody-mediated rejection of skin xenografts in the mouse. Transplantation 32: 265-70, 1981.
17. Kerr MA. The structure and function of human IgA. Biochem J 271: 285-96,1990.
18. Laus R, Ulrichs K, Müller-Rüchholtz W. Carbohydrate-specific human heterophile antibodies in normal human sera that react with xenogeneic cells. Int Arch Allergy Appl Immunol 85: 201- 7, 1988.
19. Bandien KO, Toledo-Pereyra LH, Gordon DA. Islet cell allo- and xenotransplantation-effect of collagenase-free processing and renal subcapsular site. Transplant Proc 19: 2362-3,1987.
20. Jahr H, Braun K. Effects of donor tissue or recipient treatment on the survival of pig pancreas endocrine tissue transplanted into normoglycemic rats. Transplant Proc 24: 655,1992.
21. Braun K, Jahr. Organ-specific natural antibodies in pig islet xenotransplantation. Transplant Proc 24: 2979, 1993.
22. Schaapherder AFM, Daha MR, Van der Woude FJ, et al. IgM, IgG, and IgA antibodies in human sera directed against procine islets of Langerhans. Transplantation 56: 739-41, 1993.
23. Mestecky J, McGhee JR. Immunoglobulin A (IgA): molecular and cellular interactions involved in IgA biosynthesis and immune response. Adv Immunol 40: 153-245, 1987.
24. Eckstein V, Ülrichs K, Meincke G, et al. Natural xenophile antibodies from sera of type 1 diabetic patients differ strongly in their reactivity against various porcine pancreatic cells. Transplant Proc 24: 681- 3,1992.
25. Miyagawa S, Hirose H, Shirakura R, et al. The mechanism of discordant xenograft rejection. Transplantation 46: 825-30, 1988.
26. Kumagai Braesch M, Groth CG, Korsgren O, et al. Immune response of diabetic patients against transplanted porcine fetal islet cells. Transplant Proc 24: 679-80, 1992.
27. Hallé J-P, Bourassa S, Leblond FA, et al. Protection of islets of Langerhans from antibodies by microencapsulation with alginate-poly-L-lysine membranes. Transplantation 55: 350-4, 1993.
28. Rousset B, Vialettes B, Bernier-Valentin F, et al. Anti-tubulin antibodies in recent onset type 1 (insulin-dependent) diabetes mellitus: comparison with islet cell antibodies. Diabetologia 27: 427-32, 1984.

29. Bækkeskov S, Landen M, Kristensen JK, et al. Antibodies to a 64,000 Mr human islet cell antigen precede the clinical onset of insulin-dependent diabetes. J Clin Invest 79: 926-34, 1987.
30. Bækkeskov S, Aanstoot H-J, Chistgau S, et al. Identification of the 64k autoantigen in insulin-dependent diabetes as a GABA-synthesizing enzyme glutamic acid decarboxylase.Nature (London) 347: 151- 6, 1990.
31. Palmer JP, Aspin CM, Clemons P, et al. Insulin antibodies in insulin dependent diabetics before insulin treatment. Science 222: 1337-9, 1983.
32. Hodgson RJ, Loudovaris T, Charlton B, et al. Destruction of transplanted β cells into diabetic NOD mice is not mediated by antibody alone. Transplant Proc 24: 2300, 1992.
33. French ME, Batchelor JR. Immunological enhancement of rat kidney allografts. Lancet 2: 1103-6, 1969.
34. Morris PJ. Suppression of rejection of organ allografts by antibody. Immunol Rev 49: 93-125, 1980.
35. Winearls CG, Fabre JW, Millard PR, et al. A quantitative comparison of whole antibody and F(ab')2 in kidney allograft enhancement. Transplantation 28: 36-9,1979.
36. Munn SR, Marjoribanks C. Abrogation of islet immunogenicity using an anti-MHC class 1 monoclonal antibody. Transplant Proc 24: 1038-9, 1992.
37. Munn SR, Marjoribanks. Masking donor major histocompatibility complex class 1 antigens on allogeneic islets. Transplant Proc 24: 2857, 1992.
38. Faustman D, Coe C. Prevention of xenograft rejection by masking donor HLA class I antigens. Science 252: 1700-2, 1991.
39. Snell GD. The homograft reaction. Ann Rev Microbiol 11: 439-58, 1957.
40. Lafferty KJ, Bootes A, Dart G, et al. Effect of organ culture on the survival of thyroid allografts in mice. Transplantation 22: 138-49,1976.
41. Lacy PE, Davie JM. Transplantation of pancreatic islets. Ann Rev Immunol 2: 183-98, 1984.
42. Faustman D, Hauptfeld V, Lacy P, et al. Prolongation of murine islet allograft survival by pretreatment of islets with antibody directed to Ia determinants. Proc Natl Acad Sci USA 78: 5156-9, 1981.
43. Faustman DL, Steinman RM, Gebel HM, et al. Prevention of mouse islet allograft rejection by elimination of intraislet dendritic cells. Transplant Proc 17: 420-4, 1985.
44. Gores PF, Sutherland DER, Platt JL, et al. Depletion of donor Ia+ cells before transplantation does not prolong islet allograft survival. J Immunol 137: 1482-5, 1986.
45. Reece-Smith H, Mc Shane P, Morris PJ. Pretreatment of isolated adult islets with antibody. Effect on survival in allogeneic hosts. Transplantation 36: 228-30, 1983.
46. Bretzel RG, Flesch BK, Brennenstuhl G, et al. Rat pancreatic islet pretreatmen with anti-MHC class II monoclonal antibodies and culture: in vitro MLIC test response does not predict islet allograft survival. Acta Diabetol 30: 49-56, 1993.
47. Sinclair NRStC, Panoskaltsis A. Immunoregulation by Fc signals: A mechanism of self-nonself discrimination Immunol Today 8: 76-9, 1987.
48. Harnett MM, Klaus GGB. G protein regulation of receptor signaling. Immunol Today 9: 315-20, 1988.
49. Hutchinson IV, Brent L. Effect of decomplementation with cobra venom factor on the passive immunological enhancement of mouse skin allografts. Transplantation 34: 64-7, 1982.
50. Hutchinson IV. Antigen-reactive cell opsonization (ARCO) and its role in antibody-mediated immune suppression. Immunol Rev 49: 167-97, 1980.

CHAPTER 4

Cytokines in Transplantation

Margaret J. Dallman

Cytokines are important mediators of cellular communication and have a major role in directing not only the magnitude, but also the nature of immune responses. During the immune response to transplanted tissue a wide variety of cytokines are expressed which, if unchecked, produce a leukocytic response that results in graft rejection. As if this weren't bad enough, transplanters of islet grafts must also concern themselves with the apparently directly toxic effects of certain cytokines on the islets themselves (Fig. 4.1).

The response associated with graft rejection sees the production of two types of cytokines, the proinflammatory and inflammatory cytokines such as IL-1, IL-6 and TNFα and the essentially T cell derived cytokines such as IL 2, IFNγ, IL-4 and IL-5. Whilst controlling the latter type of cytokine may be most important in the control of graft rejection itself, with respect to islet transplantation, it may be critical to control the expression of all of these cytokines as it is the inflammatory cytokines which appear to exert the directly toxic effects on islets.

CYTOKINES PRODUCED AS A RESULT OF SURGICAL PROCEDURES AND INFLAMMATION

Some time ago we and a number of other groups began to investigate the expression of cytokines following both experimental and clinical transplantation. A variety of different approaches have been taken including measurement of cytokines in the circulation or draining fluids of transplants by bioassay or enzyme-linked immunosorbant assay/radioimmunoassay (ELISA/RIA) and the direct measurement of cytokine transcripts within the grafts (for recent reviews see[1,2,3,4]). Of particular interest is that certain cytokines such as IL-1 and IL-6 are produced irrespective of there being an associated immune response. This is perhaps particularly obvious in the experimental models of transplantation where it is possible to compare cytokine expression in syngeneic grafts with that occurring in allogeneic grafts. In the former, an inflammatory but not an immune response will occur whilst in the latter, not only the inflammatory response associated with surgery, but also an immune response will occur. Using a semi-quantitative, reverse transcriptase-polymerase chain reaction (RT-PCR) we have found in syngeneic transplants, including in mouse heart or rat heart, liver

Pancreatic Islet Transplantation Volume II: Immunomodulation of Pancreatic Islets, edited by Robert P. Lanza, MD, William L. Chick, MD; ©1994 R.G. Landes Company.

and small bowel grafts, a very early increase in several cytokine transcripts, particularly those for IL-1 and IL-6[5] (and unpublished). It is likely that some of these cytokines, for instance IL-6, are expressed by parenchymal cells of the graft itself. The expression of these cytokines diminishes fairly rapidly in the syngeneic grafts. In the allografts however, we have observed the same initial burst of expression which may decline slightly, but which again rapidly increases as the graft becomes infiltrated by leukocytes of many different types and rejection begins. Of interest is that rather similar results have been obtained in clinical transplantation where serum levels of IL-6 are found to increase rapidly following kidney transplantation and to decline only in the absence of rejection.[6] Further, Yoshimura et al[6] and other workers[7] have demonstrated that serum IL-6 levels rise in association with infection but often not with rejection episodes. Studies in patients undergoing surgery that is unrelated to transplantation have also demonstrated increases in circulating IL-1 and IL-6 confirming that the expression of such cytokines may occur in the absence of an immune response.[8]

The presence of this type of cytokine in islet grafts is clearly of great interest since, as mentioned above, they may be directly toxic for islets. The evidence for direct toxicity of cytokines to islets comes mainly from cell culture systems in which IL-1β, IL-6, TNFα and IFNγ are all detrimental to islet survival and /or insulin secretion.[9,10,11,12,13,14] These cytokines appear to have somewhat varying effects on islets of different species, but are usually additive or synergistic in their damaging effects which seem to be mediated in large part through the elaboration of nitric oxide and free radicals.[15,16] Further, it has been shown that, following a variety of stimuli, islet β cells themselves can produce the very cytokines that may be damaging.[16,17,18] For instance, after exposure to

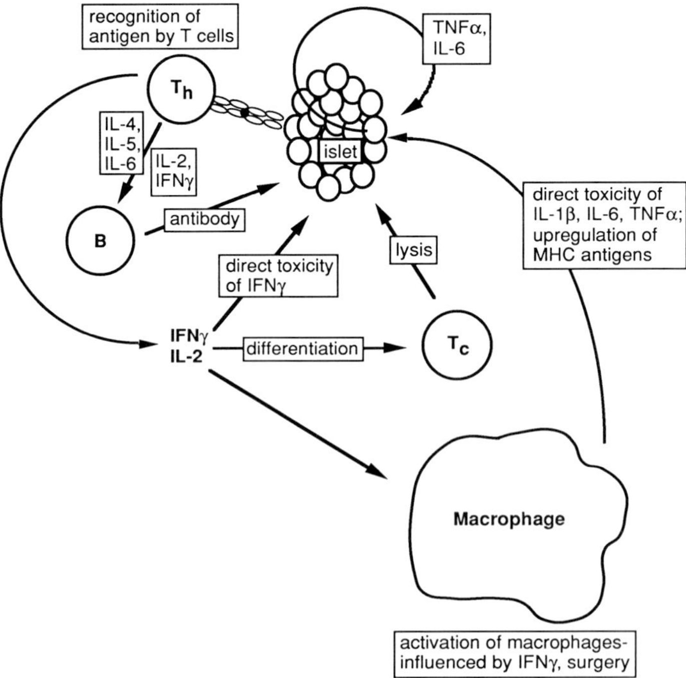

Fig. 4.1. The cytokine network and damage to islets.

IL-1β, β cells will produce quite substantial levels of TNFα.[17] There has been very little work on the expression of cytokines following islet cell transplantation and, in the only published work of this kind, the expression of IL-1, IL-6 or TNFα was not examined.[19] In this study however, IFNγ transcripts were detected in both syngeneic and allogeneic grafts and their level declined rapidly in the syngeneic grafts whilst being maintained in the allografts. It will be of great interest to islet transplanters to analyse the expression of inflammatory cytokines in such grafts and to try to assess their contribution not only to the rejection process, but also to the primary non-fuction that sometimes occurs.

CYTOKINES PRODUCED AS A RESULT OF THE ANTIGEN-SPECIFIC IMMUNE RESPONSE

Using similar techniques to those mentioned above, cytokines derived primarily from T cells, such as IL-2, IL-4, IL-5 and IFNγ have also been detected following organ grafting. It appears to be more difficult to detect such cytokines in the circulation, although this has been described during the rejection of clinical renal[20] and liver[21] transplants. Soluble IL-2 receptors (IL-2R) are clearly found in the circulation of some transplant patients, although the relationship between expression and graft rejection is not clear.[22,23,24] T cell derived cytokines are probably normally expressed in rather low amounts and primarily function at a local level, so perhaps it is not surprising that it is often difficult to find these cytokines in the circulation. Using an analysis of mRNA by RT-PCR it is possible to detect expression of these T cell cytokines within experimental allografts, but only at very low or undetectable levels in syngeneic grafts.[5,19] Of note is that the expression of most T cell associated cytokines is rather transient, peaking before loss of graft function occurs. This means that the interpretation of clinical results, where material is often only obtained from grafts on an infrequent basis, is rather difficult. In the clinical studies performed, IL-2 for instance often does not show an increase during rejection.[25] In view of the experimental data this may not be surprising and indeed in a study in which daily samples of kidney transplants were obtained by fine needle aspiration, we found expression of IL-2 before, but often not during, rejection.[26] O'Connell et al[19] in their study of experimental islet grafts also found expression of T cell derived cytokines associated with graft rejection. Of interest was that although IL-2 and IFNγ were expressed, again in transient fashion, IL-4 was undetectable in most grafts.

Although RT-PCR has been very useful for examining cytokine expression in vivo in that it is easy to analyse local events, is very rapid and requires only very small amounts of material, it clearly also has some disadvantages. First, it is not possible, unless isolated populations of cells are used, to ascribe cytokine production to any particular cell type. The problem with isolating cells before analysis is that cytokine mRNAs tend to have rather short half-lives[27,28,29] such that lengthy methods of cell purification will render results difficult to interpret. Alternatively, the methods used to isolate cells may themselves induce expression of certain cytokines. Second, the level of mRNA expression may not always directly relate to the level of protein production. Both of these problems could be addressed if antibodies could be routinely used in immunohistology to detect cytokine protein on tissue sections. This theoretically very attractive approach has been rather more difficult for many people to achieve than one might have imagined, although some groups, with judicial choice of antibodies, have been successful.[30,31,32,33] The disadvantages of this approach appear to be first, that it is difficult to distinguish cells that are synthesizing cytokine from those that have bound and/or internalized cytokine. This problem is tackled by the combined use of in situ hybridization and immunohistology,[34] but this approach should not be tackled by the faint hearted as it is very time consuming and difficult! Second, unexpected patterns of expression may be observed[35] raising questions about the specificity of staining.

CYTOKINES AND THE INDUCTION OF IMMUNOSUPPRESSION OR TRANSPLANTATION TOLERANCE

Some years ago it was noted that, depending on the nature of antigen delivery and other variables, an immune response tended towards either a cell- or antibody-mediated reaction.[36] At the time, the reasons for this apparent divergence in the immune response were not clear but more recently it has been suggested that the different responses result from the production of different cytokines. [37] Cellular immune responses tend to be driven by an IL-2 and IFNγ dominated profile, whilst antibody production is associated with IL-4, IL-5 and IL-6 production. This association is however not completely clear cut, since the production of particular subclasses of antibody seems to require the presence of IL-2 and IFNγ and cytokines such as IL-4 may be involved in the generation of cytotoxic T cells. Nevertheless, there are several examples in animals in which domination of the immune response by particular cytokines allows either progression or resolution of disease. For example, inbred mouse strains infected with *Leishmania major* may either be resistant or susceptible to disease.[38,39] In resistant strains, coincidentally with control of the disease and the appearance of delayed type hypersensitivity to parasite antigens, there is an increase in CD4+ T cells that secrete IFNγ. In comparison, the reaction to *L. major* in susceptible strains includes an increase in IL-4 secreting CD4+ T cells and in the levels of immunoglobulin, particularly of the IgE isotype. The administration of neutralizing antibodies to either IL-4 in BALB/c mice or IFNγ in C3H mice renders the animals resistant or susceptible to disease respectively, emphasising the importance of cytokines in determining disease outcome.[40,41]

The production of different cytokines has been attributed to the differentiation of distinct T cells, the so called Th1 and Th2 cells which appear to be derived from a common precursor that is able to produce a wide spectrum of cytokines.[42,43] Not only do these T cells produce different cytokines, but they appear to regulate the activity or proliferation of each other (Fig. 4.2). The Th1 cells produce primarily IFNγ, IL-2 and TNFβ, whilst the Th2 cells make mostly IL-4, IL-5, IL-6, IL-10 and IL-13. At least in cell culture systems, the presence of IL-4 or IFNγ at the beginning of the immune response ensures a Th1 or Th2 dominated response respectively.[44,45,46,47] Further, IL-10 or IFNγ inhibits the proliferation or differentiation respectively of Th2 or Th1 cells.[48,46,42,49] IL-10 appears not only to have direct effects on T cells but also to inhibit the production of IL-12 by macrophages which is required for Th1 cells.[50,51]

The possibility that disruption of the cytokine network may provide a new approach to regulation of the immune response to organ and tissue transplants is tantalizing. Given that acute graft rejection is thought primarily to be mediated by a cellular immune response, it has been tempting to conclude that diversion of the immune response away from IL-2/IFNγ production or inhibition of Th1 cells would result in acceptance of grafts and further that stimulation of Th2 cells might result in immunosuppression or tolerance. What is the evidence from experimental models that this might be the case?

BLOCKING TH1 CYTOKINES MAY RESULT IN IMMUNOSUPPRESSION OR TOLERANCE

IL-2R antibodies have been used extensively as immunosuppressive agents in murine experimental models of transplantation.[52,53,54] In some cases only a modest prologation of graft survival may be observed, but with some antibodies, notably those that effectively block functional binding of IL-2 to its receptor, indefinite graft survival may be obtained with only a short period of antibody treatment.[55] Further, with some protocols, such antibodies may allow the induction of tolerance to graft-donor antigens. In a recent study we found not only that our IL-2R antibodies were able very effectively to prevent the rejection of neuronal allografts placed in the lateral ventrical of rats, but also that they induced tolerance as a second neuronal graft, placed under the kidney capsule of the original recipents, was accepted with no immunosuppression.[56] The situation with respect to blocking IFNγ activity is more complex. In rat models of transplantation, IFNγ antibodies were unable to prolong and indeed in some cases actually shortened graft survival.[57,58] However, the results of these experiments are complicated by the fact that rather than blocking its activity a cytokine-specific antibody may sometimes promote its action by creating a long-lived pool of cytokine in the animal.[59] It would be of interest to analyse to action IFNγ receptor-specific antibodies in experimental transplant models.

Immunosuppressive or Tolerance Promoting Protocols May Result in Down-Regulation of Th1 Cytokines

A number of groups have assessed the expression of cytokines in animals that will not reject a graft following the use of tolerance-inducing protocols.[60,61,62,63,64,65] These experiments have shown a down-regulation in the ability of animals to make either IL-2 or IL-2 and IFNγ. This may be, but is not always, accompanied by either a maintained or up-regulated expression of at least some of the Th2 derived cytokines.

The Induction of Tolerance May Be Prevented by Administration of Th1 Cytokines

In a rat model in which tolerance is achieved by preoperative blood transfusion, we[60] and Bugeon et al[65] have shown not only that animals have an impaired ability to make Th1 cytokines, but also that tolerance induction may be prevented by the administration of either IL-2 or IFNγ at the time of transplantation.

The Effect of IL-4 Binding Proteins on Graft Survival

If we believe that Th2 cytokines promote graft survival, then it should follow that blocking their action will result in more

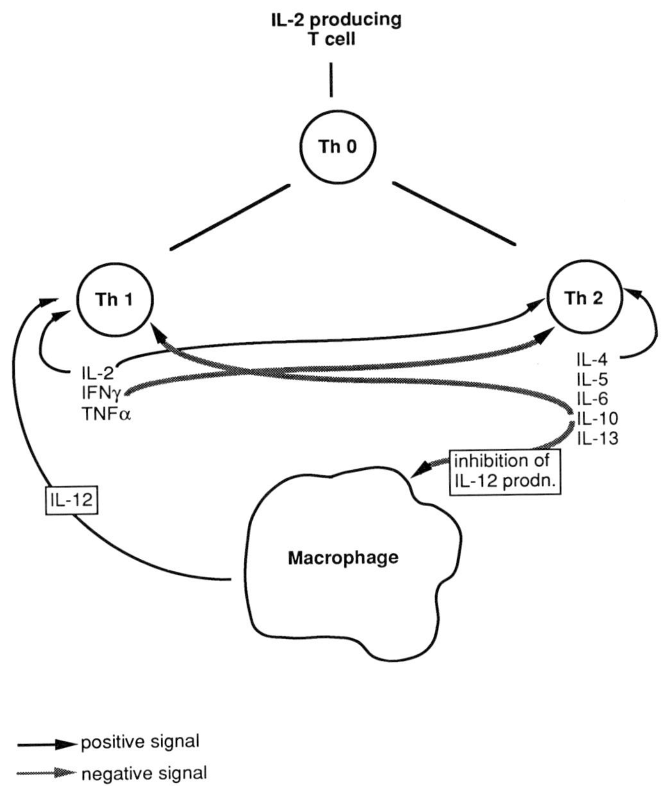

Fig. 4.2. Cytokine producing cells and their mutual regulation.

rapid graft rejection. In the only experiments that directly approach this issue it was found that in mice injected with soluble IL-4R (which will bind IL-4) or transgenic for soluble IL-4R, prolongation rather than shortening of graft survival was observed.[66,67] The interpretation of these experiments is however again complicated by the fact that soluble IL-4R may create a circulating pool of IL-4, thus promoting its function. Experiments in which blocking IL-4R antibodies are used will be of much interest.

In summary, it is clear from the experimental data that manipulation of the cytokine network resulting in blockade of Th1 cell function or cytokines will be beneficial to graft survival. However, whether this can be achieved through promoting Th2 cytokines or cells is not clear. Further, the role of the different cytokines in maintaining the tolerant state once it has been induced has yet to be investigated. None of these issues have yet been addressed for islet transplants, although it is apparent that islet rejection is associated with a Th1 cytokine pattern.[19]

Finally, perhaps a note of caution. We should approach any intervention strategies based on the gross disruption of the cytokine balance with a degree of caution—the balance between cytokine subsets is critical and any change in the equilibrium may have dire consequences such as the induction of autoimmunity.[68] Two mouse models of autoimmune disease, chronic stimulatory graft-versus-host disease and host-versus-graft disease, which are induced by injection of allogeneic lymphocytes into different mouse strains, have many features in common with human systemic lupus erythematosus. When the cytokine profile in these diseases is analysed, the most striking observation is the presence of Th2 type cytokines, IL-4 and IL-5, and an impairment in the ability of the host to produce Th1 cytokines.[69,70,71] The cross-regulatory role of cytokines such as IL-4 and IL-10 on IL-2 and IFNγ is suggested as playing a vital role in these autoimmune diseases.

Cytokine research continues to be an expanding area in transplantation biology but our knowledge of cytokine involvement in the immune response to islet grafts remains sparse. Molecular techniques have allowed a rapid accumulation of knowledge and reagents which will be invaluable to this work. As yet, the exciting potential of cytokines and their receptors in redirecting immune responses has not been fully realized, but the next few years should see major advances in this area.

References

1. Dallman MJ, Clark GJ. Cytokine and their receptors in transplantation. Curr Op in Immunology 1992; 3: 729-734.
2. Dallman MJ. The cytokine network and regulation of the immune response to organ transplants. Transplant Revs 1992; 6: 209-217.
3. Dallman MJ. Cytokines as mediators of organ graft rejection and tolerance. Curr Op in Immunol 1993; 5: 788-793.
4. Dallman MJ. Cytokine regulation of the immune response to organ transplants. in Immunology of Renal Transplantation Eds Thomson AW and Catto, GRD 1993; 97-111.
5. Dallman MJ, Larsen CP, Morris CP. Cytokine gene transcription in vascularised organ grafts-analysis using semiquantitative polymerase chain reaction. J Exp Med 1991; 174: 493-496.
6. Yoshimura N, Oka T, Kahan BD. Sequential determinations of serum interleukin 6 levels as an immunodiagnostic tool to differentiate rejection from nephrotoxicity in renal allograft recipients. Transplantation 1991; 51: 172-176.
7. Tilg H, Nordberg J, Vogel W et al. Circulating levels of interleukin 6 and C-reactive protein after liver transplantation. Transplantation 1992; 54: 142-146.
8. Baigrie RJ, Lamont PM, Dallman MJ et al. The release of IL-1 precedes that of IL-6 in patients undergoing major surgery. Lymphokine and Cytokine Res 1991; 10: 253-256.
9. Mandrup-Poulsen T, Bendtzen K, Nerup J et al. Affinity-purified human interleukin-1 is cytotoxic to isolated islets of langerhans. Diabetologia 1986; 29: 63.
10. Campbell IL, Iscaro A, Harrison LC. Interferon-γ and tumour necrosis factor-α: cytotoxicity to murine islets of Langerhans. J Immunol 1988; 141: 2325.

11. Punkel C, Baquerizo H, Rabinovitch A. Destruction of rat islet cell monolayers by cytokines. Synergistic interactions of interferon-γ, tumor necrosis factor, lymphotoxin and interleukin 1. Diabetes 1988; 37: 133.
12. Campbell IL, Cutri A, Wilson Aet al. Evidence for IL-6 production by and effects on the pancreatic β-cell. J Immunol 1989; 143: 1188-1191.
13. Soldevila G, Buscema M, Doshi M et al. Cytotoxic effect of IFN-gamma plus TNF-alpha on human islet cells. J Autoimmun 1991; 4: 291-306.
14. Eizirik DL. Interleukin-1 beta induces an early decrease in insulin release, (pro)insulin biosynthesis and insulin m RNA in mouse pancreatic islets by a mechanism dependent on gene transcription and protein sythesis. Autoimmunity 1991; 10: 107-113.
15. Yamada K, Inada C, Otabe S et al. Effects of free radical scavengers on cytokine actions on islet cells. Acta Endocinol Copenh 1993; 128: 379-384.
16. Corbett JA, Sweetland MA, Wang JL et al. Nitric oxide mediates cytokine-induced inhibition of insulin secretion by human islets of Langerhans. Proc Natl Acad Sci (USA) 1993; 90: 1731-1735.
17. Yamada K, Takane N, Otabe Set al. Pancreatic β cell-selective production of tumor necrosis factor-α induced by Interleukin-1. Diabetes 1993; 42: 1026-1031.
18. Jiang Z, Woda BA. Cytokine gene expression in the islets of the diabetic Biobreeding/Worcester rat. J Immunol 1991; 146: 2990-2994.
19. O'Connell PJ, Pacheco-Silva A, Nickerson PW et al. Unmodified Pancreatic Islet Allograft Rejection Results In The Preferential Expression Of Certain T Cell Activation Transcripts. J Immunol 1993; 150: 1093-1104.
20. Simpson MA, Madras PN, Cornaby AJ et al. Sequential determinations of urinary cytology and plasma and urinary lymphokines in the management of renal allograft recipients. Transplantation 1989; 47: 218-223.
21. Tilg H, Vogel W, Aulitzky WE et al. Evaluation of cytokines and cytokine-induced secondary messages in sera of patients after liver transplantation. Transplantation 1990; 49: 1074-1080.
22. Cohen N, Gumbert M, Birnbaum J et al. An improved method for the detection of soluble interleukin 2 receptors in liver transplant recipients by flow cytometry. Transplantation 1991; 51: 417-421.
23. Jutte NHPM, Hesse CJ, Balk AHMM et al. Sequential measurements of soluble interleukin 2 receptor levels in plasma of heart transplant recipients. Transplantation 1990; 50: 328-330.
24. Young JB, Windsor NT, Smart FW et al. Inability of isolated soluble IL-2 receptor levels to predict biopsy rejection scores after heart transplantation. Transplantation 1991; 51: 636-641.
25. Martinez OM, Villanueva JC, Lake J et al. IL-2 And IL-5 Gene Expression In Response To Alloantigen In Liver Allograft Recipients And In Vitro. Transplantation 1993; 55: 1159-1166.
26. Dallman MJ, Roake J, Hughes D et al. Sequential analysis of IL-2 gene transcription in renal transplants. Transplantation 1992; 53: 683-685.
27. Shaw G, Kamen R. A conserved AU sequence from the 3' untranslated region of GM-CSF mRNA mediates selective mRNA degradation. Cell 1986; 46: 659-667.
28. Caput D, Beutler B, Hartog K et al. Identification of a common nucleotide sequence in the 3'-untranslated region of mRNA molecules specifying inflammatory mediators. Proc. Natl. Acad. Sci. (USA) 1986; 83: 1670-1674.
29. Shaw J, Meerovitch K, Bleakley RC et al. Mechanisms regulating the level of IL-2 mRNA in T lymphocytes. J Immunol 1988; 140: 2243-2248.
30. Norohna IL, Eberlein-Gonska M, Hartley B et al. In Situ Expression Of Tumor Necrosis Factor-Alpha, Interferon-gamma, And Interleukin-2 Receptors In Renal Allograft Biopsies. Transplantation 1992; 54: 1017-1024.

31. Hoffman MW, Wonigeit K, Steinhoff G et al. Production Of Cytokines (TNF-alpha, IL-1 beta) And Endothelial Cell Activation In Human Liver Allograft Rejection. Transplantation 1993; 55: 329-335.
32. Ruan X-M, Qiao J-H, Trento A et al. Cytokine Expression And Endothelial Cell And Lymphocyte Activation In Human Cardiac Allograft Rejection: An Immunohistochemical Study Of Endomyocardial Biopsy Sample. J Heart Lung Transplant 1992; 11: 1110-1116.
33. Hancock W, Sayegh MH, Kwock CA et al. Oral, But Not Intravenous, Alloantigen Prevents Accelarated Allograft Rejection By Selective Intragraft TH2 Cell Activation. Transplantation 1993; 55: 1112-1118.
34. Morel D, Normand E, Lemoine C et al. Tumor Necrosis Factor Alpha In Human Kidney Transplant Rejection-Analysis By In Situ Hybridisation. Transplantation 1993; 55: 773-777.
35. Wanders A, Wells AF, Larsson E et al. Expression of an interferon-gamma-like substance in normal and transplanted rat heart tissue. J Heart Lung Transplant 1992; 11: 142-146.
36. Parish C. The relatioship between humoral and cell-mediated immunity. Transplant Rev 1972; 13: 35-66.
37. Mosmann TR, Coffman RL. TH1 and TH2 cells: Different patterns of lymphokine secretion lead to different functional properties. Ann Rev Immunol 1989; 7: 145-173.
38. Moll H, Rollinghoff M. Resistance to murine cutaneous Leishmaniasis is mediated by TH1 cells, but disease promoting CD4+ cells are different from TH2 cells. Eur J Immunol 1990; 20: 2067-2074.
39. Boom WH, Liebster L, Abbas AK et al. Patterns of cytokine secretion in murine Leishmaniasis: correlation with disease progression or resolution. Infect Immun 1990; 58: 3863-3870.
40. Belosevic M, Finbloom DS, van der Meide PH et al. Administration of monoclonal anti-IFN-γ antibodies in vivo abrogates natural resistance of C3H/HeN mice to infection with *Leishmania major*. J Immunol 1989; 143: 266-274.
41. Sadick MD, Heinzel FP, Holaday BJ et al. Cure of murine leishmaniasis with anti-interleukin 4 monoclonal antibody. J Exp Med 1990; 171: 115-127.
42. Fiorentino DF, Bond MW, Mosmann TR. Two types of mouse helper T cell iv. Th2 cells secrete a factor that inhibits cytokine production by Th1 clones. J Exp Med 1989; 170: 2081-2095.
43. Street NE, Schumacher JH, Fong TAT et al. Heterogeneity of mouse helper T cells: evidence from bulk cultures and limiting dilution cloning for precursors of Th1 and Th2 cells. J Immunol 1990; 144: 1629-1639.
44. Swain SL, Weinberg AD, English M et al. IL-4 directs the development of TH2-like helper effectors. J Immunol 1990; 145: 3796-3806.
45. LeGros G, Ben-Sasson SZ, Seder RA et al. Generation of interleukin 4 (IL-4)-producing cells in vivo and in vitro: IL-2 and IL-4 are required for in vitro generation of IL-4 producing cells. J Exp Med 1990; 172: 921-929.
46. Gajewski TF, Schell SR, Nau G et al. Regulation of T cell activation: differences among T-cell subsets. Immunol Rev 1989; 111: 79-110.
47. Swain SL, Huston G, Tonkonogy S et al. Transforming growth factor-β and IL-4 cause helper T cell precursors to develop into distinct effector helper cells that differ in lymphokine secretion pattern and cell surface phenotype. J Immunol 1991; 147: 2991-3000.
48. Gajewski TF, Fitch FW. Anti-proliferative effect of IFN-γ in immune regulation I. IFN-γ inhibits the proliferation of TH2 but not TH1 murine helper T lymphocyte clones. J Immunol 1988; 140: 4245-4252.
49. Mosmann TR, Moore KW. The role of IL-10 in crossregulation of TH1 and TH2 responses. Immunoparasitology Today 1991; 12: A49-A53.
50. Fiorentino DF, Zlotnik A, Mosmann TR et al. IL-10 inhibits cytokine production by activated macrophages. J Immunol 1991; 147: 3815-3822.

51. Hsieh CS, Macatonia SE, Tripp CS et al. Development of Th1 CD4+ T cells through IL-12 produced by Listeria-induced macrophages. Science 1993; 260: 547-548.
52. Kupiec-Weglinski JW, Diamantstein T, Tilney NL. Interleukin 2 receptor-targeted therapy-rationale and applications in organ transplantation. Transplantation 1988; 46: 785-792.
53. Kirkman RL, Barrett LV, Gaulton GN et al. Administration of an anti-interleukin 2 receptor monoclonal antibody prolongs cardiac allograft survival in mice. J Exp Med 1985; 162: 358-362.
54. Tellides G, Dallman MJ, Kupiec-Weglinski JW et al. Functonal blocking of the interleukin-2 receptor (IL-2R) may be important in the efficacy of IL-2R antibody therapy. Transplant Proc 1987; XIX: 4231-4233.
55. Tellides G, Dallman MJ, Morris PJ. Mechanism of action of Inteleukin-2 receptor (IL-2R) monoclonal antibody (MAb) therapy: target cell depletion or inhibition of function? Transplant Proc 1989; XXI: 997-998.
56. Wood MJA, Sloan DJ, Dallman MJ et al. Specific Tolerance To Neural Allografts Induced With An Antibody To The Interleukin-2 Receptor. J Exp Med 1993; 177: 597-603.
57. Scheringa M, de Bruin RFW, Jeekel H et al. Anti-tumour necrosis factor alpha serum prolongs heart allograft survival in rats. Transplant Proc 1991; 23: 547-548.
58. Paineau J, Priestley C, Fabre J et al. Effects of gamma interferon and interleukin-2, and of gamma-interfeon antibodies on the rat immune response against allografts. Transplant Proc 1989; 21: 999-1001.
59. Else KJ, Finkleman FD, Maliszweski CR et al. Cytoine-mediated regulation of chronic intestinal helminth infection. J Exp Med 1994; 179: 347-351.
60. Dallman MJ, Shiho O, Page TH et al. Peripheral tolerance to alloantigen results from altered regulation of the interleukin 2 pathway. J Exp Med 1991; 173: 79-87.
61. Dallman MJ, Wood KJ, Hamano K et al. Cytokines and Peripheral Tolerance to Alloantigen. Imm Rev 1993; 133: 5-18.
62. Takeuchi T, Lowry RP, Konieczny B. Heart allografts in murine systems. Transplantation 1992; 53: 1281-1294.
63. Mohler KM, Streilein JW. Lymphokine production by MLR-reactive reaction lymphocytes obtained from normal mice and mice rendered tolerant of class II MHC antigens. Transplanation 1989; 47: 625-633.
64. Mohler KM, Streilein JW. Differential expression of helper versus effector activity in mice rendered neonatally tolerant of class II MHC antigens. Transplantation 1989; 47: 633-640.
65. Bugeon L, Cuturi M-C, M-M H et al. Peripheral Tolerance Of An Allograft In Adult Rats-Characterization By Low Interleukin-2 And Interferon-g mRNA Levels And By Strong Accumulation Of Major Histocompatibility Complex Transcripts In The Graft. Transplantation 1992; 54: 219-225.
66. Fanslow WC, Clifford KN, Park LS et al. Regulation of alloreactivity in vivo by IL-4 and the soluble IL-4 receptor. J Immunol 1991; 147: 535-540.
67. Maliszewski CR, Morrissey PJ, Fanslow WC et al. Delayed Allograft Rejection In Mice Transgenic For A Soluble Form Of The IL-4 Receptor. Cell Immunol 1992; 143: 434-448.
68. Goldman M, Druet P, Gleichmann E. TH2 cells in systemic autoimmunity: insights from allogeneic diseases and chemically-induced autoimmunity. Immunology Today 1991; 12: 223-227.
69. Schurmans S, Heussen CH, Qin H-Y et al. In vivo effects of anti-IL-4 monoclonal antibody on neonatal induction of tolerance and on an associated autoimmune syndrome. J Immunol 1990; 145: 2465-2473.
70. Dobashi K, Ono S, Murakami S et al. Polyclonal B cell activation by a B cell differentiation factor, B151-TRF2. III. B151-TRF2 as a B cell differentiation factor closely associated with autoimmune disease. J Immunol 1987; 138: 780-787.
71. Abramowicz D, Oultrelepont JM, Lambert P et al. Increased expression of Ia antigens on B cells after neonatal induction of lymphoid chimerism in mice: role of interleukin 4. Eur J Immunol 1990; 20: 469-476.

CHAPTER 5

Role of Adhesion Molecules in Transplantation

Carl G. Figdor

Y. van Kooyk

In order to effectively defend the body against infectious organisms, cells of the immune system should be able to circulate as non-adherent cells in blood and lymph, and to migrate as adherent cells throughout the tissues. To arrive at sites of infection and to adhere to target cells bearing foreign antigen, cells need to cross endothelial and vessel walls. To control this rapid transition between adherent and non-adherent states, lymphocytes are equipped with different adhesion receptors (Fig. 5.1). Lymphocytes express several integrin molecules at their cell surface, which may all participate in the same intercellular interaction. Apart from integrins,[1] lymphoid cells express other adhesion receptors, which may regulate cell adhesion, or contribute to the integrin mediated cell-cell interaction. Cloning of the genes encoding these molecules and their counter receptors, revealed that they belong to distinct families of structurally related proteins: the selectins, immunoglobulin superfamily and the CD44 adhesion receptor (Fig. 5.1). Also in transplantation immunology these same adhesion receptors play an important role. The interaction of leukocytes with endothelium is mediated by adhesion molecules, but also in the initiation phase, the proliferation phase, as well as in the effector phase adhesion molecules are of major importance (Fig. 5.2).

MECHANISMS THAT REGULATE LEUKOCYTE ADHESION

Lymphocytes and other leukocytes are equipped with several mechanisms to direct and regulate adhesion to other cells and migration throughout the body (Table 5.1). First, up-regulation or down-regulation of surface expression is a major tool employed by cells to regulate cell adhesion. Upon stimulation, for instance with cytokines, several cell types are capable of increasing expression of adhesion molecules or their ligands. This is not only restricted to lymphocytes, since expression of ICAM-1, ligand of LFA-1[2] or VCAM-1, ligand of VLA-4[3] is strongly induced by inflammatory mediators on endothelial cells. IFNγ, IL-1 and TNFα strongly induce ICAM-1[4,5] or

Pancreatic Islet Transplantation Volume II: Immunomodulation of Pancreatic Islets, edited by Robert P. Lanza, MD, William L. Chick, MD; ©1994 R.G. Landes Company.

VCAM-1 expression,[6] resulting in enhanced binding of lymphocytes.[7] In contrast, other ligands of LFA-1 (ICAM-2,[8] and ICAM-3[9,10]) seem less sensitive to inflammatory cytokines.[11,12,13]

Down-regulation of L-selectin molecules has been observed on neutrophils after activation with phorbol ester altering their adhesive properties.[14] Differences in the state of glycosylation may also contribute to the capacity of adhesion receptors to bind to their ligand.[15,16,17] Furthermore, clustering of cell adhesion receptors at specific sites at the cell surface may increase the avidity of cell-cell interactions.[18] Recently we have demonstrated that certain integrins are localized in clusters at the cell surface facilitating the interaction with its ligand.[19]

Yet another mechanism to regulate cell adhesion is activation and inactivation of adhesion receptors. This holds for all integrins. Activation of integrins can be achieved through "Inside Out" signalling, whereby signals are generated from within the cell[20] (Table 5.1). Signals generated by a still increasing number of cell surface molecules on leukocytes are able to transmit signals into the interior of the cell that lead to activation of integrin molecules. Activation is thought to involve conformational changes within the receptor, which lead to a higher affinity for its ligand, establishing cell-cell interaction.[21] Binding of ligand by integrins may also result in so called "Outside In" signaling, which may affect cellular processes such as migration, proliferation, or differentiation of the cell.[22,23]

ADHESION CASCADES

A major question often raised is; why are so many adhesion molecules expressed on one and the same cell? First of all, certain adhesion receptors may operate in particular cellular interactions, but not in others. It is well known that the adhesive interaction CD2/LFA-3 is important in cytotoxic inter-

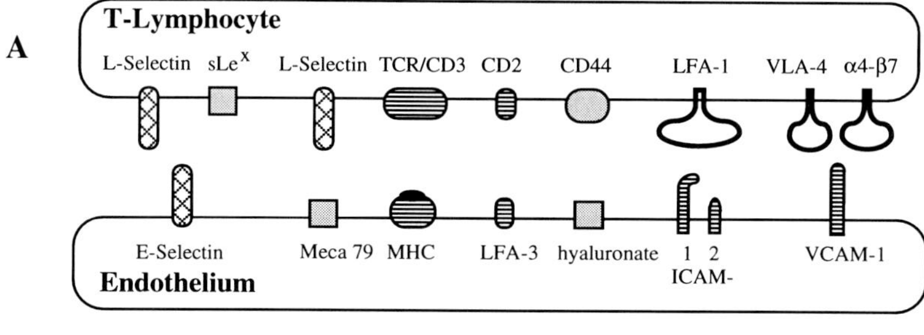

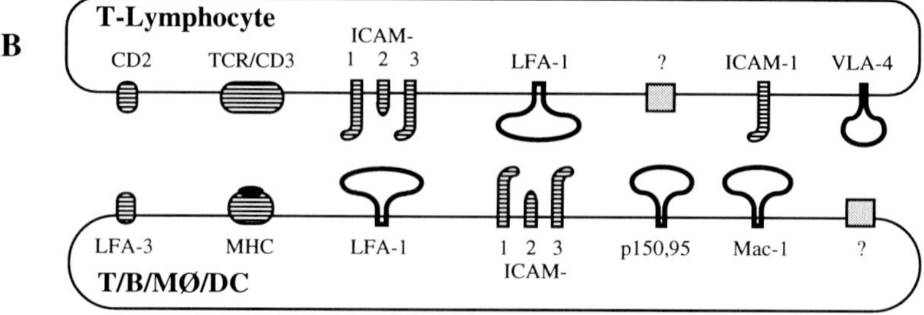

Fig. 5.1. Lymphocytes express a multitude of adhesion molecules. Depending on the type of interactions (A and B), distinct adhesion molecules are involved.

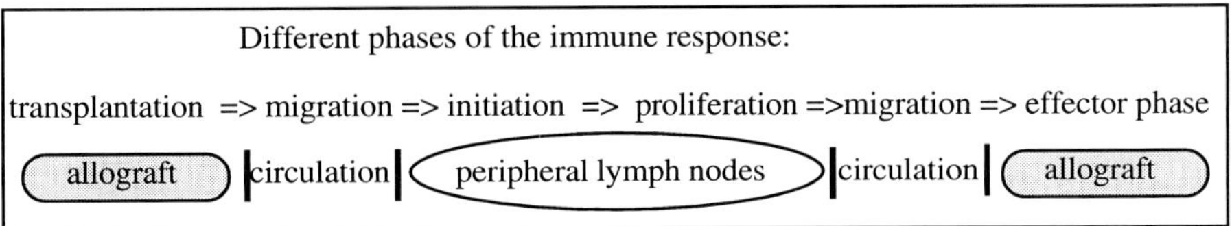

Fig. 5.2. Immune responses leading to transplant rejection can de divided into different phases. In each of these phases distinct cellular interactions, and consequently different adhesion molecules are involved.

Table 5.I. Mechanisms that regulate β2 mediated cell adhesion

Regulation at the level of:	Influenced by:
A. Expression of receptors and their ligands	Cytokines, Infectious agents, Glycosylation
B. Affinity/Avidity modulation of adhesion receptors	
- "Inside Out" signaling	(De-) Phosphorylation, Second messengers
- Conformational changes	Divalent cations, Integrin mabs
- Clustering of receptors	Divalent cations
- Adhesion cascades	?
C. Signaling through adhesion receptors	
- "Outside In" signaling	Second Messengers, Kinase activity

actions, but less important in interactions of lymphocytes with endothelium, despite the fact that LFA-3 is expressed at high levels on activated endothelium. In addition several studies have shown that adhesion molecules may operate successively in time. For example, leukocyte adhesion to endothelium at sites of inflammation is a multistep process involving initial unstable adhesion mediated by selectins, followed by stable adhesion by β2 integrins to their counter-receptors. Different examples can be given of adhesion cascades leading to stable cell-cell binding. Here we shall discuss two examples that are also relevant in transplant rejection processes.

Recognition of foreign antigen by lymphocytes is mediated by the T cell receptor-antigen/MHC interaction on T lymphocytes. Only if an antigenic peptide presented by MHC molecules is recognized by the T cell receptor, a signal is generated through the CD3 complex of molecules that are associated with the T cell receptor.[24,25] These signals result in activation of the adhesion receptor LFA-1, expressed on the same cell, which results in a high affinity interaction with its ligand ICAM-1 expressed on the target cell. This stable LFA-1/ICAM-1 interaction now guarantees strong binding of the T cell with the target cell, i.e. a virus infected cell, a tumor cell or a allogeneic cell in the case of transplantation.

The second example concerns the interaction of leukocytes with endothelial cells (Fig. 5.3). Upon infection with bacterial pathogens inflammatory mediators are produced by the bacteria and tissue macrophages. These mediators activate endothelial cells lining the blood vessels in the vicinity of the inflammation. This results in the upregulation of several adhesion receptors, notably E-selectin, P-selectin, ICAM-1 and VCAM-1.[14,27] The expression of the selectins at the cell surface results in tethering of neutrophils to the activated endothelial cells. E- and P- selectin expressed on the endothelial cells are capable of interacting with L-selectin expressed by the neutrophils.[28,29,30] The interaction by these adhesion receptors dramatically slows down the speed with which the neutrophils flow through the vessels, and starts the neutrophils to roll along the vessel wall. Therefore, the selectin molecules are also termed rolling receptors. This slow rolling of cells is a prerequisite for the integrin molecules to bind their ligand, since this interaction cannot take place at high speed. Additional intracellular signals generated by the selectin mediated interaction of the neutrophils with the endothelium results in the activation of integrin molecules at the surface of the neutrophil. These integrin mediated interactions now facilitate stable binding of the neutrophil to the vessel wall. Next, the neutrophils start to migrate into the underlying tissue. The migratory behavior is also mediated by integrins. A gradient of chemotactic compounds directs the neutrophils towards the site of inflammation as has been elegantly demonstrated by W. Smith and colleagues.[31,32] To facilitate migration the L-selectin molecules are clipped from the cell membrane, probably by surface bound protease's. Interestingly, essentially the same adhesion molecules are expressed at the endothelium of allografts which have been stored for several hours. The expression of these molecules are amongst others thought to play a major role in reperfusion injury after transplantation and subsequent restoration of the circulation. Recent findings by Winn et al[33] show that treatment witch antibodies against these adhesion molecules may overcome reperfusion injury.

ROLE OF LYMPHOCYTE ADHESION RECEPTORS IN VIVO

The importance of adhesion receptors in vivo is best illustrated in patients suffering from the leukocyte adhesion deficiency 1 (LAD-1) syndrome,[34,35,36,37,38,39] a genetic deficiency of the β2 integrin receptor caused

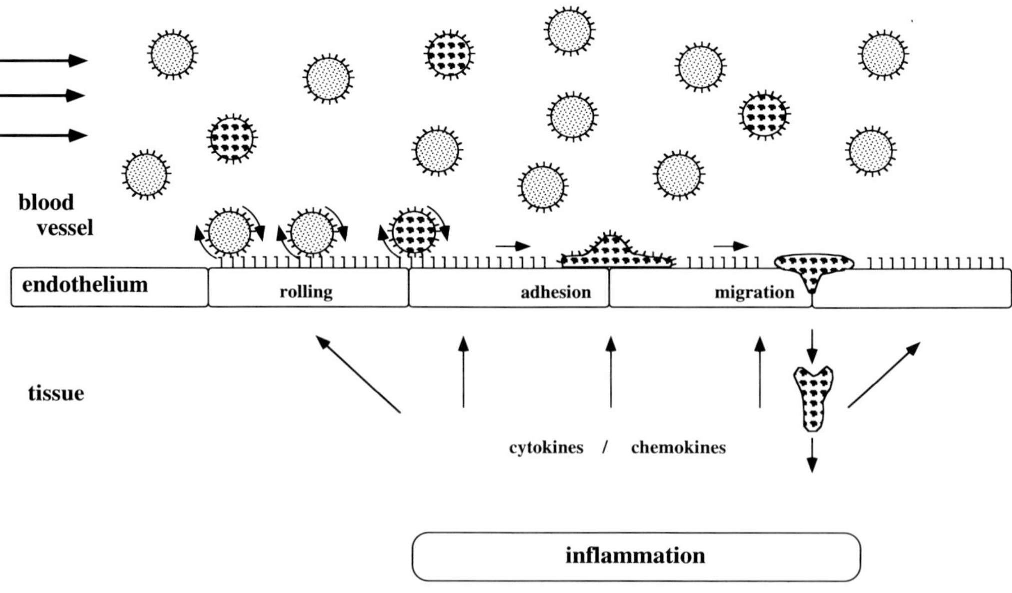

Fig. 5.3. Adhesion of leukocytes to endothelium in an inflammatory/immune response requires the coordinated interaction of selectin molecules and integrin molecules.

by mutations in the common β2 subunit. The LAD syndrome results in the absence of LFA-1, CR3 and p150, 95 on the cell surface of leukocytes. Patients have recurring, life-threatening bacterial infections, and severe defects in adhesion dependent leukocyte functions, which are often fatal in childhood, unless corrected by bone marrow transplantation.[40]

More recently a second adhesion receptor defect has been found, which has been designated LAD-2.[41] This defect concerns the absence of a fucosyltransferase resulting in the absence of sialyl lewis X, a carbohydrate group that is present on a large number of glycoproteins. E-selectin expressed by activated endothelium specifically recognizes the sialyl lewis X group on glycoproteins expressed by leukocytes. Therefore, leukocytes from LAD-2 patients are unable to roll along the endothelium. Consequently the cells are not able to extravasate because they circulate too rapid to enable integrin mediated adhesion.

Both the LAD-1 and the LAD-2 syndromes clearly demonstrate the important role of adhesion molecules in immune and inflammatory reactions. Therefore, they are expected to play also a major role in transplant reactions. Antibodies against adhesion structures may thus be of therapeutical value to prevent or inhibit transplant rejection.

The potential of mabs directed against integrins, selectins and their counter receptors, to reduce vascular and tissue damage in a variety of clinical disorders, has been examined (acute and chronic allograft rejection, rheumatoid arthritis, inflammatory skin disease, asthma and ischemia-reperfusion syndromes).

Inhibition of leukocyte adhesion processes by "anti-adhesion" therapy represents a novel approach to treat disorders in which leukocytes contribute significantly to vascular and tissue damage.[42] In vivo treatment with anti-VLA-4 antibodies inhibits migration of lymphocytes to cutaneous inflammatory sites.[43,44] Anti-ICAM-1 antibodies have

Table 5.2. Overview graft survival

Antigen	Antibody	Species	Effect on survival	Date / Author
Bone marrow				
LFA-1	25.3	human (infant)	++	86, Fischer[53]
LFA-1	M23.2 (anti-β)	human (adult)	-	89, Baume[55]
LFA-1	M7/15	mouse	+	90, van Dijken[56]
LFA-1	M17.4	mouse	+	91, Harning[73]
ICAM-1	YN1/1		+	
Kidney				
LFA-1	25.3	human	+	91,93,LeMauff[58]
ICAM-1	B1RR-1	human	+/-	92, Cosimi,[60] 93, Haug[61]
ICAM-1	R6.5	monkey	+	91, Wee et al[62]
ICAM-1		monkey	+	90, Cosimi[59]
ICAM-1		monkey	+	91, Flavin[63]
Islets				
CD2	12.15	mouse	+	92, Chavin[64]
Skin				
LFA-1	M17.4	mouse	+/-	93, van Kooyk[69]
ICAM-1	YN1/1	"	-	
LFA-1 / ICAM-1	combination	"	+	

been shown to reduce airway inflammation, hyper-responsiveness and asthma symptoms.[45] Moreover, a soluble form of ICAM-1, as well as anti-ICAM-1 antibodies inhibit rhinovirus infections, which cause 50% of common colds.[46] ICAM-1 has been identified as the cellular receptor for a subgroup of rhinoviruses[47,48] and is one of the receptors for *Plasmodium falciparum* (malaria)-infected erythrocytes.[49,50]

It has been demonstrated that anti-CD18 antibodies prevent ischemia-reperfusion injury,[51] whereas anti-CD11b antibodies reduce infarct size in a canine model.[52] Similarly, antibodies directed against E- and P selectin have been demonstrated to be extremely effective in the prevention of reperfusion injury.[27,32] Administration of anti-adhesion molecule antibodies has been effective in enhancing graft survival (Table 5.2)[53,54,55,56,57] showed that anti-CD11a/CD18 antibodies and anti-ICAM-1 antibodies inhibited allograft responses. Also in kidney transplantations anti-adhesion therapy with monoclonal antibodies seems to be beneficial.[58,59,60,61,62,63] Thus far, very limited information is available with respect to anti-adhesion therapy in islet transplantation. Chavin et al[64] studied the effects of anti-CD2 antibodies on Islet survival in a mouse model. By far the most studies have been performed in a heart transplantation model (Table 5.3). Anti-LFA-1 or anti- ICAM-1 antibodies by themselves are not very efficient in preventing graft rejection. However, when combined promising results have been obtained. Prolonged graft survival upon anti-LFA-1 and -ICAM-1 was reported by several investigators (Table 5.3), and Isobe et al. reported indefinite survival and tolerance towards a second skin transplant.[65] Also the combination of antibodies and immunosupressive drugs results in enhanced survival.[66] Combination of antibodies directed against different adhesion pathways may also be effective.[67,68]

On the other hand the promising results listed in Table 5.1 should be interpreted with

Table 5.3. Overview Graft Survival

Antigen	Antibody	Species	Effect on survival	Date / Author
Heart				
LFA-1	M17.4	mouse	++	93, Nakakusa[73]
LFA-1	WT1	rat	–	93, Komari[66]
LFA-1 / CyA	"	"	+	
ICAM-1	1A29	"	–	
ICAM-1 / CyA	"	"	+	
LFA-1	WT1 / WT3	rat	+/–	93, Kameoka[74]
ICAM-1	1A29	"	–	
LFA-1 / ICAM-1	combination	"	+	
LFA-1	KBA	mouse	+/–	92, Isobe[65]
ICAM-1	YN1/1	"	–	
LFA-1 / ICAM-1	combination	"	+++ tolerance	
LFA-1	TA-3	rat	+	93, Paul[67]
VLA-4	TA-2	"	–	
LFA-1 / VLA-4	combination	"	+	
VCAM-1	M/K-2	mouse	+	93, Pelletier[75]
LFA-1 / ICAM-1 / CD4	M17.4 /YN1/1 / GK1.5	mouse	+	93, Jendrisak[76]
CD2	12.15	mouse	+	92, Chavin[64]
CD2	12.15	mouse	+	93, Chavin[77]
CD3	145-2C11	"	+	
CD2/CD3	combination	"	++	93, Chavin[80]

caution. Not only different experimental settings were used by the various authors, but also experiments were performed in different species, or strains of the same species. Depending on the MHC barrier between host and donor, different results may be obtained. For instance, we have not been able to obtain tolerance to skin transplants with a combination of anti-LFA-1 and anti-ICAM-1 antibodies.[69,70] This finding is supported by recent data from skin transplantations in CD18 deficient cattle.[71] These animals which suffer from the LAD syndrome by a point mutation in the gene encoding the CD18 protein are completely deficient for LFA-1. When transplanted with skin from unrelated normal donors they accept the skin for a significantly enhanced period, but ultimately they reject the graft. Repeated transplantations on these animals showed the development of T cell mediated immunity against the allograft, demonstrating that blockage of the LFA-1/ICAM-1 adhesion pathway is not sufficient to obtain tolerance. These data are in contrast with the findings of Isobe et al.[65] However, it should be noted that skin grafts are not vascularized whereas heart transplants are. In addition different experimental models and antibodies were used which may explain the different results.

CONCLUSIONS

It has become clear that adhesion receptors play an important role in different immunological reactions. Leukocyte specific adhesion receptors such as LFA-1 show a dynamic nature by the presence of distinct conformational changes, which can be regulated intracellularly by the generation of distinct signals or ligand binding. The usage of monoclonal antibodies directed against adhesion receptors or their ligands in vivo by an anti-adhesion therapy demonstrates a promising reduction in tissue destruction, caused by disease or by inflammatory responses. Future experiments will determine if combinations of antibodies directed against distinct adhesion receptors will give optimal acceptance of tissue transplants.

ACKNOWLEDGEMENTS

This work is supported by a grant from the Dutch Kidney Foundation "Nierstichting" grant number C87.724. NWO 800-509-185

REFERENCES

1. Springer, T. A. Adhesion receptors of the immune system. Nature 1990. 346: 425-434.
2. Marlin, S. D. and T. A. Springer. Purified intercellular adhesion molecule-1 (ICAM-1) is a ligand for lymphocyte function-associated antigen 1 (LFA-1). Cell 1987. 51:813-819.
3. Elices, M. J., L. Osborn, Y. Takada et al. VCAM-1 on activated endothelium interacts with the leukocyte integrin VLA-4 at a site distinct from the VLA-4/fibronectin binding site. Cell 1990. 60:577-584.
4. Dustin, M. L., R. Rothlein, A. K. Bhan et al. Induction by IL1 and interferon-γ: tissue distribution, biochemistry, and function of a natural adherence molecule (ICAM-1). J. Immunol. 1986. 137:245-254.
5. Pober, J. S., M. P. Bevilacqua, D. L. Mendrick et al. Two distinct monokines, interleukin 1 and tumor necrosis factor, each independently induce biosynthesis and transient expression of the same antigen on the surface of cultured human vascular endothelial cells. J. Immunol 1986. 136: 1680-1687.
6. Osborn, L., C. Hession, R. Tizard et al. Direct expression cloning of vascular cell adhesion molecule 1, a cytokine-induced endothelial protein that binds to lymphocytes. Cell 1989. 59:1203-1211.
7. Dustin, M. L. and T. A. Springer. Lymphocyte function-associated antigen-1 (LFA-1) interaction with intercellular adhesion molecule-1 (ICAM-1) is one of at least three mechanisms for lymphocyte adhesion to cultured endothelial cells. J. Cell Biol. 1988. 107:321-331.
8. Staunton, D. E., M. L. Dustin, and T. A. Springer. Functional cloning of ICAM-2, a cell adhesion ligand for LFA-1 homologous to ICAM-1. Nature 1989. 339:61-64.

9. Fawcett, J., C. L. L. Holness, L. A. Needham et al. Molecular cloning of ICAM-3, a 3rd ligand for LFA-1, constitutively expressed on resting leukocytes. Nature 1992. 360:481-484.
10. Vazeux, R., P. A. Hoffman, J. K. Tomita et al. Cloning and characterization of a new intercellular adhesion molecule ICAM-R. Nature 1992. 360:485-488.
11. Staunton, D. E., V. J. Merluzzi, R. Rothlein et al. A cell adhesion molecule, ICAM-1, is the major surface receptor for rhinoviruses. Cell 1989. 56:849-853.
12. de Fougerolles, A. R., S. A. Stacker, R. Schwarting et al. Characterization of ICAM-2 and evidence for a third counter-receptor for LFA-1. J. Exp. Med. 1991. 174:253-267.
13. de Fougerolles, A. R. and T. A. Springer. Intercellular adhesion molecule 3, a third adhesion counter-receptor for lymphocyte function-associated molecule 1 on resting lymphocytes. J. Exp. Med. 1992. 175:185-190.
14. Anderson, D.C., O. Abbassi, J.D. Forten–berry et al. Abnormalities of LECAM-1- and Mac-1-dependent neutrophil endothelial cell adhesion in the developing host. In: Proceedings of the second international conference on structure and function and regulation of molecules involved in leukocyte adhesion. 1991.337-355.
15. Larson, R. S., A. L. Corbi, L. Bermanet et al. Primary structure of the leukocyte function-associated molecule-1 α subunit: an integrin with an embedded domain defining a protein superfamily. J. Cell Biol. 1989. 108:703-712.
16. Dahms, N. M. and G. W. Hart. Influence of quaternary structure on glycosylation. Differential subunit association affects the site-specific glycosylation of the common beta-chain from Mac-1 and LFA-1. J. Biol. Chem. 1986. 261:13186-13196.
17. Shimizu, Y., G. A. Van Seventer, K. J. Horgan et al. Roles of adhesion molecules in T-cell recognition: fundamental similarities between four integrins on resting human T cells (LFA-1, VLA-4, VLA-5, VLA-6) in expression, binding, and costimulation. Immunol. Rev. 1990. 114:109-143.
18. Detmers, P. A., S. D. Wright, E. Olsen et al. Aggregation of complement receptors on human neutrophils in the absence of ligand. J. Cell Biol. 1987. 105:1137-1145.
19. van Kooyk, Y., P. Weder, K. Heije et al. Extracellular Ca2+ modulates Leukocyte function associated antigen-1 cell surface distribution on T lymphocytes and consequently affects cell adhesion. J. Cell Biol. 1994 in press.
20. Hynes, R. O. Integrins: Versatility, modulation, and signaling in cell adhesion. Cell 1992. 69:11-25.
21. Figdor, C. G., Y. van Kooyk, and G. D. Keizer. On the mode of action of LFA-1. Immunol. Today 1990. 11:277-280.
22. Shimizu, Y. and S. Shaw. Lymphocyte interactions with extracellular matrix. FASEB. J. 1991. 5:2292-2299.
23. Pardi, R., L. Inverardi, and J. R. Bender. Regulatory mechanisms in leukocyte adhesion: flexible receptors for sophisticated travelers. Immunol. Today 1992. 13:224-230.
24. Dustin, M. L. and T. A. Springer. T-cell receptor cross-linking transiently stimulates adhesiveness through LFA-1. Nature 1989. 341:619-624.
25. van Kooyk, Y., P. van de Wiel van Kemenade, P. Weder et al. Enhancement of LFA-1-mediated cell adhesion by triggering through CD2 or CD3 on T lymphocytes. Nature 1989. 342:811-813.
26. van Kooyk, Y., Weder, P., Heije, K. et al. Role of intracellular Ca2+ levels in the regulation of CD11a/CD18 mediated cell adhesion. Cell Adh. and Comm. 1993. 1:21-32.
27. Lorant, D.E., M.K. Topham, R.E. Whatley et. al. Inflammatory roles of P-selectin. Am. Soc. for Clin.Invest. Inc. 1993. 92: 559-570.
28. Lawrence, M. B. and T. A. Springer. Leukocytes roll on a selectin at physiologic flow rates: distinction from and prerequisite for adhesion through integrins. Cell 1991. 65:859-873.
29. Lawrence, M. B., C. W. Smith, S. G. Eskin et al. Effect of venous shear stress on CD18-mediated neutrophil adhesion to cultured endothelium. Blood. 1990. 75:227-237.

30. Lo, S. K., S. Lee, R. A. Ramos et al. Endothelial-leukocyte adhesion molecule 1 stimulates the adhesive activity of leukocyte integrin CR3 (CD11b/CD18, Mac-1, alpha m beta 2) on human neutrophils. J. Exp. Med. 1991. 173:1493-1500.
31. Mayadas, T.N., R.C. Johnson, H. Rayburn et al. Leukocyte rolling and extravasation are severely compromised in P selectin-deficient mice. Cell 1993. 74:541-554.
32. Doré, M., R.J. Korthuis, N. Granger et al. P-selectin mediates spontaneous leukocyte rolling in vivo. Blood 1993. 82:1308-1316.
33. Winn, R.K., D. Liggitt, N.B. Vedder et al. Anti-P-selectin monoclonal antibody attenuates reperfusion injury to the rabbit ear. Am. Soc. for Clin.Invest. Inc.1993. 92:2042-2047.
34. Springer, T. A., W. S. Thompson, L. J. Miller et al. Inherited deficiency of the Mac-1, LFA-1, p150,95 glycoprotein family and its molecular basis. J. Exp. Med. 1984. 160:1901-1918.
35. Anderson, D. C. and T. A. Springer. Leukocyte adhesion deficiency: an inherited defect in the Mac-1, LFA-1, and p150,95 glycoproteins. Annu. Rev. Med. 1987. 38:175-194.
36. Kishimoto, T. K., K. O'Conner, and T. A. Springer. Leukocyte adhesion deficiency. Aberrant splicing of a conserved integrin sequence causes a moderate deficiency phenotype. J. Biol. Chem. 1989. 264:3588-3595.
37. Todd, R. F. and D. R. Freyer. The CD11/CD18 leukocyte glycoprotein deficiency. Hematol. Oncol. Clin. North. Am. 1988. 2:13-31.
38. Fischer, A., R. Seger, A. Durandy et al. Deficiency of the adhesive protein complex lymphocyte function antigen 1, complement receptor type 3, glycoprotein p150,95 in a girl with recurrent bacterial infections. J. Clin. Invest. 1985. 76:2385-2392.
39. Arnaout, M. A., N. Dana, S. K. Gupta et al. Point mutations impairing cell surface expression of the common beta subunit (CD18) in a patient with leukocyte adhesion molecule (Leu-CAM) deficiency. J. Clin. Invest. 1990. 85:977-981.
40. Fischer, A., B. Lisowska Grospierre, D. C. Anderson et al. Leukocyte adhesion deficiency: molecular basis and functional consequences. Immunodefic. Rev. 1988. 1: 39-54.
41. Von Andrian, U.H., E.M. Berger, L. Ramezani et al. In vivo behaviour of neutrophils from two patients with distinct inherited leukocyte adhesion deficiency syndromes. Am.Soc. for Clin.Invest.Inc. 1993. 91:2893-2897.
42. Carlos, T.M. and J.M. Harlan. Membrane proteins involved in phagocyte adherence to endothelium. In: Immunological Reviews. G. Moller, editor. Munksgaard, Copenhagen. 1990. 5-28.
43. Issekutz, T. B. Inhibition of in vivo lymphocyte migration to inflammation and homing to lymphoid tissues by the TA-2 monoclonal antibody. A likely role for VLA-4 in vivo. J. Immunol 1991. 147: 4178-4184.
44. Yednock, T.A., C. Cannon, L.C. Fritz et al. Prevention of experimental autoimmune encephalomyelitis by antibodies against $\alpha 4\beta 1$ integrin. Nature. 1992. 356:63-66.
45. Wegner, C. D., R. H. Gundel, P. Reilly et al. Intercellular adhesion molecule-1 (ICAM-1) in the pathogenesis of asthma. Science 1990. 247:456-459.
46. Marlin, S. D., D. E. Staunton, T. A. Springer et al. A soluble form of intercellular adhesion molecule-1 inhibits rhinovirus infection. Nature 1990. 344:70-72.
47. Staunton, D. E., M. L. Dustin, H. P. Erickson et al. The arrangement of the immunoglobulin-like domains of ICAM-1 and the binding sites for LFA-1 and rhinovirus [published erratum appears in Cell 1990 Jun 15;61(2):1157]. Cell 1990. 61:243-254.
48. Greve, J. M., G. Davis, A. M. Meyer et al. The major human rhinovirus receptor is ICAM-1. Cell 1989. 56:839-847.
49. Ockenhouse, C. F., R. Betageri, T. A. Springer et al. Plasmodium falciparum-infected erythrocytes bind ICAM-1 at a site distinct from LFA-1, Mac-1, and human rhinovirus. Cell 1992. 68:63-69.

50. Berendt, A. R., A. McDowall, A. G. Craig et al. The binding site on ICAM-1 for plasmodium falciparum-infected erythrocytes overlaps, but is distinct from, the LFA-1-binding site. Cell 1992. 68:71-81.
51. Vedder, N. B., R. K. Winn, C. L. Rice et al. A monoclonal antibody to the adherence-promoting leukocyte glycoprotein, CD18, reduces organ injury and improves survival from hemorrhagic shock and resuscitation in rabbits. J. Clin. Invest. 1988. 81:939-944.
52. Simpson, P. J., R. F. Todd, J. C. Fantone et al. Reduction of experimental canine myocardial reperfusion injury by a monoclonal antibody (anti-Mo1, anti-CD11b) that inhibits leukocyte adhesion. J. Clin. Invest. 1988. 81:624-629.
53. Fischer, A., C. Griscelli, Blanche et al. Prevention of graft failure by an anti-HLFA-1 monoclonal antibody in HLA-mismatched bone-marrow transplantation. Lancet. 1986. 1058-1061.
54. Heagy, W. and C. Waltenbaugh. Potent ability of anti-LFA-1 monoclonal antibody to prolong allograft survival. Transpl. 1983. 37:520-523.
55. Baume, D., M. Kuentz, J.L. Pico et al. Failure of a CD18/anti-LFA-1 monoclonal antibody infusion to prevent graft rejection in leukemic patients receiving T-depleted allogeneic bone marrow transplantation. Transpl. 1989. 47:472-474.
56. Van Dijken, P.J., T. Ghayur, P. Mauch et al. Evidence that anti-LFA-1 in vivo improves engraftment and survival after allogeneic bone marrow transplantation. Transpl. 1990. 49:882-886.
57. Harning, R., J. Pelletier, K. Lubbe et al. Reduction in the severity of graft-versus-host disease and increased survival in allogeneic mice by treatment with monoclonal antibodies to cell adhesion antigens LFA-1 and MALA-2. Transpl. 1991. 52:842-845.
58. Le Mauff, B., M. Hourmant, J.P. Rougier et al. Effect of anti-LFA-1 (CD11a) monoclonal antibodies in acute rejection in human kidney transplantation. Transpl. 1991. 52:291-296.
59. Cosimi, A. B., D. Conti, F. L. Delmonico et al. In vivo effects of monoclonal antibody to ICAM-1 (CD54) in nonhuman primates with renal allografts. J. Immunol. 1990. 144:4604-4612.
60. Cosimi, AB, Rothlein, R., Auchincloss, H., et al. Phase I clinical trial of anti-ICAM-1 (CD54) monoclonal antibody immunosuppression in renal allograft recipients. Proceedings of the second international conference on structure and function of molecules involved in leukocyte adhesion. 1991. 373-380.
61. Haug, C.E., Colvin, R.B., Delmonico, F.L., etal. A phase I trial of immunosuppression with anti-ICAM-1 (CD54) aAb in renal allograft recipients. Transpl. 1993. 55: 766-772.
62. Wee, S.L., A.B. Cosimi, F.I. Preffer et al. Functional consequences of anti-ICAM-1 (CD54) in cynomolgus monkeys with renal allografts. Transpl.Proc. 1991. 23:279-280.
63. Flavin, T., K. Ivens, R. Rothlein et al. Monoclonal antibodies against intercellular adhesion molecule 1 prolong cardiac allograft survival in cynomolgus monkeys. Transpl. Proc. 1991. 23:533-534.
64. Chavin, K.D., H.T. Lau and J.S. Bromberg. Prolongation of allograft and xenograft survival in mice by anti-CD2 monoclonal antibodies. Transpl. 1992. 54:286-291.
65. Isobe, M., H. Yagita, K. Okumura et al. Specific acceptance of cardiac allograft after treatment with antibodies to ICAM-1 and LFA-1. Science. 1992. 255:1125-1127.
66. Komari, A., M. Nagata, T. Ochiai et al. Role of ICAM-1 and LFA-1 in cardiac allograft rejection of the rat. Transpl.Proc. 1993. 25: 831-832.
67. Paul, L.C., A. Davidoff, P.W. Paul et al. Monoclonal antibodies against LFA-1 and VLA-4 inhibit graft vasculitis in rat caridiac allografts. Transpl.Proc.1993. 25:813-814.
68. Jendrisak, M., G. Jendrisak, J. Gamero et al. Prolongation in murine cardiac allograft survival with monoclonal antibodies to LFA-1, ICAM-1, and CD4. Transpl.Proc. 1993. 25:835-827.

69. van Kooyk, Y., A. de Vries-van der Zwan, L.P. de Waal et al. Efficiency of antibodies directed against adhesion molecules to prolong skin graft survival in mice. Transp.Proc. 1994. 26:401-403.
70. van Kooyk, Y. et al. submitted.
71. Müller, K. submitted.
72. Harning, R., J. Pelletier, K. Lubbe et al. Reduction in the severity of graft-versus-host disease and increased survival in allogeneic mice by treatment with monoclonal antibodies to cell adhesion antigens LFA-1α and MALA-2. Transpl. 1991.52: 842-845.
73. Nakakura, E.K., S.M. McCabe, B. Zheng et al. A non-lymphocyte-depleting monoclonal antibody to the adhesion molecule LFA-1 (CD11a) prevents sensitization to alloantigens and effectively prolongs the survival of heart allografts. Transpl.Proc. 1993. 25: 809-812.
74. Kameoka, H., M. Ishibashi, T. Tamatani et al. Comparitive immunosuppressive effect of anti-CD18 and anti-CD11a monoclonal antibodies on rat heart allotransplantation. Transpl.Proc. 1993. 25:833-836.
75. Pelletier, R., R. Ohye, P. Kincade et al. Monoclonal antibody to anti-VCAM-1 interferes with murine cardiac allograft rejection. Transpl. Proc. 1993. 25:839-841.
76. Jendrisak, G. , J. Gamero, T. Mohanakumar et al. Clonal anergy induction by monoclonal antibodies to CD4, LFA-1 and ICAM-1. Transpl. Proc. 1993. 25:828-830.
77. Chavin, K.D., L. Qin, A.J. Kaplan et al. Anti-CD2 monoclonal antibodies dynergize with anti-CD3 to prolong allograft survival and decease cytokine production. 1993. 25:823-824.
78. Chavin K.D., L. Qin, J. Lin et al. Combined anti-CD2 and anti-CD3 receptor monoclonal antibodies induce donor-specific tolerance in a cardiac transplant model. J. of Immunol. 1993. 151:7249-7259.

CHAPTER 6

IMMUNOSUPPRESSION FOR ISLET TRANSPLANTATION

Paul F. Gores

David E. R. Sutherland

The driving force responsible for the improved results of solid organ transplantation over the last three decades has been the development and refinement of immunosuppressive protocols. One year graft survival rates are now in the range of 75-90% for kidneys, hearts, livers, and pancreases. However, application of these regimens of immunosuppression to clinical islet transplantation has not resulted in significant long-term graft function in the vast majority of cases. Analysis of registry data reveals only 11 documented cases of insulin-independence in 139 attempts since 1974.[1] The reasons for failure are multifactorial but the reliable success of islet autotransplantation (in patients undergoing total pancreatectomy for benign disease)[2] implies that the failure of allotransplantation is the result of inadequate immunosuppression. However, before discussing strategies of immunosuppression, a word is in order concerning the nature of the islet preparation to be transplanted.

NATURE OF THE ISLET PREPARATION

It has generally been assumed that significant exocrine contamination of islet tissue limits engraftment and enhances immunogenicity to such an extent that clinical success is not achievable. The corollary to this is that the more highly purified the islet preparation, the less vigorous the recipient's immune response to the graft and the higher the likelihood of a successful result. As theoretical support for this argument, the passenger leukocyte theory has been invoked as a means of explaining islet allograft immunogenicity.[3] This theory predicts that if a graft is devoid of passenger leukocytes, i.e. donor antigen presenting cells, it will be non-immunogenic. Numerous experiments using inbred rodent strains lend support to this concept,[4-6] however, there are exceptions[7,8] and there is at best meager support in clinically relevant large animal models.[9-11] Although the weight of the evidence supports the conclusion that lymphoid contamination of islet tissue does increase the immunogenicity of the graft, it does not follow that purified endocrine tissue is not immunogenic. Thus, Stock, et al, have shown that

Pancreatic Islet Transplantation Volume II: Immunomodulation of Pancreatic Islets, edited by Robert P. Lanza, MD, William L. Chick, MD; ©1994 R.G. Landes Company.

rigorously purified β cells, free of contaminating leukocytes, are capable of inducing proliferation of allogeneic lymphocytes in vitro with generation of allospecific cytotoxic T lymphocytes.[12] Although purified β cells are not capable of antigen presentation, donor antigen may still be presented to recipient lymphocytes after processing by recipient antigen presenting cells (indirect pathway). In vitro, it has been shown that β cells sensitize unless both stimulator-type and responder-type antigen presenting cells have been eliminated from the system.[12] Thus, it is not surprising that the elimination of passenger leukocytes from a graft does not abolish the tissues' capacity to immunize. This has been confirmed in vivo by Pipeleers et al who, working with inbred rodent strains, showed that in the absence of immunosuppression, rigorously purified β cells are rejected when transplanted across a major histocompatibility barrier.[13] Systemic immunosuppression with cyclo–sporine is required for long-term β cell function even when purified grafts are utilized.[14]

Thus, the hope that clinical application of islet transplantation in the absence of immunosuppression will be possible once techniques are developed that yield pure populations of endocrine cells, is a futile one. Until strategies allowing the development of antigen-specific tolerance or immunoisolation devices are perfected, we are left with systemic immunosuppression in order to prevent the destruction of allogeneic islet tissue.

IMMUNOSUPPRESSION

The ideal immunosuppressive agent (or regimen) would inhibit immunologically mediated β cell damage (both the generalized inflammatory damage that occurs during the engraftment phase and classic T-lymphocyte mediated rejection occurring subsequently) and would not possess diabetogenic toxicity. It is noteworthy that conventional regimens of immunosuppression are frankly diabetogenic, with as many as 19% of previously non-diabetic kidney transplant recipients developing altered glucose metabolism after being placed on standard triple immunotherapy consisting of cyclo–sporine, azathioprine, and prednisone.[15] Those patients who maintain normal glucose disposal on triple therapy do so only because of their ability to increase insulin secretion two- to three-fold.[16,17]

The precise mechanism by which glucose metabolism is altered by immunosuppressive therapy is not known. Broadly speaking, corticosteroids are known to induce insulin resistance in experimental animals and man. Decreased receptor number and affinity,[18,19] decreased glucose transporter activity,[20] impaired suppression of hepatic glucose production by insulin,[21] and activation of the glucose/fatty acid cycle[22] have all been evoked to explain the decreased sensitivity to insulin.

Cyclosporine has also been implicated in the development of impaired glucose tolerance. It is well documented that therapeutic concentrations of cyclosporine inhibit glucose stimulated insulin secretion in vitro.[23,24] However, a detailed study of patients with multiple sclerosis treated with cyclosporine monotherapy for a year showed no adverse effect on insulin secretory kinetics during intravenous glucose tolerance testing.[25] In addition, no differences were noted between treated patients and appropriately matched control subjects.

The combination of cyclosporine (inhibition of insulin secretion) and prednisone (development of insulin resistance) may act synergistically to impair glucose metabolism. In support of this is the observation that post-transplant diabetes is significantly increased in patients receiving cyclosporine, prednisone, and azathioprine in contrast to patients on azathioprine/prednisone alone.[15]

Sustained hyperglycemia renders β cells glucose unresponsive and if hyper-glycemia is severe and prolonged, leads to direct β cell destruction.[26,27] Although the toxic effect is reversible if hyperglycemia is of short duration, prolonged exposure results in irreversible damage. Furthermore, hyper-glycemia itself has been shown both in vitro[28] and in vivo[29] to lead to insulin resistance which further exacerbates the hyperglycemia. Thus, a vicious cycle occurs in which the side effects of immunosuppressive drugs lead to hyperglycemia, which in turn causes further insulin resistance and β cell dysfunction thereby exacerbating the hyperglycemia.

It is apparent that for clinical islet transplantation to succeed under immunosuppressive therapy, molecules capable of preventing immune-mediated damage, but lacking in diabetogenic toxicity need to be employed. Several promising new drugs are currently in clinical development. Most of the experience to date has been with solid organ transplantation, particularly liver and kidney recipients. The only molecules for which any data are available in the setting of clinical islet transplantation, are 15-deoxyspergualin and FK 506.

15-DEOXYSPERGUALIN

15-Deoxyspergualin (DSG, Fig. 6.1) is the 15-dehydroxy derivative of the anti-tumor antibiotic spergualin. It is capable of prolonging the survival of skin, heart, kidney, liver, and pancreas allografts.[30-33] It has also been used to reverse established rejection[34] and has been shown to be an effective immunosuppressant for autoimmune diseases.[35] Walter et al were the first to demonstrate activity in a rodent model of islet allotransplantation.[36]

The mechanism of action is unknown, although it appears to be novel. DSG binds to a member of the heat shock protein 70 family and does not compete with the immunophilins-cyclophilin or FK binding protein.[37] In addition to inhibiting the generation of antigen-specific cytoxic T-lymphocytes, DSG has been reported to inhibit several macrophage functions.[38] It inhibits lysozomal enzyme release and superoxide production as well as class II MHC antigen induction in response to immunologic stimuli. DSG also inhibits ornithine decarboxylase activity which is associated with impaired macrophage function.

DSG is well tolerated in humans. Because of its anti-tumor activity it was initially used in Phase I studies in patients with advanced malignancies in order to assess its safety profile, maximum tolerated dose, and pharmocokinetics. Because of its structure (Fig. 6.1) DSG is degraded in the acid-peptic environment of the upper gastrointestinal tract and must be delivered via the intravenous route. Phase I studies were conducted using 3 or 24 hour intravenous infusions of DSG for 5 days.[39] A total of 123 patients were treated at doses ranging from 2 mg/kg to 69 mg/kg for the 24 hour infusion study and from .05 mg/kg to 15 mg/kg for the 3 hour infusion trial. When infused over 24 hours hypotension was the dose limiting (53 mg/kg) toxicity. Sporadic asymptomatic hypotension occurred at a dose of 42 mg/kg. These patients also complained of perioral numbness. Myelosuppression was sporadic and not clearly dose related. In the 3 hour infusion study dose limiting toxicity was perioral numbness and mild myelosuppression at a dose of 12 mg/kg. DSG has also

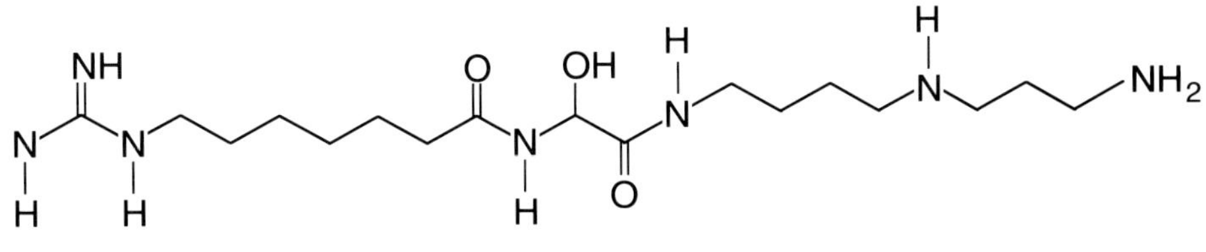

Fig. 6.1. Chemical structure of 15-deoxyspergualin.

been evaluated in Phase I/II studies for the prevention or treatment of renal allograft rejection. DSG has been delivered as a 3 hour infusion for 5 consecutive days at doses ranging from 2-6 mg/kg/d. The overall instance of significant adverse effects has been low. In addition to mild myelosuppression, toxicity observed has included facial flushing, perioral numbness, and asymptomatic increases and decreases in blood pressure at the 6 mg/kg dose level. No dose level toxicities have been encountered.

Hyperglycemia has not been noted in patients receiving DSG, nor has it been reported in animal models to date. Furthermore, DSG does not inhibit glucose-induced insulin secretion in vitro of either rat or human islets.[40] Also, normal rats treated with 1,4, or 10 mg/kg/d intraperitoneally for 1 week do not exhibit disordered glucose metabolism or insulin secretion.[40]

DSG's ability to inhibit both macrophage and T-lymphocyte functions make it a promising agent for investigation of efficacy in islet transplantation. Daily administration of DSG to C57BL/6J(H-2^b) recipients of B10.BR(H-2^k) islets at a dose of 0.625 mg/kg/d i.p. completely abrogates the phenomenon of primary non-function, as well as that of classic rejection, with all grafts surviving greater than 100 days.[41] Furthermore, once DSG is stopped a metastable situation exists with graft function continuing unabated although rejection can be induced with donor-strain splenocyte injections.

In the clinical situation, when single donors are used, we are always dealing with a marginal mass of engrafted islets after transplantation. The effectiveness of DSG in a marginal islet mass model has been investigated in mice.[42] 75% (12 of 16) of C57BL/six islet isograft recipients attained euglycemia after transplantation of 150 islets per recipient at a mean of 39 ± 6 days posttransplant. Treatment with DSG (0.625 mg/kg/d i.p.) results in earlier graft function (18 ± 3 vs 39 ± 6 days). However, the proportion of those attaining euglycemia is not altered. This suggests that mediators of non-specific inflammation present during the engraftment phase inhibit the function of freshly transplanted isologous islets. In the allogeneic setting, only 22% (2 of 9) of untreated C57 BL/ 6 recipients of B10.BR islets attain euglycemia; when DSG is administered the cure rate increases to 75% (6 of 8) at 23 ± 5 days.

DSG also appears to be active in the more difficult large animal model of canine islet transplantation. In this model, when cyclosporine is administered in clinically relevant doses, along with azathioprine and an induction course of antilymphoblast globulin, median islet allograft survival is only 4 days. Regimens including corticosteroids are even less successful. However, the addition of low dose DSG (0.5 mg/kg/d) as induction therapy for 10 days to a regimen of cyclosporine/azathioprine/antilymphoblast globulin increases the median survival of canine islet allografts to 22 days.[43] These encouraging data provided the rationale for a pilot study of the efficacy of DSG in clinical islet transplantation.

PILOT STUDY OF 15-DEOXYSPERGUALIN IN HUMAN ISLET TRANSPLANTATION

If islets are to replace whole organ pancreases as the preferred mode of endocrine replacement therapy for patients with Type I diabetes and end-stage renal disease durable success must be achievable with islets derived from a single donor. Because the number of purified islets obtained from an individual pancreas is usually insufficient to render patients insulin-independent, we have increased islet yield by omitting density gradient purification and have injected unpurified islets into the portal vein at the time of simultaneous kidney transplantation from the same cadaver donor.[44] In this pilot study, immunosuppression has consisted of induction with DSG (4 mg/kg/d i.v. for 10 days), antilymphoblast globulin (MALG) or antithymocyte globulin (ATG) at a dose of 20 mg/kg/d for 7 days and a prednisone taper beginning at 1 mg/kg/d. At the conclusion of the induction course of DSG, azathioprine (1.5 mg/kg/d) orally is instituted. Maintenance immunosuppression includes azathioprine and prednisone along with cyclosporine (8 mg/kg/d beginning on day 5). The first two patients on this regimen, despite experiencing early steroid-resistant rejection episodes, achieved long-term insulin-independence. Both have been followed for greater than 2 years and continue to have excellent islet and renal graft function with baseline serum C-peptide of 0.54 and 1.59 pm/ml, and stimulated C-peptide of 1.14 and 2.61 pm/ml. Their serum creatinine is 1.4 and 1.7 mg/dl respectively. The first patient achieved good early engraftment (Fig. 6.2) and excellent glycemic control, with Hgb A1c ranging between 5.7 and 6.1% (normal 4.3-6.0%). Exogenous insulin therapy was withdrawn 11 months posttransplant, and except for a brief period (16 months posttransplant) coinciding with a soft tissue (atypical mycobacterial infection) he has been insulin-independent. Currently he is 25 months posttransplantation with stable renal and islet allograft function and is insulin independent.

The second patient also achieved excellent early function of her islet transplant (Fig. 6.3) and despite having steroid-resistant renal allograft rejection episodes 3 weeks and 11 months posttransplantation, she has stable islet function. She was insulin-independent for 9 months; however, because of her insulin resistance, we have chosen to treat her with 15 units of exogenous insulin per day in an effort to take some of the metabolic workload off of the islet graft, and hopefully, prolong its function. Both of these patients have excellent glycemic control with hemoglobin A1c currently ranging between 6.4 and 6.6%.

Four additional fully evaluable patients have received simultaneous islet/kidney grafts (islet mass transplanted similar to the first two patients; 8,432 ± 2,120 [S.D.] versus 10,601 ± 3,845 islet equivalents) but have had ATG (Upjohn Co; Kalamazoo, MI) substituted for MALG. Although their renal function is excellent, durable engraftment of islet tissue has not occurred. This suggests that induction therapy with 15-deoxyspergualin may not be effective in the

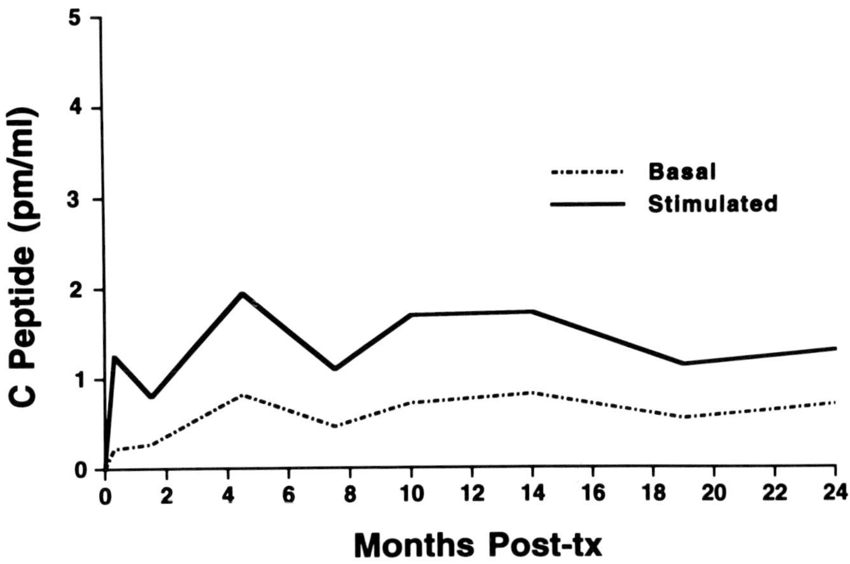

Fig. 6.2. Serum C-peptide levels in patient 1 as a function of time following simultaneous islet/kidney transplantation. Values are plotted as basal and after ingestion of 360 ml of Ensure, a liquid mixed meal containing 51 g carbohydrate, 13 g protein, and 13 g fat.

absence of MALG. Nevertheless, the first two patients demonstrate that unpurified islet tissue can engraft and function well enough to maintain an insulin-independent state for a prolonged period of time. However, the second patient illustrates again the difficulty of achieving routine success in the face of the heightened insulin-resistance engendered by the immunosuppressive regimen. In order for islet transplantation to replace pancreas transplantation as the preferred mode of therapy for the diabetic patient with end-stage renal disease who is either receiving or has already received a renal allograft, non-steroid based immunosuppressive therapy must be developed.

The role of DSG is currently limited by the need for intravenous infusion. Although the development of an oral formulation is unlikely, the development of a transdermal delivery system is possible. Of the other immunosuppressive molecules currently in the clinical investigation phase, FK506, although clearly effective in preventing solid organ graft rejection, has been shown to inhibit insulin secretion in vitro[45] and in vivo[46] and lead to new onset diabetes in up to 14% of patients during the first 6 months post-transplantation.[47] Clinical experience with this drug in the setting of islet allotransplantation in patients with Type I diabetes has been disappointing with all patients remaining insulin-dependent.[48] However, there has been long-term function noted with combined liver/islet grafts in patients undergoing foregut amputation (including pancreatectomy) for malignancy.[48,49]

FUTURE STRATEGIES

Mycophenolic mofetil (MM – a morpholinoethyl ester of mycophenolic acid, Fig. 6.4) is an inhibitor of inosine monophosphate dehydrogenase (IMP) and results in the depletion of guanosine monophosphate and hence purine synthesis.[50] Since lymphocytes, in contrast to other cell types, do not have a salvage pathway and rely exclusively on de novo purine synthesis, antiproliferative ef-

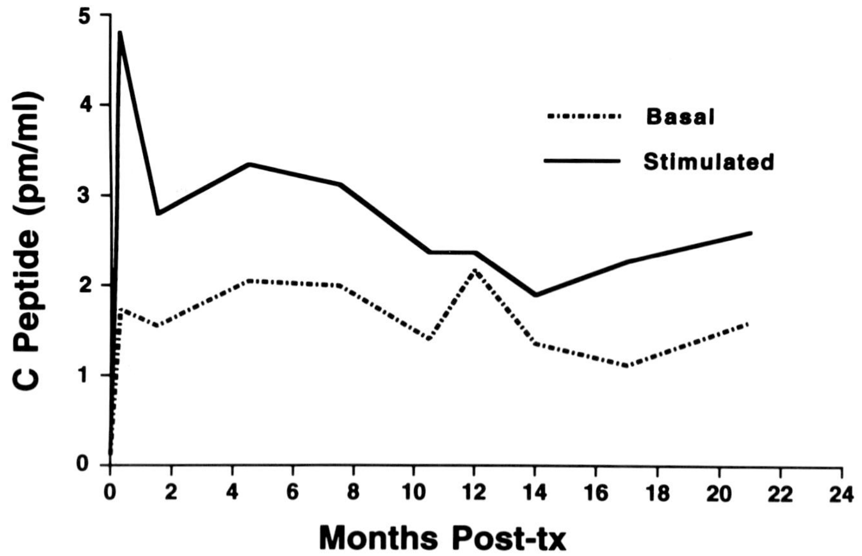

Fig. 6.3. Serum C-peptide levels in patient 2 as a function of time following simultaneous islet/kidney transplantation. Values are plotted as basal and after ingestion of 360 ml of Ensure, a liquid mixed meal containing 51 g carbohydrate, 13 g protein, and 13 g fat.

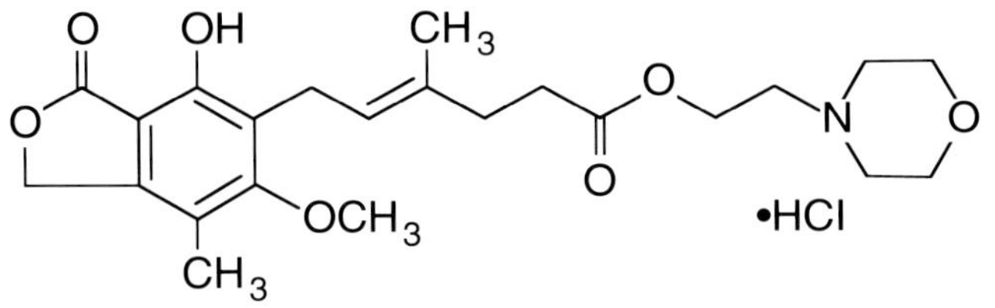

Fig. 6.4. Chemical structure of mycophenolate mofetil.

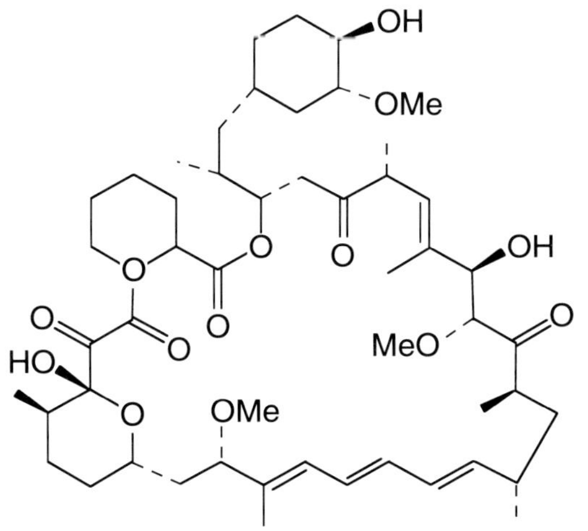

Fig. 6.5. Chemical structure of rapamycin.

fects produced by interruption of the IMP dependent de novo pathway are more potent on lymphocytes than on other cell types.

MM is effective in prolonging allograft survival in a variety of small and large animal models and is currently in advanced stages of clinical testing. In vivo, mono–therapy with MM has been shown to prolong the survival of heart allografts in rats[51] and islet allografts in mice.[52] MM treatment prevents the development of diabetes in BB rats as long as the drug continues to be administered. However, a state of tolerance is not created as diabetes ensues once the drug is withdrawn.[53] Furthermore, treatment with MM does not prevent islet graft destruction following transplantation to the spontaneously diabetic NOD mouse.[54]

MM does not appear to be diabetogenic. Hyperglycemia has not been observed in experimental or clinical use to date. However, there is a single report describing inhibition of glucose-stimulated insulin secretion in vitro after 6 days of culture in the presence of the drug.[55] There are no reports of efficacy in large animal models of islet transplantation.

Rapamycin is a macrolide antibiotic produced by *Streptomyces hygroscopicus* (Fig. 6.5). It was originally identified as an antifungal agent, however, subsequent studies have demonstrated impressive anti-tumor and immunosuppressive activities. Rapamycin belongs to a class of macrocyclic immunosuppressants that include FK506 and cyclosporine. These latter drugs inhibit transcription of the IL-2 gene in T cells by interrupting the calcium dependent signal transduction pathway initiated by antigen binding. FK506 and cyclosporine, when complexed with their respective immunophilins, form a complex which binds to calcineurin, thereby inhibiting that enzyme's ability to dephosphorylate peptide substrates essential for single transduction.[56] Rapamycin, although it binds to FKBP, has no effect on calcineurin activity. Although rapamycin-FKBP complexes are necessary for rapamycin's immunosuppressive effect, the molecular target of this complex is unknown. Rapamycin does not interfere with IL-2 gene transcription or IL-2 binding to its receptor; rather, it interrupts IL-2 dependent signaling pathways.[57]

Rapamycin exerts potent effects in several small and large animal models of islet transplantation and currently is in Phase I human studies. Chemically induced diabetic mice treated with either 0.1 or 0.3 mg/kg/d intraperitoneally of rapamycin exhibit prolonged islet allograft survival.[58] When doses of rapamycin an order of magnitude higher were used islet allograft function was not maintained, suggesting a possible diabetogenic effect of rapamycin at elevated doses. Although there is no data on islet transplantation in the rat model, the survival of pancreacticoduodenal grafts has been increased significantly by a 14 day course of rapamycin administered at a dose of 0.8 mg/kg/d iv following transplantation.[59]

Importantly, rapamycin exhibits strong therapeutic synergism with cyclosporine. This has been shown by isobologram analysis in the quantal mouse-heart allograft assay,[60] as well as by median effect analysis in the immediately vascularized rat heterotopic cardiac allograft model.[61] Rapamycin has also been shown to reverse ongoing rejection of heart, kidney, and pancreas allografts in the rat.[62] Large animal models in which rapamycin's immunosuppressive abilities have been demonstrated include the dog,[63] pig,[64] and subhuman primates.[65] The dog exhibits species-specific toxicity to macrolide immunosuppressive agents manifested by diffuse gastrointestinal vasculitis. However, in an important study by Yakimets et al, the combination of nonimmunosuppressive doses of cyclosporine and rapamycin (0.05 mg/kg) resulted in significantly prolonged survival of intrasplenically transplanted islet allografts in pancreatectomized mongrel dogs.[66]

Although the side effect profile of rapamycin is only now being chronicled in Phase I clinical studies, high doses in rodent models have suggested a tendency toward diabetogenicity. Thus, male Sprague-Dawley rats treated with rapamycin at a dose of 1.5 mg/kg/d ip or 10 mg/kg/d p.o. developed hyperglycemia. This dose is an order of magnitude above that which leads to immunosuppressive activity, particularly when rapamycin is administered in conjunction with cyclosporine.

Several other molecules are also in development. These include brequinar, mizoribine, discodermolide, and leflunomide. Experience with these drugs, particularly clinical experience, is still limited. Nevertheless, it is reasonable to expect that their differing mechanisms of selectively interfering with T-cell activation and proliferation will enable combination regimens to be developed that utilize small doses of individual agents but achieve therapeutic immunosuppressive effects. Presumably because of the pleotropic nature of the side effect profiles of individual agents, combinations can be selected that either are lacking in diabetogenic tendencies, or because of therapeutic synergy, can be used at doses below the threshold for diabetogenicity. The development of non-corticosteroid based non-diabetogenic regimens of immunosuppression should allow islet transplantation to become the preferred mode of endocrine replacement therapy in the diabetic patient with end stage renal disease who is committed to receiving or already has received a renal allograft. Such a regimen may also have a role in preventing insulin dependent diabetes mellitus from developing in patients at risk. With improvements in our ability to predict which individuals will manifest the disease, early prevention trials are being initiated. Although monotherapy with any particular agent is likely to result in unacceptable side effects at dosage levels required for immunosuppression, it is reasonable to expect that combination regimens will have a favorable side effective profile and may be used to prevent the development of the disease altogether.

References

1. Federlin KF, Bretzel RG, Hering BJ. International islet transplant registry. Newsletter 1993; No 4.
2. Farney AC, Najarian JS, Nakhleh RE, Lloveras G, Field MJ, Gores PF, Sutherland DER. Autotransplantation of Dispersed Pancreatic Islet Tissue Combined with Total or Near-Total Pancreatectomy for Treatment of Chronic Pancreatitis. Surgery 1991; 110: 427.
3. Lafferty KJ, Prouse SJ, Simeonovic CJ, Warren MS. Immunobiology of tissue transplantation: A return to the passenger leukocyte concept. Ann Rev Immunol 1983; 1: 143.
4. Faustman D, Hauptfeld V, Lacy P, Davie J. Prolongation of murine allograft survival by pretreatment of islets with antibody directed to Ia determinants. Proc Natl Acad Sci USA 1981; 78: 5156.
5. Faustman D, Steinman RM, Gebel HM, Hauptfeld V, Davie JM, Lacy PE. Prevention of rejection of murine islet allografts by pretreatment with anti- dendritic cell antibody. Proc Nat Acad Sci USA 1984; 81: 3864.
6. Lau H, Reemtsma K, Hardy MA. Prolongation of rat islet allograft survival by direct ultraviolet irradiation of the graft. Science 1984; 223: 607.
7. Gores PF, Sutherland DER, Platt J, Bach FH. Depletion of donor Ia+ cells before transplantation does not prolong islet allograft survival. J of Immunol 1986; 137: 1482.
8. Naji A, Woehrle M, Markmann JF. Influence of physical parameters of tissue culture on the fate of islet allografts. In van Schilfgaarde R, Hardy MA (eds): Transplantation of the endocrine pancreas." Amsterdam 1988; Elsevier, pp 292.
9. Kenyon NS, Strasser S, Alejandro R. Ultraviolet light immunomodulation of canine islets for prolongation of allograft survival. Diabetes 1990; 39: 305.
10. Stegall MD, Chabot J, Weber C, Reemtsma K, Hardy MA. Pancreatic islet transplantation in cynomolgus monkeys. Initial studies and evidence that cyclosporine impairs glucose tolerance in normal monkeys. Transplantation 1989; 48: 944.
11. Warnock GL, Dabbs KD, Cattral MS, Rajotte RV. Improved survival of in vitro cultured canine islet allografts. Transplantation 1994; 57: 17.
12. Stock PG, Ascher NL, Chen S, Field J, Bach FH, Sutherland DER. Evidence for direct and indirect pathways in the generation of the alloimmune response against pancreatic islets. Transplantation 1991; 52: 704.
13. Pipeleers DG, Pipeleers-Marichal M, Vanbrabandt B, Duys S. Transplantation of purified islet cells in diabetic rats. II Immunogenicity of allografted islet B-cells. Diabetes 1991; 40: 920.
14. Pipeleers-Marichal M, Zhi-Dong L, Teng M, Pipeleers DG. Transplantation of purified islet cells in diabetic rats. III Immunosuppressive effect of cyclosporine. Diabetes 1991; 40: 931.
15. Boudreaux JP, McHugh L, Canafax DM. The impact of cyclosporine and combination immunosuppression on the incidence of posttransplant diabetes in renal allograft recipients. Transplantation 1987; 44: 376.

16. Katz H, Homan M, Velosa J, Robertson P, Rizza P. Effects of pancreas transplantation on postprandial glucose metabolism. N Engl J Med 1991; 325: 1278.
17. Scharp DW, Lacy PE, Santiago JV et al. Results of our first nine intraportal islet allografts in Type I, insulin-dependent diabetic patients. Transplantation 1991; 51: 76.
18. Cigolini M, Smith U. Human adipose tissue in culture VIII. Studies on the insulin-antagonistic effect of glucocorticoids. Metabolism 1979; 28: 502.
19. Kahn CR, Goldine ID, Neville DM, Demeyts P. Alteration in insulin binding induced by changer in vivo in the levels of glucocorticoids and growth hormone. Endocrinology 1987; 103: 1054.
20. Gagano G, Cavallo-Perin P, Cassader M. An in vivo and in vitro study of the mechanism of prednisone-induced insulin resistance in healthy subject. J Clin Invest 1983; 72: 1814.
21. Cahill G. Action of adrenal cortical steroids on carbohydrate metabolism. In Christy N (eds) 1971. "The human adrenal cortex." New York: Harper Row 1971; pp 205.
22. Randle PJ, Garland PB, Maler CN, Newsholme EA. The glucose fatty-acid cycle – its role in insulin sensitivity and the metabolic disturbances of diabetes mellitus. Lancet 1963; 1: 785.
23. Andersson A, Borg H, Hallberg A, Hellerstrom C, Sandler S, Schnell A. Long-term effects of cyclosporine A on cultured mouse pancreatic islets. Diabetologia 1984; 27: 66.
24. Martin F, Bedoya FJ. Short-term effects of cyclosporine on secretagogue-induced insulin release by isolated islets. Transplantation 1990; 50: 551.
25. Robertson RP, Franklin G, Nelson L. Glucose homeostasis and insulin secretion during chronic treatment with cyclosporine in nondiabetic humans. Diabetes 1989; 38: 99.
26. Dohan FC, Lukens FEW. Lesions of the pancreatic islets produced in cats by administration of glucose. Science 1947; 105: 183.
27. Leahy JL, Bonner-Weir, Weir GC. B-cell dysfunction induced by chronic hyperglycemia. Current ideas on mechanism of impaired glucose-induced insulin secretion. Diabetes Care 1992; 15: 442.
28. Garvey WT, Olefsky JM, Matthaei S, Marshall S. Glucose and insulin correlate the glucose transport system in primary cultured andipocytes: a new mechanism of insulin resistance. J Biol Chem 1987; 262: 189.
29. Kahn BB, Shulman GI, Defronzo RA, Cushman SW, Rossetti L. Normalization of blood glucose in diabetic rats with phlorizin treatment reverses insulin-resistant glucose transport in adipose cells without restoring glucose transporter gene expression. J Clin Inv 1991; 87: 561.
30. Shorlemmer HU, Dickneite G, Siler FR. Treatment of acute rejection episodes and induction of tolerance in rat skin allot–ransplantation by 15-deoxyspergualin. Transplant Proc 1990; 22: 1626.
31. Reichenspurner H, Hilebrandt A, Human PA et al. 15-Deoxyspergualin for induction of graft nonreactivity after cardiac and renal allotransplantation in primates. Transplantation 1990; 50: 181.
32. Inagaki K, Fukuda Y, Sumimoto K et al. Effects of FK 506 and 15-deoxyspergualin in rat orthotopic liver transplantation. Transplant Proc 1989; 21: 1069.
33. Schubert G, Stoffregen C, Timmermann W, Schang T, Thiede A. Comparison of the New Immunosuppressive Agent 15-Deoxy–spergualin and Cyclosporine A after Highly Allogeneic Pancreas Transplantation. Transplant Proc 1987; 19: 3978.
34. Fukao K, Ofsuka M, Iwasaki H, Yuzawa K, Iwasaki Y. Immunosuppressive effect of Deoxyspergualin on Acute Renal Allograft Rejection in Dogs. Transplant Proc 1989; 21: 1090.
35. Newmoto K, Abe F, Takita T, Nakamure T, Takeuchi T, Umezawa H. Suppression of Experimental Allergic Encephalomyelitis in Guinea Pigs by Spergualin and 15-Deoxy–spergualin. J Antibiotics 1987; 40: 1193.
36. Walter PK, Dickneite G, Schorlemmer HU et al. Prolongation of graft survival in allogenic islet transportation by 15-deoxyspergualin in the rat. Diabetologia 1987; 30: 38.

37. Nadler SG, Tepper MA, Schacter B, Mazzucco CE. Interaction of the immunosuppressant deoxyspergualin with a member of the HSP 70 family of heat shock proteins. Science 1992; 258: 484.
38. Tepper MA. Deoxyspergualin - Mechanism of Action Studies of a Novel Immunosuppressive Drug. Annals NY Acad Sci 1993; 696: 123: 132.
39. National Cancer Institute. Annual Report to the Food and Drug Administration; Deoxyspergualin NSC356894: (IND 28053), 1990.
40. Xenos ES, Casanova D, Sutherland DER, Farney AC, Lloveras JJ, Gores PF. The in vivo and in vitro effect of 15-deoxy–spergualin on pancreatic islet function. Transplantation 1993; 56: 144.
41. Kaufman DB, Field MJ, Gruber SA, Farney AC, Stephanian E, Gores PF, Sutherland DER. Extended functional survival of murine islet allograft with 15-deoxyspergualin. Transplant Proc 1992; 24: 1045.
42. Kaufman DB, Farney AC, Field MJ et al. Effect of 15-Deoxyspergualin on Immediate Function and Long-term Survival of Transplanted Islets in Recipients of a Marginal Islet Mass. Diabetes 1994; (in press).
43. Stephanian E, Lloveras JJ, Sutherland DER et al. Prolongation of canine islet allograft survival by 15-deoxyspergualin. J Surg Res 1992; 52: 621.
44. Gores PF, Najarian JS, Stephanian E, Lloveras JJ, Kelley SL, Sutherland DER. Insulin independence in Type I diabetes after transplantation of unpurified islets from single donor with 15-deoxyspergualin. Lancet 1993; 341: 19.
45. Ishizuka J, Gugliuzza KK, Wassmuth Z et al. Effects of FK 506 and cyclosporine on dynamic insulin secretion from isolated dog pancreatic islets. Transplantation 1993; 56: 1486.
46. Ricordi C, Zeng Y, Alejandro R et al. In vivo effect of FK 506 on human pancreatic islets. Transplantation 1991; 52: 519.
47. Tabasco-Minguillan J, Mieler L, Carroll P et al. Insulin requirements after liver transplantation and FK 506 immunosuppression. Transplantation 1993; 56:862.
48. Ricordi C, Tzakis AG, Carroll PB et al. Human islet isolation and allotransplant–ation in 22 consecutive cases. Transplantation 1992; 53:407.
49. Tzakis AG, Ricordi C, Alejandro R, et al. Pancreatic islet transplantation after upper abdominal exenteration and liver replacement. Lancet 1990; 336:402.
50. Eugui EMK, Almquist SJ, Muller CD et al. Lymphocyte selective cytostatic and immunosuppressive effects of mycophenolic acid in vitro: role of deoxyguanosine nucleotide depletion. Scand J Immunol 1991; 33: 175.
51. Morris RE, Hoyt EG, Murphy MP, Eugui EM, Allison AC. Mycophenolic acid morpholinoethylester (RS-61443) is a new immunosuppressant that prevents and halts heart allograft rejection by purine synthesis. Transplant Proc 1990; 22: 1659.
52. Hao L, Calcinero F, Gill RG, Eugui EM, Allison AC, Lafferty KJ. Facilitation of Specific Tolerance Induction in Adult Mice by RS-61443. Transplantion 1992; 53. 590.
53. Hao L, Chan SM, Lafferty KJ. Mycophe–nolate mofetil can prevent the development of diabetes in BB rats. Ann NY Acad Sci 1993; 696: 328.
54. Hao L, Wang Y, Chan SM, Lafferty KJ. Effect of mycophenolate mofetil on islet allografting to chemically induced or spontaneously diabetic animals. Transplant Proc 1992; 24: 2843.
55. Sandler S, Sandberg JO, Anderson A. Exposure of rat pancreatic islets to RS-61443 inhibits B-cell function. (Abstract) Fourth International Congress on Pancreas and Islet Transplantation. Amsterdam, The Netherlands, June 1993.
56. Liu J, Farmer Jr JD, Lane WS, Friedman J, Weissman I, Schreiber SL. Calcineurin is a common target of cyclophilin-cyclosporine A and FKBP-FK 506 complexes. Cell 1991; 66: 807.
57. Sehgal SN, Molnar-Kimber K, Ocain TD, Weichman BM. Rapamycin: A novel immunosuppressive macrolide. Medicinal Research Reviews 1994; 14: 1.
58. Fabian MC, Lakey JFT, Kneteman NM. Rapamycin prolongs murine islet allograft survival. Transplantation 1994 (in press).

59. Chen HF, Wu JP, Luo HY, Daloze PM. The immunosuppressive effect of rapamycin on pancreaticoduodenal transplants in the rat. Transplant Proc 1991; 23: 2239.
60. Morris RE, Meiser BM, Wu J, Shorthouse R, Wang J. Use of Rapamycin for the suppression of alloimmune reactions in vivo: schedule dependence, tolerance, induction, synergy with cyclosporine and FK 506, and effect on host-versus-graft and graft-versus-host reactions. Transplant Proc 1991; 23: 521.
61. Kahan BD, Gibbons S, Tejpal N, Stepkowski SM, Chou TC. Synergistic interactions of cyclosporine and rapamycin to inhibit immune performances of normal human peripheral blood lymphocytes in vitro. Transplantation 1991; 51: 232.
62. Chen HF, Wu JP, Luo HY, Daloze PM. Reversal of ongoing rejection of allografts by rapamycin. Transplant Proc 1991; 23: 2241.
63. Knight R, Ferraresso M, Serino F, Katz S, Lewis R, Kahan BD. Low-dose rapamycin potentiates the effects of subtherapeutic doses of cyclosporine to prolong renal allograft survival in the mongrel canine model. Transplantation 1993; 55: 947.
64. Calne RY, Lim S, Samaan A et al. Rapamycin for immunosuppression in organ allografting. Lancet 1989; 2: 227.
65. Collier DS, Calne RY, Pollard SG, Friend PJ, Thiru S. Rapamycin in experimental renal allografts in primates. Tranplant Proc 1991; 23: 2246.
66. Yakimets WJ, Lakey JRT, Yatscoff RW, et al. Prolongation of canine pancreatic islet allograft survival with combined rapamycin and cyclosporine therapy at low doses. Transplantation 1993; 56: 1293.

CHAPTER 7

Islet Transplantation to Immunoprivileged Sites

Helena P. Selawry

An immunologically privileged site can be defined as a site in which an immune response is either impaired or absent. Since pancreatic islets were shown to be unusually prone to rejection, attempts to protect grafted islets against immunologic destruction have included, among others, the transplantation of isolated cells into immunologically favored sites.

The mechanisms for immunological privilege are diverse and not all of the factors are operative in every privileged site. The basic mechanisms, however, are the same and may involve one or more of the following: (1) The organ site is devoid of lymphatic drainage causing an afferent block of the immune response. (2) Absence of vascular supply to the transplant site leading to failure of the efferent or effector limb of the immune response. (3) The local environment is antagonistic to an immune reaction due to the local production of immunosuppressive factors.

The following immunologically privileged sites have been explored for purposes of pancreatic islet transplantation:

(1) The anterior chamber of the eye.
(2) The cheek pouch of the hamster.
(3) The brain and CSF-space.
(4) The testis, especially when translocated into the abdominal cavity.

For obvious reasons, the first two sites are not directly applicable to man but will be described for their research interest. The latter two sites have direct clinical potential.

ANTERIOR CHAMBER OF THE EYE: [AC]

The implantation of fetal or neonatal pancreatic fragments into the anterior chamber allowed close observation of the growth and development of grafted cells potentially uninfluenced by immunosuppressive drugs. Coupland[1] showed that fetal pancreatic tissue grafted into the mother's eye undergo specific morphologic changes over time: Acinar tissue degenerates and completely disappears during the first 2 weeks of transplantation. The duct epithelium then grows and large numbers of islets are produced containing both β and α cells. After one year's residence in the anterior chamber the bulk of the grafted tissue consists of pure islets containing both α and

Pancreatic Islet Transplantation Volume II: Immunomodulation of Pancreatic Islets, edited by Robert P. Lanza, MD, William L. Chick, MD; ©1994 R.G. Landes Company.

β cells. Browning and Resnick[2] made similar observations upon grafting of embryonic, newborn, and adult mouse pancreas into the AC but detected only β cells within the islets: A cells were not found. Donath and Adeghate[3] examined the ultrastructural characteristics of pancreatic light and clear cells in transplanted tissue fragments in the anterior eye-chamber of rats. In these studies it was apparent that light β, α, and δ cell-types survived in transplanted pancreatic tissue, of which the light α cell was the most abundant. Morphologically all three cell types appeared normal. The author did not explore the functional integrity of the grafts. Evidence that the cells can also be functionally intact was provided by the studies of Arburosa and co-workers[4] who examined the impact of grafted embryonic pancreatic tissue on glucose homeostasis in alloxan diabetic rats. Their data demonstrated that anterior chamber grafted islets were able to release insulin into the systemic circulation with marked improvement of the diabetic condition in rat recipients.

The mechanism for the immunologically privileged status of the anterior chamber was thought to be due to an absence of lymphatic drainage with a consequent blockade in the afferent limb of the immune response.[5] But studies by Kaplan and Stevens[6] failed to show evidence for either an afferent or efferent defect in the immunologic reflex arc. Rather, it was demonstrated that small venules serve as afferent arm permitting escape of alloantigens and immunogenic cells to the spleen via the systemic circulation. The resulting aberrant immune reaction in the spleen is credited with adaptive growth of transplanted tissue in the AC.[7] Specifically, radiolabeled cells injected into the AC exit rapidly via small venules into the systemic circulation and from there into the spleen. Detection of circulating antibodies to injected lymphocyte suspensions occurs soon after the injection of alloantigens into the anterior chamber. But whereas the humoral immune response is intact systemic expression of cell-mediated immunity is suppressed.[7] The authors postulated that processing of alloantigen in the spleen results in the generation of suppressor T cells, resulting in an inhibition of immune destruction of AC allografts. The latter phenomenon was described as a "lymphocyte-induced immune deviation".[7] Additional studies on grafted malignant cells into the AC demonstrated that hosts with extended survival of MHC-incompatible tumor cells were unable to reject orthotopic skin grafts from the same donor.[8] AC-associated immune deviation was shown to be dependent not only on an intact spleen at the time of grafting, but also on the continuous presence of antigenic material in the anterior chamber.[9] These data are in support of the contention that protection of AC allografts is most likely due to tolerance induction to the graft secondary to an intravenous delivery of the alloantigen.

THE CHEEK POUCH OF THE HAMSTER

The primary function of the cheek pouch is the storage of food. The inner lining of the pouch has a rich network of blood vessels and nerve endings, but no evidence for any lymphatic channels.[10] Studies by Barker and Billingham[10] showed that the cheek pouch affords a safe environment for not only tissue allografts, but to some extent, xenografts, provided the recipients are given concomitant immunosuppression. The mechanism for immunologic privilege of the hamster cheek pouch is credited to a lack of lymphatic drainage to regional lymph nodes. In presensitized hamsters grafted tissues are not protected against rejection suggesting that the efferent arc of the immune response is intact.[10]

THE BRAIN

During the 1950s, the studies of Greene[11] showed that tumor homo- and heterotransplants survived longer in the brain than in conventional organ sites. Medawar[12] demonstrated that intracerebrally implanted homologous skin grafts failed to elicit either a typical primary or secondary set reaction by histological examination of the tissues. But not all tissues grafted into the brain thrived equally as well. Head and Griffin[13] showed that while parathyroid glands survived almost indefinitely in the brain cortex fragments of skin did not. The data suggested that tissues of lower immunogenicity fare better following transplantation into the brain.

The brain as an organ site for the grafting of pancreatic islets was first explored by McEvoy and Leung.[14] These authors set out to determine viability of transplanted syngeneic and allogeneic fetal rat pancreas in the lateral ventricles of diabetic Lewis rats and compared their survival with that of similar tissues grafted into the liver. Only the grafted syngeneic pancreas survived, while pancreas grafted against histocompatibility barriers were rejected. In rats with functional syngeneic islet grafts, insulin secreted into the cerebral spinal fluid did traverse the blood-brain barrier causing an amelioration of diabetes mellitus. The authors concluded that the cerebral ventricles cannot serve as a privileged site for allogeneic islet grafts.[14]

We owe most of our understanding of the brain as an organ site for the transplantation of endocrine pancreas to the extensive studies by Tze and his associates. Tze and Tai[15] were the first to report that the intracerebral injection of suspensions of single pancreatic cells of Lewis donors into diabetic ACI rats, induced normoglycemic for periods exceeding 176 days. In a follow-up study the same authors compared the survival of intact islets with that of dispersed pancreatic cells, grafted intracerebrally against major histocompatibility barriers.[16] Various regions within the brain were explored for the injection of endocrine pancreas. Normoglycemia was induced in diabetic ACI rats following transplantation of dispersed islet cells from Lewis rats donors without immunosuppression of the recipients. In contrast, grafted whole islets failed to induce normoglycemia for any prolonged period of time. Also, the frontal lobe appeared a more suitable site for the grafting of the cells than the lateral ventricle area. Histologic examination of the grafts revealed lymphocytic infiltrates associated only with whole islets and not with the dispersed cells. The rapid rejection of intact islets was presumed to be due to a larger mass of contaminating passenger lymphocytes associated with these preparations: The break-up of the islets into single cells apparently led to the removal of contaminating leukocytes.

The observation that the dispersion of islets into single cells results in a more purified preparation was important since it suggested that a similar approach might be used for the pretreatment of islet xenografts, for instance, to reduce their immunogenicity prior to transplantation. Or alternatively, similar preparations could be used for the grafting of islet cells into more conventional organ sites. Such a study was undertaken by Tze and his co-workers.[17] They compared the survival of islets and dispersed cells grafted into ten different organ sites with some interesting results: Dispersed cells prepared from Wistar islets and grafted either intramuscularly, or intravenously, or intraportally into ACI rats showed no evidence of survival. Disappointing results were likewise obtained when cells were grafted either underneath the renal capsule or into the omentum. In contrast, indefinite survival of cells injected into the cerebral cortex occurred in all recipients. Islet cells injected into the testis, in it's original scrotal position, improved the diabetic state only temporarily. Assessment of survival of the cells in the abdominal testis was not done. The lack of survival of cells in the testis in it's scrotal position is in accordance with the results of Selawry and Whittington.[18] They discovered that the testis transferred to the abdominal cavity proved to be a much more suitable site for grafting of islets with close to 100% survival rate. In retrospect, a more relevant comparison would have been to assess the survival of dispersed islet cells in the cerebral cortex with that of similar preparations grafted into the abdominal testis.

As a further extension of their work Tze and Tai[19] examined the survival of endocrine cells grafted into the subarachnoid space of rats. The authors demonstrated that injection of suspensions of their purified islet preparations directly into the cisterna magna led to the induction of prolonged normoglycemia in ACI recipients. Intrathecal transplantation with stained cells revealed that they were found mainly in the cisterna magna and subarachnoid space on the dorsal aspects of the cerebellum and ventral surface of the brain. The grafted rats showed no change in either appearance or in behaviour. Similar results were recently obtained with the grafting of whole islets into the cisterna magna of diabetic rats.[20] The observation that the intrathecal injection of cells caused no brain damage coupled with the simplicity of the procedure, makes this approach very appealing for clinical application in the future.

One of the main reasons proposed for failure of islet allograft survival is that the transplanted cells are susceptible to destruction by the original autoimmune reaction. Tze and his associates designed a study to examine this problem in BB/Wor rats with spontaneous diabetes mellitus.[21] These rats develop typical type 1 diabetes and the islet lesions that lead to the destruction of β cells resemble those found in humans with the disease. Dispersed islet cells, isolated from histoincompatible hosts were injected intracerebrally in non-immunosuppressed BB/Wor rats. The results were impressive: All of the recipients became normoglycemic and no longer required insulin therapy. IVGTT data suggested a near normal insulin release pattern to IV glucose. Taken together, the data accrued over a period of 5 years by this group provide persuasive evidence that suspensions of islet cells grafted into the brain are protected against destruction by both a rejection reaction and to recurrence of an autoimmune disease process.

A critical question in diabetes research is whether complete normalization of plasma glucose levels early on would prevent the secondary complications of the disease. An advantage of the transplant model of Tze and his associates was that the animals became successfully transplanted without the need for immunosuppression. In a follow-up study Tze and Tai[22] set out to investigate the impact of islet transplantation on the development of nerve dysfunction in diabetic rats. In earlier studies they demonstrated that diabetic rats show a 19% reduction in motor nerve conduction velocity (MNCV) and muscle evoked potential amplitude (EMPA) was reduced to 72% of control values. Streptozotocin-induced ACI rats were grafted intracerebrally with dispersed islet cells isolated from Lewis rats. Studies on rats who became normoglycemic showed almost complete amelioration of the typical nerve lesions, clearly demonstrating that complications can be prevented by early successful transplantation of rats. The effect of intracerebrally transplanted islet cells on the reversal of established or chronic nerve defects should provide additional important information.

For the most part earlier studies were done on the adult brain as organ site for the transplantation of islet allografts. In more recent work Huxlin et al[23] used the neonatal rat brain in attempts to study the growth and development of iso-, allo-, and xenograft fetal pancreas injected into the left cerebral hemisphere. It was postulated that the neonatal brain might be a more suitable site for grafting of islets due to immunologic immaturity of the recipient. Interestingly, none of the neonatal hosts rejected their grafts and survival rates of iso-, allo-, and xenografts were similar and lasted about 6 weeks. A minor degree of lymphocytic infiltration in neonatal allo- and xenografts was found although the immune reaction was greater for allo- than for xenografts. None of the grafts were rejected even after the hosts had reached immunologic maturity. The significance of these observations awaits clarification.

The mechanisms that offer privileged survival of islets allografts in the brain are not clear. Classically it has been believed that immune privilege is attributable to a decrease or absence of lymphatic drainage to regional lymph nodes. Another theory holds that a shortage of Ia+ cells or antigen presenting cells in the brain plays a role in the protection of grafted cells against rejection.[24] It is important to resolve the problem since the brain may be used as a site for the grafting of human islet allografts. However, information which has steadily been accrued over the past decade is beginning to shed light on the problem. Tze and Tai[25] examined the immunological status of the brain and showed that intracerebrally grafted islets could sensitize the recipient. Conversely, presensitization of host rats led to rapid rejection of islet cells subsequently grafted into the brain. Cytotoxic antibody titers were shown to be measurable following intracerebral islet allografts although the levels were much higher in rats who rejected their grafts compared to those with long-term functioning allografts. Donor skin grafts were shown to induce rejection of intracerebral islet cells suggesting that these grafts retain their antigenicity even after a year's survival in the brain. Rats with established, intracerebral islet allografts failed to develop systemic tolerance to their grafts. Taken together their data are in accord with those of Head and Griffin[26] who suggested that a deficient antigen presenting mechanism rather than the absence of an afferent or efferent immune response arc is the most likely mechanism of immune privilege of the brain.

THE TESTIS

The recognition that the testis is an immunologically privileged site was made many decades ago. During the 1940s Greene[27] reported that intratesticular transplants of malignant human breast sarcoma cells remained alive for variable periods of time in 3 of 20 guinea pig recipients without immunosuppression of the hosts. Subsequent studies have shown that fragments of skin,[28] and parathyroid,[29] glands can successfully be transplanted against major histocompatibility barriers. Even parathyroid xenografts were shown to survive for about 25 days following intratesticular transplantation.[30] Ferguson and Scothorne[31] showed microscopic survival of intratesticular pancreatic islet allografts in guinea pigs. While the functional status of the transplants was not evaluated, important other information was gained: Intratesticular allograft survival was shown to depend on the size of the antigenic dose; the larger the dose the more vigorous the rejection reaction.[32] Furthermore, protection of grafts against rejection was not absolute and intratesticular islets were rejected in an accelerated fashion in hosts presensitized by a previous skin graft from the same donor.[32]

Functional documentation of grafted intratesticular islets was made by Gonet and Renold[33] who studied the survival of fetal pancreas in the testis of rats and observed a decrease in serum glucose levels in some of the recipients for as long as 60 days. Akimura et al[34] were the first to show that an insulinoma could be successfully transplanted into the testis. Of 19 grafted recipients, 3 became normoglycemic for a mean of 27 days whereas none of the recipients of similarly grafted cells beneath the skin showed evidence of alleviation of the diabetic state.

Bobzien and co-workers[35] were the first to assess the survival of islet xenografts (rat to mouse) in the testis. Freshly isolated islet xenografts were shown to survive in 3 of 12 diabetic mice for periods of up to 60 days; by contrast, similar islet preparations grafted either into the spleen, or liver, or kidney capsule, did not survive for longer than a mean of about 11 days. Morphologic examination of the intratesticular islet xenografts revealed the presence of well granulated β cells.

There is little doubt that the earlier studies suggested that the testis is a more suitable organ site for the transplantation of both islet allo- and xenografts compared to the more conventional sites. On the other hand, survival in most instances was not permanent and eventually all of the grafts showed signs of failure. Whether graft failure was caused by a slow rejection reaction or whether β cells become "exhausted" due to increased demands for insulin as the grafted animal gains weight has not been clarified.

In a study to assess the comparative survival of islets of ACI donor rats in a number of different organ sites in Wistar-Lewis recipients, Selawry and Whittington[18] made a surprising discovery: Rats with islets grafted into the testis, in its original scrotal position, remained hyperglycemic. In contrast, if the grafted testes were immediately anchored into the abdominal cavity, the rats became normoglycemic within 24 hours and remained so virtually indefinitely. No immunosuppression was given to the hosts and when islets were grafted into more conventional sites such as the liver or into the renal, subcapsular space the rats became normoglycemic only briefly. Orchiectomies done on rats with testes anchored in the abdominal cavity, resulted in rapid reversal to hyperglycemia within 24 hours. Microscopic examination of the allografts revealed the presence of viable and well granulated β cells.

The remarkable aspect of this finding is that thermal injury to the testis leads to the induction of a series of pathologic changes including atrophy of the seminiferous tubules and aspermatogenesis.[36] Yet, functional and ultrastructural analyses of both islet allo-and xenografts showed that the cells seemed to thrive in this environment: Islets transplanted against major histocompatibility barriers remained viable indefinitely without the need for sustained immunosuppression.[18] In BB/Wor dp rats with diabetes of spontaneous origin, intratesticular islet grafts from either MHC -compatible or -incompatible hosts led to rapid reversal of the diabetic process.[37,38] The grafted rats no longer needed insulin injections and sustained immunosuppression was not required. Microscopic examination of grafts obtained from normoglycemic BB/Wor dp rats showed the presence of viable β cells, in close association with necrotic seminiferous tubules. The interstitial areas showed evidence of an increased vascular supply without evidence of an inflammatory reaction. Thus intratesticular islet allografts were protected from destruction by both a rejection reaction and by recurrence of the original disease process.[39] Of interest in this regard was a recent report by Linn et al[40] who showed that abdominal testis transplantation prevented rejection of islet isografts in low-dose streptozotocin-induced diabetes. The authors have previously shown that rejection of islets occurred when isotransplantation was performed in mice with low-dose streptozotocin-induced diabetes. This phenomenon was described as typical for an autoimmune process.

Since successful transplantation in the BB/Wor dp rat uniformly resulted in normalization of glucose levels without need for immunosuppression,[37] this model provided a unique opportunity to investigate several critical questions related to islet transplantation research. Studies were first initiated to examine the effect of known insulin secretagogues on insulin release patterns. This investigation was considered important also from the standpoint that insulin was being released into the sytemic circulation rather than into the portal venous sytem which is more physiologic: Oral glucose tolerance tests which were done in BB/Wor dp rats with long surviving grafts in excess of 100 days showed that the pattern of release of insulin was identical to the control group with a peak measured at 15 min.[41] In addition, liver enzymes associated with glycogenesis and glycogenolysis, glycogen synthase, and glycogen phosphorylase, respectively, were restored to normal levels in diabetic rats.[42] Microscopic and biochemical analyses of the grafted testes showed that the islets contained not only β cells but considerable amounts of glucagon and α cells.[41] Of three islet cell secretagogues tested, glucose by mouth was the most potent insulin releasing agent. Glipizide, given by mouth, had a minor effect on insulin but produced a significant suppression of glucagon. Arginine, infused IV, was the most potent glucagon releasing agent with only a minor effect on insulin release. Thus abdominal, intratesticular islet allografts were shown to contain both β and α cells which had the capacity to respond to insulin and glucagon secretagogues in a distinct and independent manner. Furthermore, there was no evidence of either graft failure or of development of side effects caused by systemic delivery of insulin.

The abdominal, intratesticular islet graft model made possible also an investigation of the impact of islet transplantation on secondary complications associated with diabetes. The objectives of a study initiated by Murray et al[43] were to investigate the effects of abdominal, intratesticular allografts in BB/Wor dp rats on prevention of kidney disease and nerve lesions. At intervals following transplantation urine total protein was quantitated and sural nerve morphometry and sexual function assessed. BB/Wor dp rats were transplanted within a week following the onset of hyperglycemia without immunosuppression or other therapy. Induction of longterm normoglycemia occurred in 9 of 16 rats for a period of at least six months. In the successfully grafted rats glycosylated hemoglobin levels were not different from controls. Likewise, total urinary protein was significantly less than untreated diabetic rats and not different from controls. Penile reflexes and serum testosterone levels remained normal in islet-transplanted rats. Sural nerve morphometry was normal with 29% fewer abnormalities (paranodal swelling, paranodal demyelination, myelin wrinkling, Wallerian degeneration). In contrast, conduction velocity in the dorsal penile nerve remained abnormal in some of the transplanted rats. Taken together, the data suggested that certain diabetic complications might respond differently to islet implantation even in the case of only mild hyperglycemia.

To assess whether the abdominal testis is an appropriate site also for the grafting of islet xenografts, Selawry and co-workers[44] initiated a comparative study on survival of islet xenografts (hamster to rat) in BB/Wor dp rats with spontaneous diabetes and in ACI and Wistar-Lewis rats with streptozotocin-induced diabetes. The grafted rats were immunosuppressed either with ALS or with cyclosporine (CsA) for 30 days. Interestingly, islet xenografts were rejected in all three groups of rats treated with ALS. In contrast, CsA treated ACI and Wistar-Lewis rats remained normoglycemic for a mean of more than 130 days whereas BB/Wor dp rats reverted to diabetes within 2 days after withdrawal of the drug. One possible explanation for these results was that ACI and Wistar-Lewis rats developed a state of unresponsiveness to their xenografts. Graft survival in the presence of CsA was shown to lead to a state called "CsA-induced tolerance".[45] This tolerance involves the generation or programming of antigen-specific suppressor cells, which in turn was shown to require a normally functioning thymus.[46] In a recent report Georgiou et al[47] provided evidence that T-lymphocyte dysfunctions in the BB/Wor dp rat might be due to a thymus-derived defect.[47] Such a thymus derived defect was clearly consistent with the data of Selawry et al: Prolonged survival of islet xenografts occurred only in ACI and Wistar-Lewis rats and not in BB/Wor dp rats.

Although the induction of tolerance was an attractive explanation for the extended survival of intratesticular islet xenografts in ACI and Wistar-Lewis rats, it still had to be demonstrated by further studies. In a follow-up study Bellgrau and Selawry[48] thus transplanted secondary islet xenografts either into the renal subcapsular space, or into the liver, or into the contralateral testis in rats who had established intratesticular islet xenografts of longer than 200 days duration. The durations of normoglycemia in the grafted rats that were given a second xenograft injected into the renal subcapsular space, into the portal vein, and into the contralateral testis were 22 ± 6, > 48–± –11, and > 99 ± 26, days, respectively. In contrast, a prompt rejection occurred when primary islet xenografts were implanted either into the renal, subcapsular space or into the liver. The results strongly supported the contention that the rats had developed systemic tolerance to their xenografts.

As an additional proof Selawry and Bellgrau recently showed that "tolerance" could be adoptively transferred to naive rats by means of a single intravenous injection of a total of 5 million splenic lymphocytes obtained from rats with long surviving intratesticular islet xenografts. Similar populations of lymphocytes obtained from rats that rejected their xenografts led to rapid rejection of islet xenografts subsequently implanted into the abdominal testis (Selawry and Bellgrau, unpublished observations). Identification of the cell responsible for adoptive transfer of tolerance awaits further investigation.

The mechanism of action which allows extended intratesticular islet allo- and xenograft survival has not been elucidated. The immunologically protective mechanism of the brain and AC seems to involve primarily deficient lymphatic drainage. The testis, however, has an excellent lymphatic drainage system.[49] Antigens grafted into the testis stimulate both humoral and cellular immune responses indicating the presence of an intact afferent limb of the immune response.[50] Evidence for an intact efferent limb was provided by the the earlier studies by Ferguson and Scothorne[32] who demonstrated that intratesticular islet allografts are susceptible to immunologic destruction in presensitized recipients. These studies led to the hypothesis that local factors produced within the testis might be responsible for the inhibition of the immune response. Head and Billingham[51] investigated the effects of local factors produced by the testis on parathyroid allograft survival. They demonstrated that functional survival of these grafts were impaired in rats who were pretreated with estrogen, which lowered serum testosterone levels. Testicular concentrations of testosterone were not measured.

Extended abdominal, intratesticular islet allograft survival made possible additional investigations of effects of local factors on immune responses in the testis. Selawry and Whittington[52] designed a study to assess islet allograft survival in testes in which Leydig cell function had been selectively destroyed. In order to accomplish this a GnRH agonist, leuprolide, known to cause severe depression of testosterone biosynthesis, was used.[53] Male, diabetic, Sprague-Dawley rats were pretreated with leuprolide and were then transplanted with islets isolated from Wistar Lewis rats. The grafted rats were not immunosuppressed. Continuous treatment of grafted rats with leuprolide assured prolonged inhibition of Leydig cell function. In the grafted rats serum testosterone levels decreased rapidly to below detectable levels; testicular testosterone fell to castrate levels. But despite evidence of depressed Leydig cell function intratesticular islet grafts remained viable without loss of function over the lifespan of the rat. More recent data reported by Cameron et al[54] were in support of these findings. These investigators used a substantially more potent drug, ethanedimethylsulfanate, known to completely eliminate all Leydig cell functions. The data thus indicated that the abdominal testis provided immunoprotection of islet allografts by factors other than steroid hormone production.

The testis consists of three major cell components, germ, Leydig and Sertoli. Since neither Leydig cell function nor sperm cells appeared necessary for the protection of islet allografts against rejection attention was focused on the third component, Sertoli cells. Selawry and her co-workers[55] set out to evaluate the contribution of the Sertoli cell toward producing an immunologically privileged site. Unlike germ cells, Sertoli cells are resistant to thermal injury, and are responsible for the synthesis of a wide variety of secretory products some of which might have immunosuppressive qualities.[56] In order to test the hypothesis a series of experiments were initiated in vitro to examine the effects of Sertoli cell factors on T lymphocyte proliferation. Sertoli cells were cultured under a variety of conditions, including changes in temperature and exposure to hormones known to influence their function. The effect of the Sertoli-cell conditioned media on proliferation of T lymphocytes was then determined. These studies showed that Sertoli cells produced a factor which had the capacity to inhibit Con A stimulated lymphocyte proliferation in a dose-dependent manner. The factor was produced primarily at 37° C and its production was stimulated by FSH. The most striking finding of the study was that the inhibition of T-lymphocyte proliferation by Sertoli cell media was caused by an inhibition of production of IL-2 . The addition of exogenous IL-2 was not able to reverse this inhibition, suggesting that the inhibitory factor suppressed both IL-2 production and IL-2 responsiveness of T-cells. The isolation and identification of the inhibitor produced by Sertoli cells requires further investigation.

A major concern with regard to the use of the abdominal testis as an organ site for islet transplantation is that germ cells might undergo malignant transformation. In addition, since only males have Sertoli cells this transplanatation approach cannot be used in half of the population which is female. Because of these objections, and because previous observations showed that Sertoli cells produce a factor which inhibits IL-2 production in vitro, studies were undertaken by Selawry and Cameron[57] in an attempt to create an immunologically privileged site in a heterotopic site in vivo, other than the testis. In order to achieve this goal Sertoli cells were isolated from young male rats and were then grafted simultaneously with isolated islets into the renal subcapsular space of both male and female diabetic rats. Each rat was given only three injections of 25 mg/kg of CsA on days -0,+1, and +2 relative to the graft. PVG female rats were grafted with islets obtained from Sprague Dawley rats along with Sertoli cells procured from either young PVG, or from Sprague Dawley male, rats. The results showed that up to 63% of the recipients of a combination of islets and Sertoli cells grafted into the renal, subcapsular space became normoglycemic for periods exceeding 200 days. Control rats who were grafted with islets alone remained hyperglycemic. Ultrastructural analysis of the grafts showed the presence of well granulated β cells. Adjacent to the β cells was a high density of cells which when observed by electron microscopy, were similar in ultrastructure to Sertoli cells. There was no evidence of a lymphocytic infiltration. Additional studies done on these rats showed that grafted females were able to conceive and to carry pregnancies to fullterm. The data suggested that Sertoli cells retain the capacity to secrete immunosuppressive factor(s) in an organ site other than the testis and that the presence of these secretions are neither androgenic nor inhibitory to ovulation.

Finally, the question was asked whether the testis would be a suitable organ site also for the grafting of higher animals. This was a critical issue since if intratesticular islet allografts were shown to be viable in an animal model such as the non-human primate, then similar approaches might become feasible in clinical trials. The objective of a study planned by Selawry and co-workers[58] was to investigate the survival of islet allografts in the testis of the male Rhesus monkey, *Macaca mulatta*. Six male monkeys were made diabetic by means of a near-total pancreatectomy and a single dose of streptozotocin, 30 mg/kg, administered on the same day as the surgery. Islets were isolated from female donor animals. Each of six diabetic male monkeys were given a total of approximately 10,000 islets per Kg body weight injected slowly into both testes. The grafted organs were immediately anchored underneath the skin in the inguinal canal to expose the testes to a core body temperature of 37° C. Immunosuppression of the grafted primates consisted of a total of seven, IM injections of cyclosporine, 20 mg/kg, on days -3 to +3 relative to the graft. Oral sustacal tolerance tests were done prior to pancreatectomy, following pancreatectomy, but before grafting, and at regular intervals after transplantation. Of six grafted primates three became normoglycemic within a week following transplantation. One of the grafted animals reverted to hyperglycemia eight months following transplantation. Two of the three monkeys have been normoglycemic now for periods exceeding 2 years. The fasting serum glucose levels prior to transplantation but after pancreatectomy were in excess of 350 mg/dl in both animals. The fasting serum glucose levels after 2 years of transplantation vary between 45 and 65 mg/dl. Prior to transplantation during their diabetic phase serum C-peptide levels were less than 1.0 ng/ml. Following transplantation the C-peptide levels showed a marked increase to a mean of 5.5 ng/ml two years following transplantation (Selawry and Gaber, unpublished observations).

It can be concluded that intratesticular islet allografts remain functional for periods exceeding 2 years in successfully transplanted Rhesus monkeys. In addition, release of insulin into the systemic, rather into the portal venous system, appeared not to have led to the development of sustained hyperinsulinemia in this larger animal model.

CONCLUSIONS

To date, the two most promising immunological privileged sites for islet transplantation for type I diabetes mellitus in experimental animals include the testis in it's abdominal translocation and the brain or CSF. Transplantation to the inguinal testis was advanced to monkeys. Immuno-protection is provided by a substance or substances secreted by Sertoli cells. This substance is also operative when islet allografts are transplanted underneath the renal capsule of rats in the presence of Sertoli cells. This might well clear the way for initial clinical trials.

Much additional work needs to be done such as an investigation of the survival of dispersed islet cells in the brains and CSF of higher animals. In addition, attempts should be made to isolate the immunosuppressive factor(s) secreted by Sertoli cells, and to further identify their physiologic and immunologic properties. Allotransplants of islets plus Sertoli cells under the renal capsule should be advanced to larger animals, preferably primates, and, if successful, could then be advanced to clinical trials.

References

1. Coupland, RD. Survival and growth of pancreatic tissue in the anterior chamber of the eye, J Endocrinol 1960; 20: 69-78.
2. Browning, H and Resnick P. Homologous and heterologous transplantation of pancreatic tissue in normal and diabetic mice. Yale J Biol Med 1951; 24: 141-53.
3. Donath T, Adeghate E. Ultrastructure of pancreatic light and clear cells in normal and transplanted tissue fragments in the anterior eye-chamber of rats. Acta Morphologica Hungarica 1990; 38: 217-24.
4. Arburosa MI, Kulikov AV, Tret'iak TM. Levels of immunoreactive insulin in the pancreas and allograft to anterior chamber of the eye in experimental diabetes. Probl Endokrinol (Mosk) 1991; 39 (1): 42-4.
5. Barker CF, Billingham RE. The role of afferent lymphatics in the rejection of skin homografts. J Exp Med 1968; 128: 197-221.
6. Kaplan HJ, Stevens TR. A reconsideration of immunological privilege within the anterior chamber of the eye. Transplantation 1975; 19: 302-09.
7. Kaplan HJ, Streilein JW. Immune response to immunization via the anterior chamber of the eye. 1. F1 Lymphocyte-induced immune deviation. J Immunol 1977; 118: 809-14.
8. Niederkorn JY and Streilein JW. Induction of anterior chamber-associated immune deviation (ACAID) by allogeneic intraocular tumors does not require splenic metastases. J Immunol 1982; 128: 2470-74.
9. Streilein JW, and Niederkorn JY. Induction of anterior-associated immune deviation requires an intact, functional spleen. J Exp Med 1981; 153: 1058-67.
10. Barker CF and Billingham RE. Immunologically privileged sites. Adv Immunol 1977; 25: 1-54.
11. Greene HSN. Transplantation of tumors to brains of heterologous species. Cancer Res 1951; 11: 529-34.
12. Medawar PB. Immunity to homologous grafted skin. 111. Fate of skin homografts transplanted to brain, to subcutnaous tissue, and to anterior chamber of eye. Brit J Exp Path 1948; 29: 58-69.
13. Head JR, Griffin WST. Functional capacity of solid tissue transplants in the brain: evidence for immunological privilege. Proc R Soc Lond [Biol]. 1985; 224: 375-87.
14. McEvoy RC, Leung PE. Transplantation of fetal rat islets into the cerebral ventricles of alloxan-diabetic rats. Amelioration of diabetes by syngeneic but not allogeneic hosts. Diabetes 1983; 32: 852-57.
15. Tze WJ and Tai J. Successful intracerebral allotransplantation of purified pancreatic endocrine cells in diabetic rat. Diabetes 1983; 32:1185-87.
16. Tze WJ and Tai J. Intracerebral allotransplantation of purified endocrine cells and pancreatic islets in diabetic rats. Transplantation 1984; 38: 107-11.
17. Tze WJ and Tai J. Allotransplantation of dispersed single pancreatic endocrine cells in diabetic rats.Diabetes 1988; 383-92.
18. Selawry HP, Whittington K. Extended allograft survival of islets grafted into intraabdominally placed testis. Diabetes 1984; 33: 405-06.
19. Tze WJ and Tai J . Intrathecal allotransplantation of pancreatic endocrine cells in diabetic rats. Transplantation 1986; 41:531-34.

20. Lee HC, Ahn KJ, Lim SK et al. Allotransplantation of rat islets into the cisterna magna of streptozotocin-induced diabetic rats. Transplantation 1992; 513-16.
21. Tze WJ and Tai J. Successful intracerebral allotransplantation of pancreatic endocrine cells in spontaneous diabetic BB rats without immunosuppression. Metabolism 1984; 33: 785-89.
22. Tze WJ, Sima AAF, and Tai J. Effect of endocrine pancreas allotransplantation on diabetic nerve function. Metabolism 1985; 34: 721-25.
23. Huxlin KR, Tuch BE, Sefton AJ, Dixon G. Iso-, allo-, and xenografting of fetal pancreas into neonatal rat brain. Transplant Proc 1989; 21: 3807-08.
24. Hart DNJ and Fabre JW. Demonstration and characterization of Ia-positive dendritic cells in the interstitial connective tissues of rat heart and other tissues, but not brain. J Exp Med 1981; 347-61.
25. Tze WJ and Tai J. Immunological studies in diabetic rat recipients with a pancreatic islet cell allograft in the brain. Transplantation 1989; 47: 1053-57.
26. Head JR, Griffin WST. Functional capacity of solid tissue transplants in the brain: evidence for immunological privilege. Proc R Soc Lond [Biol] 1985; 224: 375-87.
27. Greene HSN. Familial mammary tumors in the rabbit. IV. The evolution of autonomy in the course of tumor development as indicated by transplantation experiments. J Exp Med 1940; 71: 305-24.
28. Whitmore WF, Gittes RF. Studies on the prostate and testis as immunologically privileged sites. Cancer Treatm Reports 1977; 61: 217-22.
29. Naji A, Barker CF. The influence of histocompatibility and transplant site on parathyroid allograft survival. J Surg Res 1976; 20: 261-67.
30. Dib-Kuri A, Revilla A, Chavez-Peon F. Successful rat parathyroid allografts and xenografts to the testis with and without immunosuppression. Transplant Proc 1975; 7: 753-58.
31. Ferguson J, Scothorne RJ. Extended survival of pancreatic islet allografts in the testis of guinea pigs J. Anat 1977; 124: 1-8.
32. Ferguson, Scothorne RJ. Further studies on the transplantation of isolated pancreatic islets. J Anat 1977; 124: 9-20.
33. Gonet AE, Renold AE. Homografting fetal pancreas. Diabetes 1965; 1:91-96.
34. Akimaru K, Stuhlmiller GM, Seigler HF. Allotransplantation of insulinoma into testis of diabetic rats. Transplantation 1981; 32: 227-32.
35. Bobzien B, Yasunami Y, Majercik M, et al. Intratesticular transplants of islet xenografts (rat to mouse). Diabetes 1983; 32: 213-16.
36. de Kretser DM, Sharpe RM, Swanton IA. Alterations in steroidogenesis and human chorionic gonadotropin binding in the cryptorchid rat testis. Endocrinol 1979; 105: 135-8.
37. Selawry H, Fajaco R, Whittington K. Extended survival of incubated MHC-compatible islet isografts in the spontaneously diabetc BB/W rat. Diabetes 1987; 36: 1061-67.
38. Selawry H, Fajaco R, Whittington K. Intratesticular islet allografts in the spontaneously diabetic BB/W rat. Diabetes 1985; 34: 1019-23.
39. Naji A, Silvers WK, Bellgrau D, et al. Prevention of diabetes in rats by bone marrow transplantation. Ann Surg 1981; 194: 328-38.
40. Linn T, Romann D, Voges S, et al. Abdominal testis transplantation prevents rejection of islet isografts in low-dose streptozotocin-induced diabetes. Transplant Proc 1992; 24: No 3: 998.
41. Whittington KP, Solomon SS, Selawry HP. Islet allografts in the cryptorchid testes of spontaneously diabetic BB/Wor dp rats: Response to glucose, glipizide, and arginine. Endocrinol 1991; 128: 2671-77.
42. Margolis RN, Holup JJ, Selawry, HP. Effects of intratesticular islet transplanation on hepatic glycogen metabolism in the rat. Diab Res Clin Practice 1986; 2: 291-99.
43. Murray FT, Beyer-Mears A, Johnson RD, et al. Assessment of proteinuria and neuropathy in the nonimmunosuppressed BB diabetic rat after abdominal intratesticular islet transplantation. Transplantation 1993; 56: 680-86.

44. Selawry, HP, Whittington K, Bellgrau, D. Abdominal, intratesticular islet-xenograft survival in rats. Diabetes 1989; 38: Suppl 1, 220-23.
45. Kupiec-Weglinski JW, Filho MA, Strom TB, et al. Sparing of suppressor cells: a critical action of cyclosporine. Transplantation 1984; 38: 97-101.
46. Beschorner WE, Namnoum JD, Hess AD. Immunopathology of rat thymus after cyclosporine A. Transplant Today 1986; 19: 1230-35.
47. Georgiou HM, Lagarde AC, Bellgrau D. T cell dysfunction in the diabetes prone BB rat: a role for thymic migrants that are not T cell precursors. J Exp Med 1988; 167: 132-48.
48. Bellgrau D, Selawry H. Cyclosporine-induced tolerance to intratesticular islet xenografts. Transplantation 1990; 50: 654-57.
49. Head JR, Neaves WB, Billingham RE. Reconsideration of the lymphatic drainage of the rat testis. Transplantation 1983; 35: 91-5.
50. Head JR, Neaves WB, Billingham RE. Immune privilege in the testis.I basic parameters of allograft survival. Transplantation 1983; 36:423-31.
51. Head JR, Billingham RE. Immune privilege in the testis. II. Evaluation of potential local factors. Transplantation 1985; 40: 269-75.
52. Selawry H, Whittington K. Prolonged intratesticular allograft survival is not dependent on local steroidogenesis. Horm Metab Res 1988; 20: 562-65.
53. Rivier C, Rivier J, Vale W. Antireproductive effects of gonadotropin-releasing agonist in the male rat. Science 1980: 210:93-95.
54. Cameron DF, Whittington K, Schultz, RE, et al. Successful islet/abdominal testis transplantation does not require Leydig cells. Transplantation 1990; 50: 649-53.
55. Selawry HP, Kotb M, Herrod HG, et al. Production of factor, or factors, suppressing IL-2 production and T cell proliferation by Sertoli cell-enriched preparations. Transplantation 1991; 52: 846-50.
56. Forti G, Barni T, Vannelli BG, et al. Sertoli cell proteins in the human seminiferous tubule. J Steroid Biochem 1989; 32: 135-44.
57. Selawry HP, Cameron DF. Sertoli cell-enriched fractions in successful islet transplantation. Cell Transplantation 1993; 2: 123-29.
58. Selawry HP, Gaber O, Whittington K, et al. Intratesticular islet allograft in the Rhesus monkey. Diabetes 1992: 41: 155A.

CHAPTER 8

INTRATHYMIC ISLET TRANSPLANTS AND SYSTEMIC TOLERANCE

George L. Mayo
Andrew M. Posselt
Louis Campos
Barbara C. Deli
Clyde F. Barker
Ali Naji

The restoration of normal glucose homeostasis achieved by the transplantation of pancreatic islets offers the most specific treatment for insulin-dependent diabetes mellitus. The demonstration that in rodents prevention or reversal of the microvascular complications of diabetes follows successful islet transplantation argues that a similar outcome would be achieved in human recipients of islet grafts.[1] The recent results of DCCT demonstrating that intensive insulin therapy can slow the progression of secondary complications of diabetes has put to rest the longstanding debate on whether attempts to optimize glycemic control are worthwhile and add further incentive to perfecting islet transplantation for the treatment of human diabetes.[2] However, despite these encouraging findings the practical application of this therapy for treatment of diabetes has been hampered by the vulnerability of transplanted islets to both allograft rejection and damage by anti beta cell autoimmunity.[3-6] In animal models chronic administration of potent immunosuppressive agents has been shown to promote the survival of islet allografts; however the results remain inferior when compared to the efficacy of these agents in promoting survival of vascularized whole organ allografts including pancreas.[3] Consequently, efforts in experimental pancreatic islet transplantation have recently focused on the development of the strategies that can permit long-term graft function without the need for chronic immunosuppression. One approach has been to reduce the immunogenicity of islet grafts prior to transplantation by depletion or inactivation of the immunogenic cells contained within the islet complex, intra-islet antigen presenting cells (APCs). This can be achieved by subjecting islet tissuc to low temperature in vitro culture, UV irradiation, or treatment with anti class II or anti-dendritic cell monoclonal antibodies.[7-9] Transplantation to naturally occurring or artificially constructed immunologically privileged sites offers another means by which the immune destruction of allogeneic islets may be circumvented.[11,12] In rodents, temporary restoration of

Pancreatic Islet Transplantation Volume II: Immunomodulation of Pancreatic Islets, edited by Robert P. Lanza, MD, William L. Chick, MD;

normoglycemia and modest prolongation of islet graft survival have been achieved by the implantation of islet grafts into the cerebral cortex or the abdominally displaced testicle, sites with limited practical utility. Finally, the induction of donor specific tolerance would be the ideal method of securing long-term islet allograft survival while protecting the host from the deleterious effects of immunosuppression. The feasibility of promoting acquired immunological tolerance of foreign tissue was first demonstrated by the ingenious experiments of Billingham, Brent, and Medawar who achieved donor specific tolerance in mice inoculated at birth with lymphohematopoietic cells.[12] This strategy is highly effective in that it establishes a state of life-long tolerance permitting the recipients to accept donor strain grafts of any tissue. The tolerant state achieved in this model is likely the result of several mechanisms; however the prevailing view is that the intrathymic deletion/inactivation of high avidity donor reactive T-cells is most important.[13] However, a disadvantage of the model is that the successful induction of tolerance is only feasible during the tolerance permissive period of the neonatal age. Application of this strategy to induce tolerance in immunocompetent adult hosts is unsuccessful unless accompanied by intensive lymphoid cytoablative regimen to facilitate the engraftment of donor lymphohematopoietic cells.

In the following studies we describe the thymus as a site of pancreatic islet transplantation which provides a hospitable environment for islet endocrine function and is capable of preventing destruction of islet allografts without the need for chronic host immunosuppression. Our rationale for employing the thymus is based on several morphologic and functional attributes of this lymphoid organ. First, ultrastructural and kinetic studies utilizing particulate dyes have demonstrated the presence of a blood-thymus barrier surrounding thymic cortical vessels.[14] This barrier, consisting of epithelial cell sheets connected by tight junctions, prevents extravasation of radiolabeled cells as well as low molecular weight proteins. In addition, although the thymus possesses well developed efferent lymphatics, it lacks an afferent lymphatic supply.[15] Together these anatomic attributes suggest that the thymic parenchyma is relatively sequestered from peripheral immune surveillance, a characteristic that may favorably influence survival of implanted allografts. Second, the thymus is known to play a central role in the acquisition of T-cell tolerance to self-major histocompatibility complex (MHC) and non-MHC antigens.[16] The intrathymic process of T-cell tolerance is thought to be mediated by deletion or functional inactivation of T-cell precursors bearing receptors with a high affinity for antigens expressed on the stromal and bone-marrow derived cellular components of the thymus. Thus it could be reasoned that if cells bearing foreign alloantigens are introduced directly into the thymus, they could exert similar effect on maturing thymocytes, possibly by promoting specific deletion or functional silencing of antigen reactive clones. Evidence that intrathymic inoculation of antigen can alter immune responses of the recipient originates from the studies using both soluble and cellular antigens.[17,18] More recent studies have demonstrated that intrathymic injection of prothymocytes into lethally irradiated bone marrow reconstituted mice induces a marked decrease in the fequency of cytotoxic T lymphocyte precursors towards donor alloantigens suggesting the occurrence of deletion and/or inactivation of alloreactive clones.[19]

INTRATHYMIC ISLET TRANSPLANTATION IN CHEMICALLY DIABETIC RECIPIENTS

Initial characterization of the thymus as a site for transplantation of pancreatic islets was performed utilizing rat recipients rendered diabetic with the β cell toxin streptozotocin.[20] Islets were isolated from Lewis ($RT1^l$) or DA ($RT1^a$) donor strains and transplanted to histoincompatible Wistar Furth (WF, $RT1^u$) recipients. As shown in Table 8.1, islets transplanted to conventional sites such as the liver or renal subcapsule were rapidly rejected by non-immunosuppressed recipients. Transplantation into the thymus approximately doubled the survival of islet grafts and one of seven such rats remained permanently normoglycemic, suggesting that even in fully immunocompetent hosts, the thymus can afford some protection from alloimmune rejection. However considerably more pronounced differences in graft survival were noted in recipients treated with a single dose (1 ml) of ALS at the time of islet transplantation. Although ALS therapy prolonged function of both intraportal and renal subcapsular islet allografts, all but two animals given subcapsular grafts rejected the islets within 60 days. Transplantation to an abdominally displaced testicle, a well-characterized immunologically privileged site, similarly failed to secure permanent graft acceptance with only 2 of 6 animals remaining normoglycemic beyond 200 days. In marked contrast were the findings obtained when the thymus was used as a transplant site: 10 of 13 ALS-treated recipients of intrathymic Lewis islets remained euglycemic beyond 200 days. Taken together, these results indicate that the thymus provides a favorable environment for islet endocrine function and, when combined with a brief period of immunosuppression, can facilitate permanent acceptance of allogeneic islets without the need for chronic immunosuppression.

Given the role of the thymus in induction of T-cell tolerance, and the profound influence of the repertoire of antigens expressed in the thymic microenvironment on T-cell mediated immune responses we next determined whether persistence of the allogeneic islets in the thymus might induce specific unresponsiveness to extrathymic alloantigens of the same donor strain. Therefore, WF rats that had harbored intrathymic Lewis islet allografts for >100 days were challenged with Lewis islets transplanted to an extrathymic site (renal subcapsule) without concomitant immunosuppression. In no instance were either the primary intrathymic or the renal subcapsular grafts rejected. Graft survival was confirmed by thymectomy 30 days after the second transplant (which did not cause hyperglycemia), followed eventually by removal of the islet-bearing kidney (which did result in hyperglycemia). The donor specificity of this unresponsive state was demonstrated by prompt rejection of third party renal subcapsular DA ($RT1^a$) islet allografts in WF recipients of long-term intrathymic Lewis islets (Fig. 8.1).

We next sought to determine whether the unresponsiveness we observed could be attributed solely to the prolonged residence of the graft irrespective of site or whether it was due to the persistance of the graft in the unique microenvironment of the thymus. In the animals which had retained intratesticular Lewis islets for >200 days, second Lewis islet allografts were transplanted beneath the renal capsule. These animals, unlike the recipients of intrathymic islets, were not unresponsive but reverted to hyperglycemia in 10 and 15 days after the second transplant, indicating rejection of both the intratesticular

Table 8.1. Survival of fresh Lewis islet allografts in WF recipients

Site of Islet Transplantation	Days of Islet Allograft Survival Without ALS	With ALS
Liver (intraportal)	5, 8, 8, 9, (8)*	6, 22, 29, 35, 36, (29)
Renal subcapsule	9, 9, 10, 13, (9.5)	27, 33, 38, 47, 61, > 200 x 2, (47)
Testicle	–	50, 50, 76, 110, > 200 x 2, (76)
Thymus	13, 13, 16, 17, 17, 18, > 200, (17)	28, 33, 57, > 200 x 10, (> 200)

* Numbers in parentheses denote median survival time (MST).

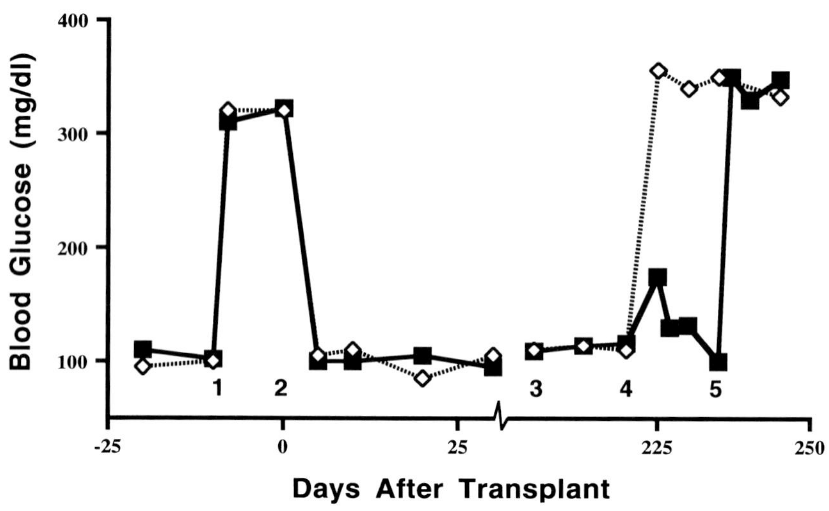

Fig. 8.1. Representative blood glucose profiles of WF rats transplanted with freshly isolated pancreatic islets. (1) Induction of diabetes. (2) Intrathymic transplantation of Lewis islets with concomitant intraperitoneal administration of ALS. (3) Extrathymic (renal subcapsule) transplants of either Lewis (■) or DNA (◆) islets. (4) Islet-bearing thymectomy. (5) Removal of extrathymic islet-bearing kidneys.

and renal subcapsular islets. We and others have previously noted that pretransplant in vitro culture of islets at 24° C depletes intraislet APCS and permits their long-term survival under the renal capsule of rats treated with a single injection of ALS.[7,21] Therefore, this model was employed as an additional control to assess the effect that long-term residence of allogeneic islets may have on peripheral immune responsiveness of the recipient. In WF recipients that had maintained successful cultured Lewis islet allografts beneath the renal capsule for >200 days, non-cultured Lewis islets were transplanted to the opposite kidney. Although all rats remained normoglycemic after this procedure, removal of the kidney bearing cultured islets 30 days later resulted in hyperglycemia, demonstrating that rejection of the second uncultured graft had occurred.

We speculated that several mechanisms might be responsible for promoting the unresponsive state exhibited by long-term recipients of intrathymic allogeneic islets to subsequent extrathymic transplants. These include: (1) nonspecific immunosuppression resulting from disruption of thymic function; (2) deletion or inactivation within the thymus of donor reactive T-cell populations which could otherwise be expected to destroy extrathymic grafts; and (3) generation of suppressor/regulatory T-cells. Immunofluorescent analysis showed no differences in the phenotypic composition of lymphocyte subpopulations between thymic allograft recipients and naive controls, demonstrating that the trauma and disruption of the thymic parenchyma caused by the inoculation had not caused global T-cell immunodeficiency. To assess the second possibility, mixed lymphocyte cultures (MLC) and limiting dilution analyses (LDA) of donor-specific cytotoxic T lymphocyte precursors (pCTL) were performed using lymphoid cells from long-term recipients of intrathymic islets. The proliferative responses of lymph node cells from islet allograft acceptors to donor-strain and third party stimulator cells were no different than the responses of naive animals. However, LDA analysis of lymph node cells from these animals showed significantly reduced (40 to 60%) pCTL frequencies to donor-strain alloantigens (Lewis) as compared with those from untransplanted controls (Fig. 8.2). In the same recipients, the pCTL frequencies for DA alloantigens were unchanged.

To assess active suppression by a population of regulatory T cells as a possible cause of the tolerant state, we performed adoptive transfer studies in which 250-300 x 10^6 spleen cells from either non-transplanted WF controls or WF rats harboring established (> 200 days) intrathymic Lewis islet allografts were transferred to sublethally irradiated WF hosts. Twenty-four hours later, these animals received islets from Lewis donors beneath the renal capsule. Islet survival in rats given splenocytes from intrathymic recipients was not significantly different from that of the control group and thus provided no evidence for the presence of suppressor cells in tolerant animals. Together, these results support the conclusion that the unresponsive state induced by long-term residence of the intrathymic allograft is the result of intrathymic deletion or inactivation of T-cell precursors recognizing alloantigens expressed on the graft.

Pancreatic islets are complex structures comprised of endocrine cells and non-endocrine bone marrow-derived cells of dendritic/macrophage lineage, which are endowed with antigen presenting capability. To study which cell population was responsible for inducing the tolerant state observed after intrathymic islet transplantation, we examined the capacity of intrathymic inocula of islets depleted of APCs by in vitro culture to promote survival of secondary donor-strain grafts transplanted beneath the renal capsule.[22] These intrathymic islets were protected from rejection both by the pretransplant culture (which deleted APCs) and because of the privileged site properties of the thymus. WF rats in which long-term (>120 days) normoglycemia had been achieved by intrathymic transplantation of cultured Lewis

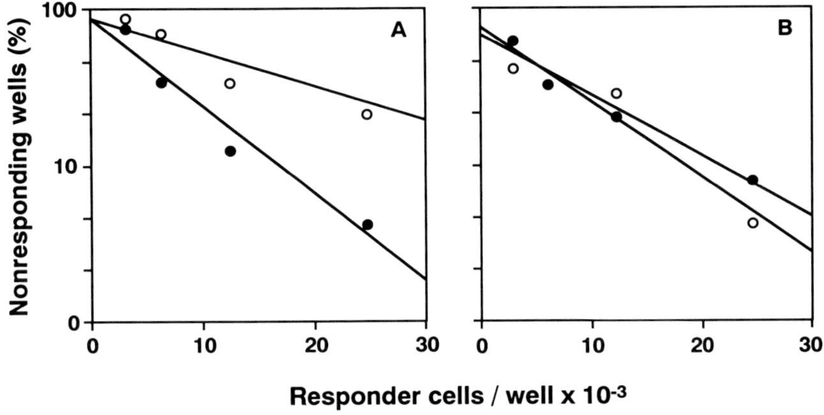

Fig. 8.2. Effect of intrathymic islet transplantation of pCTL frequencies. (A) Anti-Lewis pCTL of lymph node cells from control WF (●-●), l/f = 6,240) and WF recipienct of intrathymic Lewis islets (O-O, l/f = 16,000). (B) Anti-DA pCTL of lymph node cells from control WF (●-●, l/f = 6,930) and WF recipients of intrathymic Lewis islets (O-O, l/f = 6,500).

islets in conjunction with a single intraperitoneal dose of ALS received freshly isolated Lewis islets beneath the renal capsule 120 days after thymic inoculation. All animals promptly developed hyperglycemia, demonstrating that retransplantation had provoked the rejection of both the primary intrathymic and subsequent extrathymic test grafts. The inability to induce unresponsiveness in rats bearing in vitro cultured intrathymic islets indicates that islet endocrine cells per se are ineffective as tolerogens and demonstrates the importance of intraislet APC populations in intrathymic tolerance induction.

INTRATHYMIC ISLET TRANSPLANTATION IN SPONTANEOUSLY DIABETIC BB RATS

The spontaneously diabetic BB rat is a model with many features similar to human type I diabetes mellitus. In both the human disease and the BB rat, damage to pancreatic β cells appears to be mediated by diabetogenic T cells responding to a putative islet β cell autoantigen(s). This contention is supported by experiments in which pancreatic islets from normal diabetes resistant donors were found to be destroyed promptly if transplanted to acutely diabetic BB rats.[3] This destruction occurred just as rapidly in circumstances in which the contribution of islet directed alloreactivity was precluded by either rendering the BB recipients tolerant to islet donor alloantigens or reducing the immunogenicity of islets by pretransplant in vitro culture.[5,21] These findings convinced us that recurrent anti-β cell autoimmunity could in itself damage the islet graft, just as was later shown to be the case for human pancreatic isografts to diabetic patients.[6]

To determine whether the favorable influence of the thymus on allograft survival could also protect islets from damage by anti-β cell autoimmunity, we examined survival of MHC incompatible (Lewis) islets in acutely diabetic BB rats.[23] Pancreatic islets isolated from Lewis donors and transplanted by portal vein inoculation into spontaneously diabetic BB rats were rejected promptly in every instance (Table 8.2). In contrast to the results in extrathymic sites, BB rat recipients of intrathymic Lewis islets remained normoglycemic permanently.

To determine whether intrathymic islets transplanted to diabetic BB rats would induce an unresponsive state that could protect subsequent extrathymic islets from either rejection or autoimmunity, BB rats which had harbored an intrathymic Lewis islet transplant for >120 days received secondary Lewis islets intraportally. All animals

Table 8.2. Survival of MHC compatible and incompatible islet allografts in spontaneously diabetic BB rats

Site of Islet Transplantation	Donor Strain	Days of Islet Allograft Survival
Liver (intraportal)	Lewis	8, 9, 9, 19, 24, (9)
Thymus	Lewis	> 120 x 11, (> 120)
	WF	> 120 x 5, (> 120)

Table 8.3. Effect of intrathymic transplantation on islet xenograft survival

Site of Islet Transplantation	Days of Islet Xenograft Survival Without ATS	With ATS
Renal subcapsule	12 x 3, 14, 20, 21 x 2, 26, (17.3)	31, 39, 43, 43, 53, (41.8)
Thymus	11, 12 x 3, 13, 22 x 2, 39, (17.9)	39, 40, 57, 59, 68, 70, 90, > 100 x 7, (>94.5)

remained normoglycemic, and remained so after removal of the islet bearing thymus confirming the functional survival of the extrathymic islet transplants.

INTRATHYMIC ISLET XENOGRAFTS (RAT TO MOUSE)

The advantage of the thymus as a transplant site for pancreatic islet allografts led us and others to evaluate the capability of this organ to promote survival of islets from alien species.[24,25] In these experiments, WF ($RT1^u$) rat islets were transplanted to the thymus of streptozotocin induced diabetic C57BL/6 mice (Table 8.3). In the absence of immunosuppression, intrathymic islet xenografts did not fair significantly better than those transplanted to a control transplant site, the renal subcapsule. However, treatment of the recipients with a single dose (0.5 ml) of rabbit anti-mouse thymocyte serum at the time of intrathymic islet transplantation led to significant prolongation of islet xenograft survival. Similar to the situation observed in recipients of intrathymic islet allografts, recipients harboring long-term intrathymic islet xenografts were found unresponsive to subsequent donor-strain rat islets transplanted to an extrathymic site without further immunosuppression at the time of the second transplant. The donor specificity of the unresponsive state was demonstrated by the prompt rejection of third party (Lewis) islets in recipients harboring intrathymic WF islet xenografts. Thus, the thymus of briefly immunosuppressed mice provides sanctuary to concordant islet xenografts of rat origin and renders the recipients unresponsive to extrathymic xenogeneic islets if they are from the same rat strain donor.

SYSTEMIC TOLERANCE FOLLOWING INTRATHYMIC INOCULATION OF LYMPHOHEMATOPOIETIC CELLS

In several experimental models of transplantation tolerance, such as acquired neonatal tolerance and adult radiation chimeras the use of bone marrow as the tolerance inducing inoculum has proven particularly effective in establishing a high degree of donor specific tolerance.[12,13,26] Therefore we examined the capacity of intrathymic inocula of donor lymphohematopoietic cells in promoting the survival of cellular or vascularized organ allografts in allogeneic hosts. In addition, as our results using in vitro cultured islets demonstrated, the component of the islets which appears to be crucial for tolerance induction is antigen presenting cells within the islets rather than endocrine cells.[22] Therefore, we predicted that bone marrow, which contains precursors capable of differentiating into antigen presenting cells, might be especially efficient in promoting tolerance after intrathymic inoculation.[27]

Induction of Tolerance to Islets by Intrathymic Inoculation of Donor Bone Marrow

The protocol employed in these experiments involved treatment of prospective recipients with donor strain lymphohema-topoietic cells and concomitant administration of a single dose of ALS. Unlike the previous experiments in which the intrathymic inoculum was followed only months later by the extrathymic islet grafts, the recipients received the islet allografts within 7-14 days after the intrathymic inoculation.[28]

Normal WF recipients not pretreated with intrathymic Lewis bone marrow cells or ALS rapidly rejected Lewis islet grafts (Table 8.4). Similarly, WF recipients that were pretreated with intrathymic injections of saline in conjunction with ALS 2 weeks prior to islet transplantation also promptly rejected Lewis islet allografts. In another control group intravenous injection of Lewis bone marrow cells in conjunction with ALS two weeks prior to islet grafting led to modest prolongation of Lewis islet allograft survival; however all allografts eventually underwent rejection within 32 days. In contrast, in the experimental group in which Lewis bone marrow cells were inoculated intrathymically, 5 of 7 WF recipients of Lewis islet allografts remained permanently normoglycemic. Histologic examination of extrathymic grafts at the conclusion of the experimental period revealed numerous clusters of well-granulated islets devoid of cellular infiltration. The specificity of the tolerant state induced by inoculation of Lewis bone marrow cells was assessed by grafting WF rats which had received intrathymic or intravenous Lewis bone marrow with islets from DA ($RT1^a$) donors. These third party grafts were all rejected within 10 days.

Prolonged residence of allogeneic tissue in other immunologically privileged sites has sometimes been found to weaken the host's immune responsiveness to subsequent donor-strain allografts transplanted to conventional sites.[11] Since the thymic parenchyma is relatively inaccessible to the peripheral immune system, it was conceivable that the unresponsiveness observed in intrathymically treated rats was solely due to the presence of the conditioning marrow inoculum and that the special immunologic functions of the thymus were not relevant, i.e. its role in T lymphocyte maturation and induction of self-tolerance. To evaluate this possibility, we inoculated allogeneic Lewis bone marrow cells into another immunologically privileged site, the testicle, of WF recipients given a single injection of ALS. Two weeks following intratesticular bone marrow inoculation, these recipients were rendered diabetic and transplanted with Lewis islet allografts. All animals rapidly rejected the islets, indicating that the protective influence of the intrathymic bone marrow inoculum on subsequent allografts was unlikely to be explained entirely by the persistance of alloantigen bearing cells in a privileged site.

Mechanisms of Systemic Tolerance by Intrathymic Bone Marrow Transplantation

In accordance with the in vivo findings, intrathymic inoculation of allogeneic Lewis bone marrow cells was found to have a marked influence on T cell-mediated responses to donor alloantigens in vitro.[28] In mixed lymphocyte culture the responder cells from recipients in which long-term Lewis islet allograft survival was achieved by intrathymic bone marrow inoculation proliferated normally to third-party DA stimulators; however proliferation of these cells to Lewis stimulators was consistently decreased as compared with responses of unmanipulated controls (Fig. 8.3). Analysis of pCTL frequencies in a majority of the recipients bearing established islet allografts as a result of pretreatment with intrathymic bone marrow demonstrated significant reductions in pCTL frequencies toward donor (Lewis) alloantigens; although in some animals the frequencies were similar to those of unmanipulated animals. All animals had similar pCTL frequencies to third party DA alloantigens.

In several models of unresponsiveness induced by conditioning with allogeneic bone marrow cells, tolerance has been shown to be correlated with the presence of donor microchimerism in the thymus and peripheral lymphoid organs of the recipients.[26] To determine whether a similar chimeric state was present in our model, the lymphoid organs of WF rats that had received

Table 8.4. Survival of Lewis islet allografts in WF recipients

Site of Lewis Bone Marrow Cell Innoculation	ALS Treatment	Days of Islets Allograft Survival
None	None	9, 9, 10, 13, (9.5)
None	+	8, 9, 14, 15, 18, > 173*, (14.5)
Intravenous	+	13, 16, 21, 23, 32, 32, (22)
Thymus	+	12, 28, > 130 x 2, > 148, > 159, > 183, (> 130)
Testicle	+	7, 8, 8, 10, (8)

* Animal reverted to hyperglycemia after removal of islet-bearing kidney.

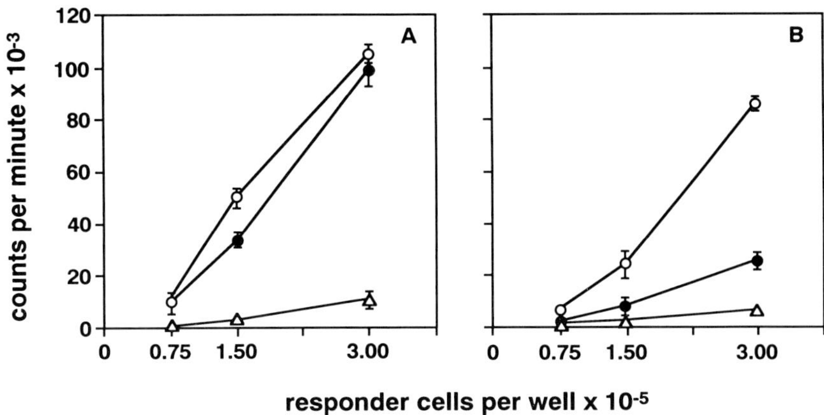

Fig. 8.3. Mixed lymphocyte culture proliferative responses of lymph node cells from (A) WF controls and (B) WF recipients in which long-term Lewis islet allograft survival was achieved by intrathymic inoculation of Lewis BMC. Graded numbers of responder cells were cultured alone (Δ–Δ) or with irradiated Lewis (●–●) or DA (O–O) lymph node stimulators for 3 days, and pulsed with tritiated thymidine for an addtional 24 hours prior to harvesting. Values are depicted as the arithmetic mean ± SD of triplicate cultures.

intrathymic Lewis bone marrow (without subsequent islet grafts) were examined at various intervals after inoculation by immunofluorescence (FACS) and immunohistochemistry utilizing a murine monoclonal antibody specific for Lewis class I alloantigens.[28,29] Using the FACS analysis, chimerism could be detected in the thymus for only 4-5 days after intrathymic inoculation and was never demonstrated in the lymph nodes. However, by the immunohistochemical method we routinely demonstrated the presence of donor strain cells scattered throughout the thymus in animals inoculated with Lewis bone marrow cells 2 to 45 days earlier. Similarly, in animals which had accepted Lewis islet grafts after conditioning with intrathymic Lewis bone marrow cells, donor-strain cells were found in the thymus when it was examined 140-170 days after inoculation, although the number of allogeneic cells appeared to decrease progressively with time. In contrast, donor-strain cells were not detected in the thymus or lymph node of animals given inoculation of intravenous or intratesticular bone marrow cells. Thus, it appears that the thymic microenvironment can support the long-term survival of implanted allogeneic hematopoietic cells and is capable of protecting them (or their descendants) from elimination by immune mechanisms.

The basis of the failure to detect intrathymic microchimerism in some animals rendered tolerant by intrathymic inoculation of donor lymphoid cells is not entirely clear. It is possible that the absence of intrathymic microchimerism may be due to the low frequency of chimeric cells or the suboptimal sensitivity of immunohistological techiniques to detect donor cells in the microenvironment of the thymus. However a more plausible explanation is that the induction of tolerance in this model may be mediated through a multi-step process involving both direct and indirect pathways of antigen recognition by T-cells. The direct pathway invites interaction of the host prothymocytes with donor chimeric cells whereas the indirect pathway requires presentation of donor alloantigens by thymic antigen presenting cells leading to induction of unresponsiveness via a self-restricted T-cell immune response. In support of the latter view is the recent finding that intrathymic inoculation of sub-cellular elements including membrane enriched fragments of donor lymphoid cells promote unresponsiveness to islet allografts.[30] Recent insight into the physiology of T-cell differentiation has demonstrated that within the thymic microenvironment a diverse repertoire of T-cell receptors recongnizing foreign antigens are developed and self-tolerance is achieved by physical elimination (clonal deletion) or functional inactivation (clonal anergy) of prothymocytes bearing self-reactive T-cell receptors. Moreover, intrathymic tolerance induction can be profoundly influenced by the repertoire of antigens expressed on non-lymphoid epithelial components of the thymus. In the above studies we exploited these findings for the purpose of inducing tranaplantation tolerance to histocompatibility antigens by employing the strategy of direct inoculation of foreign antingens into the thymus. The demonstration that intrathymic inoculation of donor cells into the thymus is efficient in promoting the induction of specific tolerance to allogeneic and xenogeneic histocompatibility antigens provides encouragement that intrathymic cellular implantation might eventually prove useful in inducing unresponsiveness in other species possibly allowing successful human transplantation without chronic immunosuppression.

References

1. Mauer SM, Sutherland DER, Steffes MW, et al: Pancreatic islet transplantation. Effects on the glomerular lesions of experimental diabetes in the rat. Diabetes 23:748, 1974.
2. The Diabetes Control and Complications Trial Research Group: The effect of intensive treatment of diabetes on the development and progression of long-term complications in insulin-dependent diabetes mellitus. N Engl J Med 329:977-986, 1993.
3. Barker CF, Naji A, and Silvers WK: Immunological problems in islet transplantation. Diabetes 29:86-92, 1980.
4. Federlin KF, Bretzel RG, Hering BJ: Islet transplant registry. In: Pancreatic islet cell transplantation. ed. C. Ricordi, R.G. Landes. 42:462-472, 1992.
5. Naji A, Silvers WK, Bellgrau D, Barker CF: Spontaneous diabetes in rats: destruction of islets is prevented by immunological tolerance. Science 213:1390-1392, 1981.
6. Sutherland DE, Goetz FC, Sibley RK: Recurrence of disease in pancreas transplantation. Diabetes 38 (suppl 1):85-87, 1989.
7. Lacy PE, Davie JM, and Finke EH: Prolongation of islet allograft survival following in vitro culture (24°) and a single injection of ALS. Science 204:312-313, 1979.
8. Faustman DL, Steinman RM, Gebel HM, Hauptfeld V, Davie JM, and Lacy PE: Prevention of rejection of murine islet allografts by pretreatment with anti-dendritic cell antibody. Proc Nat Acad Sci 81:3864-3868, 1984.
9. Lau H, Reemtsma K, and Hardy MA: Prolongation of rat islet allograft survival by direct ultraviolet irradiation of the graft. Science 223:607-609, 1984.
10. Bellgrau D, Selawry HP: Cyclosporine-induced tolerance to intratesticular islet allografts. Transplantation 50:654, 1990.
11. Barker CF, Billingham RE: Immunologically privileged sites. In: Kunkel HG, Dixon FJ, eds. Advances in immunology: Vol. 25, New York, Academic Press, 1977.
12. Billingham RE, Brent L, Medawar PB: "Actively acquired tolerance" of foreign cells. Nature (Lond.) 172:603-606, 1953.
13. Streilein JW: Neonatal tolerance of H-2 alloantigens. Procuring graft acceptance the "old-fashioned" way. Transplantation 52: 1-10, 1991.
14. Raviola E, Karnovsky MJ: Evidence for a blood-thymus barrier using electron-opaque tracers. J Exp Med 136:466-, 1972.
15. Weiss L, ed.: The blood cells and hematopoietic tissues. McGraw-Hill, pp. 503-522, 1977.
16. Schwartz RH: Acquisition of immunological self-tolerance. Cell 57:1973, 1989.
17. Vojtiskova M, Lengerova A: Thymus mediated tolerance to cellular alloantigens. Transplantation 6:13, 1968.

18. Staples PJ, Gery I, Waksman BH: Role of the thymus in tolerance. III. Tolerance to bovine gamma globulin after direct injection of antigen into the shielded thymus of irradiated rats. J Exp Med 124:127-139, 1966.
19. Shimonkevitz RP, Bevan MJ: Split tolerance induced by the intrathymic adoptive transfer of thymocyte stem cells. J Exp Med 168:143-156, 1988.
20. Posselt AM, Barker CF, Tomaszewski JE, Markmann JF, Choti MA, Naji A: Induction of donor-specific unresponsiveness by intrathymic islet transplantation. Science 249:1293-1295, 1990.
21. Woehrle M, Markmann JF, Silvers WK, Barker CF, Naji A: Transplantation of cultured pancreatic islets to BB rats. Surgery 100:334-340, 1986.
22. Campos L, Posselt AM, Mayo GL, Pete K, Deli BC, Barker CF, Naji A: The failure of intrathymic transplantation of non-immunogenic islet allografts to promote induction of donor-specific unresponsiveness. Transplantation (In Press).
23. Posselt AM, Naji A, Roark JH, Markmann JF, Barker CF: Intrathymic islet transplantation in the spontaneously diabetic rat. Annals of Surgery 214:363-373, 1991.
24. Mayo GL, Posselt AM, Campos L, Barker CF, Naji A: Intrathymic transplantation promotes survival of islet xenografts (rat to mouse). Transplant Proc (In Press).
25. Zeng JA, Bluestone ST, Ildstad MA, Torres AG, Montag RJ, Thistlethwaite Jr: Long-term functional xenograft tolerance after intrathymic islet transplantation (Lewis rat to B6 mouse). Transplant Proc 25:438-439, 1993.
26. Sharabi Y, Sachs DH: Mixed chimerism and permanent specific transplantation tolerance induced by a nonlethal preparative regimen. J Exp Med 169:493-502, 1989.
27. Bowers WE, Berkowitz MR: Differentiation of dendritic cells in cultures of rat bone marrow cells. J Exp Med 163:872-883, 1986.
28. Posselt AM, Odorico JS, Barker CF, Naji A: Promotion of pancreatic islet allograft survival by intrathymic transplantation of bone marrow. Diabetes 41:771-775, 1992.
29. Odorico JS, Barker CF, Posselt AM, Naji A: Induction of donor-specific tolerance to rat cardiac allografts by intrathymic inoculation of bone marrow. Surgery 112: 370-377, 1992.
30. Qian T, Schachner R, Brendel M, Kond SS, Alejandro R: Induction of donor-specific tolerance to rat islet allografts by intrathymic inoculation of solubilized spleen cell membrance antigens. Diabetes 42:1544-1546, 1993.

CHAPTER 9

Immunomodulation of Pancreatic Islets by Culture

Pierre Y. Benhamou

Yoko Mullen

Survival of endocrine tissue allografts can be prolonged in rodents by culturing donor tissue, under certain conditions, prior to transplantation. The main physical parameters that influence the outcome of cultures are the duration, temperature and oxygen tension. Both high oxygen tension and low temperature exert deleterious effects on passenger leukocytes carried in a graft.[1-3] Hence, these properties have been shown to reduce the immunogenicity of donor tissue. The use of high oxygen culture for mouse thyroid gland was the first such attempt,[1,3] resulting in long-term graft survival without additional immunosuppressive agents. Beneficial effects of pretransplant culture have also been demonstrated with pancreatic islet allo- and xenografts.[4-6] However, culture methods using high oxygen tension or low temperature may affect not only passenger leukocytes but also islet viability. Furthermore, culture requirements for altering islet immunogenicity appear to be different between species, thus complicating the practical use of these properties. In addition, whether these pretransplant cultures have an impact on the protection of donor islets from autoimmune destruction has not been carefully investigated in either animal models or human patients with type I diabetes. Since these culture parameters have been extensively studied and validated in rodents, we now need to examine their effectiveness with adult and fetal human islets, as well as islets of other large animal species that may be potential candidates as donor tissue for clinical transplantation. The following two issues are important in order to evaluate the implication of these pretransplant culture methods for clinical islet transplantation: (1) standardization of culture procedures based on their optimal efficiency in reducing tissue immunogenicity and toxicity for islets and (2) further understanding of the immunomodulatory mechanisms of these parameters in order to identify and select the best strategy for clinical islet transplantation.

ISLET VIABILITY UNDER DIFFERENT CULTURE CONDITIONS

The aim of islet culture in transplantation is two-fold: (1) to facilitate survival of endocrine tissue awaiting transplantation and (2) to reduce the

Pancreatic Islet Transplantation Volume II: Immunomodulation of Pancreatic Islets, edited by Robert P. Lanza, MD, William L. Chick, MD; ©1994 R.G. Landes Company.

immunogenicity of donor islets in order to minimize host rejection reactions. For the latter objective, periods of culture at 37° C or at room temperature (22-24° C, low temperature culture) in air plus 5% CO_2, or at 37° C in 95% O_2 have been the major methods used so far. Viability and survival of islets under these conditions are the first issues that need to be addressed.

Low Temperature Culture

A predominant feature of adult or fetal islets cultured at low temperature is a reduction of insulin released into the culture medium and an increase of insulin stored in β cells. If the duration of culture does not exceeds 7-28 days, this resting state is reversible within 24 hours, in vitro, when islets are returned to 37° C culture, or, in vivo, when islets are transplanted.[7] Earlier studies in rats showed that adult islets remained morphologically and functionally intact after 24° C culture for 1-4 wk.[7] However, studies with fetal porcine and human adult islets have indicated a limit of 7 days in 24° C culture. With fetal pig islets, Yoneda at al[8] demonstrated a reasonable recovery of viable β cells, when collagenase-digested fetal pancreatic tissue was cultured at 24° C for less than 8 days. These fetal β cells functioned normally, as tested in vitro by various functional tests[8] (and Mullen at al unpublished results), and grew progressively in vivo following transplantation.[9] Extended culture beyond 8 days at this low temperature was deleterious to fetal porcine β cells.[8] Similarly, a short-term culture at 24° C has minimal effect on the viability and function of isolated, adult human islets. In an in vitro perifusion system, human islets cultured for 4 to 7 days at 24° C adequately respond to a glucose challenge with insulin release[10] (and Mullen at al unpublished results). In vivo, these islets reverse streptozotocin-induced diabetes in athymic mice.[11] Scharp at al have used islets cultured at 24° C for 7 days in clinical transplantation and demonstrated amelioration of glucose metabolism in long-term type I diabetic patients for up to 10 months.[12]

Other Culture Parameters

Using murine thyroid gland, Lafferty at al[3] and Talmage and Dart[1] have shown that organ culture under high oxygen concentrations effectively reduces graft immunogenicity. However, subsequent studies with adult rat islets have revealed a rapid loss of viable β cells in high O_2 culture. Fetal β cells from mouse and human pancreas are also destroyed, in less than 5 days, under this culture condition.[13-14] Bowen at al[15] have reported that the toxic effect of oxygen can be reduced by forming large islet aggregates, "mega-islets", prior to culture. To date, the utilization of this procedure (a 7-day culture at 37° C in 95% O_2) has been limited in islet allo- and xenotransplantation in rodents[15-17] probably due to its toxicity for β cells. It is especially interesting to note that high oxygen and low temperature, when the two parameters were combined for culturing murine fetal islets, did not act synergistically in reducing immunogenic cell numbers.[14] No data are available for adult human islets.

Hyperthermia was another parameter applied to mouse thyroid allografts. A treatment protocol exposing the thyroid gland to 43° C for 2 to 4 hours prevented allograft rejection.[18] Our experience with hyperthermic treatment of fetal porcine pancreas revealed deleterious effects on β cells (unpublished results).

Culture in acidified Hanks balanced salt solution (HBSS) for 24 hours was also reported to promote islet allograft survival in mice.[19] This study was based on the finding that lymphoid cells, when used as stimulators after overnight culture in non-buffered HBSS, failed to induce generation of alloreactive cytotoxic T cells in mixed lymphocyte reactions (MLR).[20] This treatment protocol used a culture of islets for 72 hours in RPMI 1640 medium under 95% oxygen at 37° C and then for 24 hours in air and 5% CO_2 in HBSS without $NaHCO_3$, at an initial pH of 7.2. After 24 hours, the pH of HBSS dropped to 6.6. Although the shift of pH appears to have adverse effect on lymphocytes, it did not affect islet viability.[19]

This was one of the first studies addressing the importance of biochemical and, perhaps, nutritional features of culture medium on antigen presenting cells (APC) and islet viability. Further studies using larger animal models and functional tests are needed.

Other parameters of culture that may affect intraislet passenger leukocytes include the amount of medium in culture dishes and selection of serum supplement. A low level of culture medium, that barely covers the islets and maintains them at the gas-liquid interface, appears to favor efficient oxygen exchange of islet cells, minimize central necrosis of islets, and may have toxic effects on passenger leukocytes.[21] Bovine serum, but not horse serum, contains polyamine oxidase that can convert intracellular polyamines, which are released at a high level during pancreas digestion, into cytotoxic compounds.[22]

IMMUNOMODULATING EFFECTS OF VARIOUS CULTURE CONDITIONS

The relevance of immunological manipulation by culturing islets prior to transplantation has been validated in various animal species including the pig and dog. The reduction of immunogenicity has also been demonstrated with isolated, adult human islets following low temperature culture.

Studies in Rodents

The effect of low temperature culture was more extensively studied in rats than mice. Since passenger leukocytes primarily responsible for eliciting strong allograft reactions express major histocompatibility complex (MHC) class II antigens, the presence of these antigens in islets is often used as an in vitro marker for assessment of islet immunogenicity. This assumption may be valid since under normal conditions, endocrine islet cells are class II-antigen negative, as is the vascular endothelium of rodents. It was reported that class II antigen expression was more significantly reduced in rat islets following 22° C culture than 37° C culture.[23] In this report, 90% of freshly prepared islets were found to contain more than four class II antigen-positive cells, 20% of 37° C cultured islets contained such cells, and only 5% in 22° C cultured islets. Furthermore, this reduction was irreversible when islets were placed back into 37° C-culture. However, this is a controversial issue, as others did not find any difference in class II antigen expression in islets cultured at either 37° C or 24° C.[24]

A more direct method to determine the effectiveness of various culture conditions in alterating the immunological properties of islets is provided by islet allograft survival. In rats, culturing islets for 7 days at 24° C prior to transplantation was sufficient to induce long-term survival of intratesticular allografts.[25] When 24° C-cultured islets were transplanted into the liver or in the space beneath the renal capsule, only a peritransplant immunosuppression with anti-lymphocyte serum (ALS) or cyclosporine (CsA) was sufficient to induce prolonged allograft survival.[5] An important finding was that 24° C-cultured allogeneic islets also survived for a long period in the BB rat, a model of autoimmune diabetes, when a short course of immunosuppression was used.[26]

Hegre at al reported long-term survival of culture-derived perinatal rat islets in fully allogeneic recipients without immunosuppression.[22,27] These islets were produced by culturing collagenase-digested newborn pancreata for 10 days at 37° C in air plus 5% CO_2. This prolonged graft survival was correlated with the depletion of MHC class II positive cells.[22,27-30] in certain strains of rats. This strain-dependent observation may suggest the involvement of mechanisms other than depletion of class II-positive passenger leukocytes for prolonged graft survival, as discussed in the subsequent section.[31]

Successful allotransplantation was also achieved in non-immunosuppressed mice, following culture of islets in 95% oxygen for 7 days.[15,17] It was found that prolonged survival of islet allografts was achieved in donor-recipient combinations incompatible at the MHC, but not in those incompatible only at minor histocompatibility loci.[17] These results suggest an involvement of host APCs in islet rejection processes. The impact of donor islet culture on allograft survival has not been thoroughly examined in the NOD mouse, another model for autoimmune diabetes which does not have lymphopenia and which responds strongly to allogeneic and syngeneic islet transplants.[32]

All three culture procedures, 7 day-culture in air and 5% CO_2 at either 24° C or 37° C, and in 95% O_2 at 37° C, effectively prolonged concordant islet xenografts from rat to mouse.[6,16,21] Low temperature culture was also effective in prolonging discordant islet xenografts from hamster to mouse[33] and from human to mouse.[34-35] However, xenografts from discordant donors required two additional treatments for prolonged islet survival: treatment of low temperature-cultured islets with ALS directed to the donor species, and recipient immunosuppression with anti-mouse ALS. ALS treatment of donor islets probably assisted the elimination of residual passenger leukocytes in the islets. ALS treatment may also have aided in the elimination of lymphoid cells contaminating donor islet preparations, since highly purified, hand-picked human islets survived for a prolonged period after pretreatment with low temperature culture alone.[34] All these studies used mice as xenograft recipients. Further investigations are necessary in other animal species in order to determine whether pretransplant treatment of donor islets would facilitate xenograft survival.

Large Animal Species

The effects of low temperature culture have been studied on fetal porcine pancreatic tissues prepared by collagenase digestion.[8] Immunogenicity of pancreatic preparations was assessed, in vitro, by mixed islet-lymphocyte culture (MILC), performed by a method similar to MLR. Immunogenicity of collagenase-digested fetal pig pancreatic tissue was reduced after one day (pancreas from <70 day fetal pigs) or one week (pancreas from >70 day fetal pigs) in culture.[8] Culture of pancreatic tissue at 37° C also sufficiently reduced immunogenicity of younger pancreata, while longer culture periods (>30 days) were required for older pancreata. This reduced immunogenicity was not correlated with the number of MHC class II-positive cells detected in the tissue.[8] These results agreed with observations made in some rat strains.[31] MHC class II antigens are expressed, in the fetal porcine pancreas, by dendritic-like cells and by vascular endothelium. Dendritic-like cells are detected in the pancreas earlier than 40 days of gestation (the gestation period of pigs is 114 days). The number of these cells increases rapidly as gestation advances. Vascular endothelium of the pancreas becomes positive for class II antigens beginning at approximately 50 days of gestation. The percentage of class II-positive endothelial cells increases rapidly, reaching the level of adult pig pancreas at 65-70 days. In the pancreas at this developmental stage, a majority of class II-positive cells are endothelial cells.[36] Vascular endothelium of human fetal pancreas also becomes DR antigen positive beginning at approximately 16-18 weeks of gestation.[37] Although endothelium is capable of eliciting alloimmune responses in vitro,[38] the effect of various culture parameters on vascular endothelium has not been investigated.

Despite reduced immunogenicity shown in vitro by MILC, pretreatment of islets with low-temperature culture has little effect on allograft survival in pigs. Without additional recipient immunosuppression, allografts are acutely rejected (<3 weeks). As an exception, a favorable effect of low temperature culture was suggested in MHC-compatible fetal pancreas allografts in NIH miniature pigs. In this combination, 7 day-24° C culture resulted in detection of some insulin-positive cells scattered in the background of strong lymphocytic infiltration 90 days after transplantation.[8]

Islet allografts performed between mongrel dogs demonstrated the ineffectiveness of 37° C culture alone for prolonging graft survival. Islet manipulation combining culture and anti-class II antibody treatment, and temporary recipient immunosuppression with CsA for ≥30 days, was required to achieve a prolonged, but limited graft survival.[39] Immunohistochemical studies revealed a decreased number of class II antigen-bearing cells within islets cultured at 37° C for 5-8 days, but surprisingly this effect was absent when islets were cultured at 24° C.[40]

Studies with Human Islets

As previously mentioned, human islets cultured up to 7 days at 24° C retain their functional integrity.[10-12] Abrogation of allogeneic stimulation in MILC assays was reported in human insulinoma cells after one month in culture at 37° C.[41] We recently documented a 63% reduction of allostimulatory capacity of adult human islets in MILC after 3-4 day culture at 24° C as compared to 37° C.[42] Furthermore, cultured islets have been successfully used in clinical transplantation.[12] However, only in vitro studies have documented the immunomodulatory effects of culture on human islets, and the advantages of culture in clinical transplantation are still unclear.

Mechanisms Involved in Islet Immunomodulation by Various Culture Methods

The following mechanisms have been proposed to explain the beneficial effects of various culture procedures that alter islet immunogenicity.

Effect on Antigen-Presenting Cells

A well accepted hypothesis, initially proposed by Snell[43] and later strengthened by Lafferty,[44] postulated that various culture parameters act on MHC class II-positive APCs carried in islets. These APCs mostly consist of bone marrow-derived dendritic cells and macrophages. Studies in the NOD mouse have demonstrated that intraislet MHC class II-positive cells are exclusively CD45-positive, indicating their origin from the bone marrow.[45] In addition to allo-class II antigens, these donor APCs are also capable of providing a costimulatory signal necessary for the effective presentation of foreign antigens to recipient T helper lymphocytes.[44] This passenger leukocyte theory has been validated by many studies with mouse and rat islet allografts.[5,22,24,27-29] Passenger leukocytes appear to play a role in initiating xenogeneic responses as well.[30] These reports correlated the reduction in islet immunogenicity with the loss of MHC class II-positive APCs obtained by culturing. The concept of donor tissue APC depletion, using various culture methods, has successfully been applied to immunomodulate other endocrine allografts, including thyroid, parathyroid, pituitary, adrenal, and ovary.[44]

Methods for depletion of passenger leukocytes from donor tissue are not limited to culture procedures alone. Ultraviolet light irradiation, treatment by anti-class II antibody and complement, and dietary fatty acid manipulation appear to exert similar effects, and have been used successfully for prolongation of islet allograft survival. The role played by passenger leukocytes in initiating alloimmune responses is further supported by evidence that well established allografts are promptly rejected after a challenge with donor peritoneal cells[46] or splenocytes.[22]

The concept of low temperature culture derived from the earlier finding by Opelz and Terasaki[2] that human lymphocytes cultured at 22° C for more than 4 days failed to stimulate allogeneic lymphocytes in vitro, in MLRs, although they were viable and even proliferated when used as responders. Macrophages cultured in 600 mm O_2 survive less than 2 days at 26° C.[47] Histological evaluations performed on mouse and rat islets have shown that, after culturing islets for 7 days at 24° C or 37° C, MHC class II-positive cells, including lymphocytes, macrophages, and capillary endothelial cells, were no longer detectable.[24,48] In fact, quantitative detection of class II antigens indicated that Ia antigens were reduced but not totally eliminated after 7 days of culture.[24] However, there are some discrepancies between those results depending on the methods used for detecting MHC class II antigens, i.e., immunofluorescence vs peroxidase staining procedures.[49] It has also been reported that cultured rat islets were negative for surface but positive for intracytoplasmic MHC class II antigens.[49]

Species Differences in the Effectiveness of Culture Treatments for Islet Allograft Survival

It is well known that long-term survival of allografts is more easily achieved in mice than in rats.[50] In mice, prolonged, often indefinite survival of islet allografts can be achieved just by culturing donor tissue prior to transplantation. However, the same islet treatment does not extend islet graft survival in rats without short-term, peritransplant immunosuppression.[5,26,51-52] In larger animal species, the effects of such islet pretreatment on graft survival are minimal, and recipients must be treated by continuous immunosuppression for islets to survive.[39] Although these species differences are attributable to a number of physiological and immunological differences, the distribution of APCs and the cell types that express class II antigens in islets are different from one species to another.[53] In fetal pancreas, the gestation or developmental stage of the donor adds additional variables. We have found that during fetal development, dendritic-like cells migrate from the peripancreatic lymph nodes into the adjacent pancreatic tissue. These cells appear in islets about one month after birth in mice, at the time of birth in rats, by 40 days of gestation in pigs and by 12 weeks in humans.[53] Only 2-5 class II-positive cells per section were counted in fresh newborn rat islets, and up to 10 to 20 in adult rat islets.[28,49,53] The effects of 37° C culture for 10 days were compared in canine and porcine islets. Canine islets were markedly depleted of class II-positive cells, with 85% of islets completely free of class II-staining. Porcine islets also exhibited a total loss of class II reactivity on endothelial cells, but leukocytes and macrophages remained class II-positive.[54] A similar difference in class II expression was found between endothelial cells and macrophages in cultured human islets.[55] Thus, a complete depletion of passenger leukocytes from the islets cannot be expected in some animal species by culture procedures that allow endocrine cell survival. A different susceptibility of intraislet APCs to various culture conditions may exist between species, as was evidenced by different dose requirements for ultraviolet light treatment of islets.[56]

Effect on Vascular Endothelium

In addition to passenger leukocytes, the vascular endothelium is also known to express class II antigens and to stimulate allogeneic T cells.[38] MHC class II expression on endothelium varies between species. As discussed above, endothelium is class II negative in the mouse and rat, but positive in the pig.[36,53] In adult human islets, endothelial cells, including intraislet capillaries, are the major site of DR expression in adult islets, whereas endocrine, acinar and ductal cells are DR-negative under normal conditions.[55] Human fetal pancreata of 18 weeks or older also express DR antigens on the endothelium of small and medium-sized vessels, and cryptic DR antigens can be induced on endothelial cells by the addition of recombinant interferon-γ to the culture medium.[37] Culture of islets markedly depletes endothelial cells in the mouse and rat.[24,48] However, it is not clear how strongly immunogenic these class II-positive endothelial cells are in vivo when islets are transplanted.

Depletion of donor APCs is neither necessary,[31] nor sufficient[57] for the survival of culture-treated islet allografts. Thus a reduced immunogenicity was achieved with extended culture of ACI rat perinatal islets, even though these islets were already MHC class II-negative at the beginning of the extended-culture period.[31] Conversely, treatment of islets with antibodies directed against donor class II antigens failed to prolong graft survival in some studies.[57] Based on these observations, it has been suggested that at earlier stages of culture, MHC class II antigen expression is down-regulated on APCs, although these cells retain their ability to present antigens. As the culture period is prolonged, APCs are eliminated.[31]

Although passenger leukocytes play a major role in the initiation of allograft responses, alloantigens are also recognized by host APCs. Different modes of antigen presentation may lead to different modes of host immune reactions, i.e., immunity vs. tolerance, and this shift of reactions may significantly differ from one animal species to another.

Effect on MHC Class I Expression

A reduced expression of MHC class I antigens was reported on rat islet endocrine cells cultured at 24° C as compared to those cultured at 37° C.[58] Similarly, the decreased immunogenicity of thyroid allografts after culture in a high oxygen environment was correlated with reduced expression of class I antigens.[59] Moreover, 24° C cultured islets were refractory to MHC antigen expression induced in vitro by the addition of lymphokine to the culture medium.[58] The down-regulation of class I antigens may also influence the intensity of rejection reactions and thus graft survival. Purified β cells, which are class I-positive and class II-negative, stimulated a strong cytotoxic T lymphocyte (CTL) response.[60] Furthermore, depletion of islet APCs by an anti-class II antibody did not eliminate the generation of CTL.[61] In contrast, islets from MHC class I-deficient mutant mice failed to elicite CTL responses in vitro.[62] These class I- deficient islets exhibited prolonged survival in fully allogeneic recipients.[62,63] These results may provide some explanations for the beneficial effect of low temperature culture.

It is interesting to find out that MHC class I-deficient islets are fully susceptible to autoimmune destruction when transplanted into diabetic NOD mice.[63] Since class I-deficient islets escape from allograft rejection, these islets must be destroyed by autoimmune attack directed against islets in NOD mice. Thus, it may suggest a predominant role of MHC class II-restricted CD4 T cells over MHC class I-restricted CD8 cells in autoimmunity directed against allogeneic islets. However, this islet destruction may not be directed toward class II antigens, since the effective arm of the NOD's autoimmunity appears to have both MHC-restricted and MHC-non-restricted properties.[64]

The down-regulation of MHC class I antigens after 24° C culture needs confirmation in larger animals. Furthermore, the reversibility of antigenic expression following transplantation should be investigated. Indeed, de novo expression of class II antigens, as well as increased expression of class I antigens were demonstrated on rat islet endocrine cells incubated with interferon-γ in vitro.[65] Class II antigens are also induced in human islet endocrine cells, but require simultaneous exposure to TNF and interferon-γ.[66] Importantly, the beneficial effect of culture on rat islet allograft survival was lost when islets were exposed, in vitro, to interferon-γ for one week prior to transplantation.[67] Other studies using transgenic mice suggested that the deleterious effect of lymphokine exposure was related to the increase in class I expression and that de novo expression of class II antigens on endocrine cells did not confer them the ability to trigger the immune response as with accessory cells.[68]

Other Putative Effects

Histological examination of long-term surviving islet xenografts (rat to mouse) following 24° C culture revealed periinsulitis composed primarily of T cells of the Ly2$^+$ phenotype.[51] Periinsulitis was also reported in long-term surviving islet allografts from MHC class I-deficient mice (62-63). Focal accumulation of lymphocytes and plasma cells was observed at the peripheral margins of long-term surviving human-to-mouse xenografts following room temperature culture.[34] Similarly, thyroid allografts cultured under hyperbaric O_2 conditions exhibited a decreased expression of MHC class I antigens, prolonged survival, and elicited a lymphocytic periinfiltrate composed mostly of CD8 cells lacking the message for TNF-α, interferon-γ and perforin.[69] The induction of regulatory cells by culture, through an undefined mechanism, is a tempting hypothesis.

Although most allografts of cultured islets in rats require short-term immunosuppression for prolonged survival, one study reported that culture at 22° C resulted in indefinite graft survival under the kidney capsule in the majority of recipients. In contrast, grafts were rejected if islets were cultured at 37° C or first cultured at 22° C and then placed at 37° C, although similar numbers of class II antigens were expressed in both cases.[23] One possible explanation may be that the low metabolic activity of islets cultured at 22° C, and directly transplanted, could be beneficial for improving graft survival. A resting state may down-regulate the expression of various antigens, including targets for autoreactive T cells such as glutamic acid decarboxylase, on the β-cell surface. This slow metabolism may also explain the decrease of MHC class I expression. Reduction of antigenic expression may possibly reduce effector activities that destroy the graft. These hypotheses await confirmation. Recent investigations in organ recipients have shown that transplantation tolerance may depend on a state of balanced lymphodendritic cell chimerism between the host and the donor graft.[70] Whether islet culture may allow the achievement of such a chimerism remains to be tested.

CONCLUSION

The effectiveness of islet culture differs depending on animal species and strains, site of transplantation, duration and temperature of culture. Taken together, the available data suggest a predominant advantage for low-temperature culture, enabling the depletion or inactivation of intraislet APCs that trigger recipient T helper response, as well as down-regulating class I expression on endocrine cells and thus reducing CTL-mediated lysis. Immunogenicity of human islets can be reduced, without detrimental effects on islet viability and function, by a short culture period, i.e., 3-4 days, at 24° C, or 7 days at 37° C, as suggested by in vitro testing. The simplicity of this procedure reduces the risk of the adverse effects of islet manipulation (contamination, loss of islets). The relevance of combining islet culture with other approaches of graft and recipient immunomodulation will be clarified with future clinical trials.

REFERENCES

1. Talmage DW, Dart GA. Effect of oxygen pressure during culture on survival of mouse thyroid allografts. Science 1978; 200: 1066-7.
2. Opelz G, Terasaki PD. Lymphocyte antigenicity loss with retention of unresponsiveness. Science 1974; 184: 464-6.
3. Lafferty KJ, Cooley MA, Woolnough J, et al. Thyroid allograft immunogenicity is reduced after a period in organ culture. Science 1975; 188: 259-61.
4. Kedinger M, Haffen K, Grenier J, et al. In vitro culture reduced immunogenicity of transplanted endocrine islets. Nature 1977; 270: 736.
5. Lacy PE, Davie JM, Finke EH. Prolongation of islet allograft survival following in vitro culture (24° C) and a single injection of ALS. Science 1979; 204: 312-13.
6. Lacy PE, Davie JM, Finke EH. Prolongation of islet xenograft survival without continuous immunosuppression. Science 1980; 209: 283-85.
7. Ono J, Lacy PE, Michael HEB, et al. Studies of the functional and morphologic status of islets maintained at 24° C for four weeks in vitro. Am J Pathol 1979; 97: 489-97.
8. Yoneda K, Mullen Y, Stein E, et al. Fetal pancreas transplantation in miniature swine. II. Survival of fetal pig pancreas allografts cultured at room temperature. Diabetes 1989; 38, (Suppl 1): 213-6.
9. Mullen Y, Nagata M, Matsuo S, et al. Effective treatment regimes against fetal islet rejection in miniature swine with or without a combined kidney allograft. Horm Metab Res 1990; 25 (suppl): 190-2.
10. Scharp DW, Lacy PE, Finke EH, et al. Low-temperature culture of human islets isolated by the distension method and purified with Ficoll or Percoll gradients. Surgery 1987; 102: 869.
11. Ricordi C, Scharp DW, Lacy PE. Reversal of diabetes in nude mice after transplantation of fresh and 7-day-cultured (24° C) human pancreatic islets. Transplantation 1988; 45: 994-6.
12. Scharp DW, Lacy PE, Santiago JV, et al. Results of our first nine intraportal islet allografts in type I, insulin-dependent diabetic patients. Transplantation 1991; 51: 76-85.
13. Mandel TE, Hoffman L, Collier S, et al. Organ culture of fetal mouse and fetal human pancreatic islets for allografting. Diabetes 1982; 31 (Suppl 4): 39-47.
14. Mandel TE, Koulmanda M. Effect of culture conditions on fetal mouse pancreas in vitro and after transplantation in syngeneic and allogeneic recipients. Diabetes 1985; 34: 1082-87.

15. Bowen KM, Andrus L, Lafferty KJ. Successful allotransplantation of mouse pancreatic islets to nonimmunosuppressed recipients. Diabetes 1980; 29 (Suppl.1): 98-104.
16. Lacy PE, Finke EH, Janney CG, et al. Prolongation of islet xenograft survival by in vitro culture of rat megaislets in 95% O_2 Transplantation 1982; 33: 588-92.
17. Bartlett ST, Naji A, Silvers WK, Barker CF. Influence of culturing on the functioning of major-histocompatibility-complex-compatible and incompatible islet grafts in diabetic mice. Transplantation 1983; 36: 687-90.
18. Bartlett ST, Ward RE. Pretransplant hyperthermia promotes permanent survival of murine thyroid allografts. J Surg Res 1989; 46: 370.
19. La Rosa FG. Abrogation of mouse pancreatic islet allograft rejection by a four-day culture. Transplantation 1988; 46: 330-33.
20. Moreland AF, Mullbacher A. Enhancement of murine thyroid allograft survival after 16 to 20 hours' organ culture. Transplantation 1987; 43: 417-421.
21. Yasunami Y, Lacy PE, Davie JM, et al. Prolongation of islet xenograft survival (rat to mouse) by in vitro culture at 37° C. Transplantation 1983; 35: 281-84.
22. Serie JR, Hegre OD. Long-term survival of cultured islet allografts without the use of immunosuppression. Transplantation 1985; 39: 684-87.
23. Woehrle M, Beyer K, Bretzel RG, et al. The influence of the culture temperature on insulin release, antigen expression and allograft survival of islets of Langerhans. Horm Metab Res 1990; 25 (suppl): 96-100.
24. Rabinovitch A, Alejandro R, Noel J, et al. Tissue culture reduces Ia antigen-bearing cells in rat islets and prolongs allograft survival. Diabetes 1982; 31 (Suppl 4): 48-54.
25. Ricordi C, Kraus C, Lacy PE. Effect of low-temperature culture on the survival of intratesticular rat islet allografts. Transplantation 1988; 45: 234-36.
26. Woehrle M, Markmann JF, Barker CF, et al. Transplantation of cultured pancreatic islets to BB rats. Surgery 1986; 11: 334-41.
27. Hegre OD, Hickey GE, Marshall S, et al. Modification of allograft immunogenicity in perinatal islets isolated and purified in vitro. Transplantation 1984; 37: 227-233.
28. Meloche M, Ketchum RJ, Serie JR, et al. Elimination of IA-bearing cells by in vitro isolation and culture of neonatal rat pancreatic islets. Transplantation 1988; 46: 614-16.
29. Hegre OD, Ketchum RJ, Popiela H, et al. Allotransplantation of culture-isolated neonatal rat islet tissue. Absence of MHC class II positive antigen-presenting cells in nonimmunogenic islets. Diabetes 1989; 38: 146-51.
30. Serie JR, Hickey GE, Schmitt RV, et al. Prolongation of culture isolated neonatal islet xenografts without immunosuppression. Transplantation 1983; 36: 6-11.
31. Ketchum RJ, Moore WV, Hegre OD. Increased islet allograft survival after extended culture by a mechanism other than depletion of donor APCs. Lack of correlation between the elimination of donor MHC class II-positive accessory cells and increased transplantability. Transplantation 1992; 54: 347-51.
32. Terada M, Salzler M, Lennartz K, et al. The effect of H-2 compatibility on pancreatic β cell survival in the nonobese diabetic mouse. Transplantation 1988; 45: 622-7.
33. Sullivan FP, Ricordi CI, Hauptfeld V, et al. Effect of low-temperature culture and site of transplantation on hamster islet xenograft survival (hamster to mouse). Transplantation 1987; 44: 465-8.
34. Ricordi C, Lacy PE, Sterbenz K, et al. Low-temperature culture of human islets or in vivo treatment with L3T4 antibody produces a marked prolongation of islet human-to-mouse xenograft survival. Proc Natl Acad Sci USA 1987; 84: 8080-84.
35. Falqui L, Finke EH, Carel JC, et al. Marked prolongation of human islet xenograft survival (human-to-mouse) by low-temperature culture and temporary immunosuppression with human and mouse anti-lymphocyte sera. Transplantation 1991; 51: 1322-24.
36. Motojima K, Mullen Y. Interferon-γ stimulates cryptic class II antigen expression in human and pig fetal pancreata. Transplant Proc 1987; 19: 214.

37. Motojima K, Matsuo S, Mullen Y. DR antigen expression on vascular endothelium and duct epithelium in fresh or cultured human fetal pancreata in the presence of gamma-interferon. Transplantation 1989; 48: 1022-5.
38. Pober JS, Collins T, Gimbrone MA Jr, et al. Lymphocytes recognize human vascular endothelial and dermal fibroblast Ia antigens induced by recombinant immune interferon. Nature 1983; 305: 726.
39. Alejandro R. Latif Z, Noel J, et al. Effect of anti-Ia antibodies, culture, and cyclosporin on prolongation of canine islet allograft survival. Diabetes 1987; 36: 269-73.
40. Gebel HM, Yasunami Y, Diekgraefe B, et al. Ia-bearing cells within isolated canine islets. Transplantation 1983; 36: 346-8.
41. Demidem A, Thivolet CH. Absence of allogeneic T cell response to human insulin-secreting cells following long-term culture. Transplantation 1988; 45: 953-7.
42. Stein E, Mullen Y, Benhamou PY, et al. Reduction in immunogenicity of human islets by 24° C culture. Transplant Proc. 1994; 26:755.
43. Snell GD. The homograft reaction. Annu Rev Microbiol 1957; 11: 439-58.
44. Lafferty KJ, Prowse SE, Simeonovic CJ, et al. Immunobiology of tissue transplantation: a return to the passenger leukocyte concept. Annu Rev Immunol 1983; 1: 143-73.
45. McInerney MF, Rath S, Janeway Jr CA. Exclusive expression of MHC class II proteins on $CD45^+$ cells in pancreatic islets of NOD mice. Diabetes 1991; 40: 648-51.
46. Lacy PE, Davie JM, Finke EH. Induction of rejection of successful allografts of rat islets by donor peritoneal exudate cells. Transplantation 1979; 28: 415-20.
47. Talmage DW. Effects of oxygen, temperature, and time of culture on the survival of mouse thyroid and pancreas allografts Diabetes 1980; 29 (Suppl.1): 105-6.
48. Parr EL, Bowen KM, Lafferty KJ. Cellular changes in cultured mouse thyroid glands and islets of Langerhans. Transplantation 1980; 30: 135-41.
49. Pipeleers DG, Pipeleers-Marichal M, Hannaert JC, et al. Transplantation of purified islet cells in diabetic rats. I. Standardization of islet cell grafts. Diabetes 1991; 40: 908-19.
50. Morrow CE, Sutherland DE, Steffes MW, et al. H-2 antigen class: effect on mouse islet allograft rejection. Science 1983; 219: 1337-39.
51. Terasaka R, Lacy PE, Bucy RP, et al. Effect of cyclosporine and low-temperature culture on prevention of rejection of islet xenografts (rat-to-mouse). Transplantation 1986; 41: 661-62.
52. Terasaka R, Lacy PE, Hauptfeld V, et al. The effect of cyclosporin-A, low-temperature culture, and anti-Ia antibodies on prevention of rejection of rat islet allografts. Diabetes 1986; 35: 83-88.
53. Fujiya H, Danilovs J, Brown J, Mullen Y: Species differences in dendritic cell distribution in pancreas during fetal development. Transplant Proc 1985; 17: 414-6.
54. Bretzel RG, Flesch BK, Hering BJ, et al. Impact of culture and cryopreservation on MHC class II antigen expression in canine and porcine islets. Horm Metab Res 1990; 25 (suppl): 128-132.
55. Alejandro R, Shienvold FL, Hajek SV, et al. Immunocytochemical localization of HLA-DR in human islets of Langerhans. Diabetes 1982; 31 (Suppl 4): 17-22.
56. Kenyon NS, Strasser S, Alejandro R. Ultraviolet light immunomodulation of canine islets for prolongation of allograft survival. Diabetes 1990; 39: 305-11.
57. Gores PF, Sutherland DER, Platt JL, et al. Depletion of donor Ia^+ cells before transplantation does not prolong islet allograft survival. J Immunol 1986; 137: 1482-5.
58. Markmann JF, Tomaszewski I, Posselt AM, et al. The effect of islet cell culture in vitro at 24° C on graft survival and MHC antigen expression. Transplantation 1990; 49: 272-7.
59. Hullett DA, Landry AS, Leonard DK, et al. Enhancement of thyroid allograft survival following organ culture. Transplantation 1989; 47: 24-7.

60. Stock PG, Meloche M, Ascher NL, et al. Generation of allospecific cytotoxic T-lymphocytes stimulated by pure pancreatic β-cells in absence of Ia+ dendritic cells. Diabetes 1989; 38 (Suppl.1): 161-4.
61. Stock PG, Ascher NL, Platt JL, et al. Effect of immunodepletion of MHC class II-positive cells from pancreatic islets on generation of cytotoxic T-lymphocytes in mixed islet-lymphocyte coculture. Diabetes 1989; 38 (Suppl.1): 157-60.
62. Osorio RW, Ascher NL, Jaenisch R, et al. Major histocompatibility complex class I deficiency prolongs islet allograft survival. Diabetes 1993; 42: 1520-27.
63. Markmann JF, Bassiri H, Desai NM, et al. Indefinite survival of MHC class I-deficient murine pancreatic islet allografts. Transplantation 1992; 54:1085-89.
64. Matsuo S, Mullen Y, Wicker LS, et al. Islet destruction by the NOD mouse may be mediated by both MHC-restricted and MHC-non restricted mechanisms. Transplant Proc 1991; 23: 743-4.
65. Markmann JF, Hickey WF, Kimura H, et al. Gamma interferon induces novel expression of Ia antigens on rat pancreatic islet endocrine cells. Pancreas 1987; 2: 258-61.
66. Borrell RP, Todd I, Doshi M, et al. HLA class II induction in human islet cells by interferon plus tumor necrosis factor of lymphotoxin. Nature 1987; 326: 304-6.
67. Markmann JF, Jacobson JD, Kimura H, et al. Modulation of the major histocompatibility complex antigen and the immunogenicity of islet allografts. Transplantation 1989; 48: 478-486.
68. Markmann J, Lo D, Naji A, et al. Antigen presenting function of class II MHC expressing pancreatic β cells. Nature 1988; 336:476-79.
69. Everlith KM, Landry AS, Sollinger H, et al. Induction of recipient tolerance by HOC may be mediated by anergic CD8+ T cells (Abstract). Symposium on Tolerance Induction, Breckenridge, Colorado, January 17-20, 1993.
70. Starzl TE, Demetris AJ, Murase N, et al. Cell migration, chimerism, and graft acceptance. Lancet 1992; 339: 1579-82.

CHAPTER 10

Immunomodulation by Ultra-Violet B Irradiation

Mark A. Hardy
Eleni S. Athan
Elliot R. Goodman
Soji F. Oluwole

Ultraviolet irradiation is electromagnetic energy which is divided into UV-A (320-400nm), UV-B (290-320nm), and UV-C (180-190nm). All wave lengths may be toxic to lymphocytes in vitro, but their respective toxicities depend on their relative dose and absorption by cells. The effects of UV-B irradiation on donor/host immunogenicity and on the down-regulation of host immune responses have recently been reviewed.[1,2] The state of hyporesponsiveness or anergy induced by UV-B irradiation suggests that UV-B may be beneficial in reducing graft immunogenicity and in the induction of tolerogenic signals to allografts. This review will discuss the effects of UV-B on the immune response with special attention to the induction of specific unresponsiveness to islet allografts (Table 10.1).

INDUCTION OF UNRESPONSIVENESS BY DIRECT UV-B IRRADIATION OF ISLET CELLS

Rat Islet Allografts

Since Snell[3] suggested that lymphoid cells present in a graft potentiate the immune response against transplanted tissue, many studies examined the effect of transfer of such "passenger leukocytes" during transplantation.[4,5] Passenger leukocytes are presumably MHC-class II expressing interstitial dendritic cells (DC) and macrophages. Based on the hypothesis that passenger leukocytes are important in recipient sensitization, donor pretreatment protocols were designed to deplete or modulate the passenger leukocytes in the donor organ with the expectation that such treatments would prolong graft survival. Such donor pretreatment has been very effective in prolongation of isolated endocrine cellular grafts.[4-6] It appears from these studies that prevention of the initial recognition of an allograft may be achieved by the elimination or modulation of MHC class II positive cells within the graft which is critical to successful transplantation without the use of chronic immunosuppression.

Our studies have focused on the use of UV-B irradiation in the pretreatment of isolated islets to modulate the MHC-class II antigen presenting

Pancreatic Islet Transplantation Volume II: Immunomodulation of Pancreatic Islets, edited by Robert P. Lanza, MD, William L. Chick, MD; ©1994 R.G. Landes Company.

Table 10.1. Experimental models of induction of immunologic tolerance to islet grafts in adult animals by UV-B irradiation

Transplant model	Species	Peritransplant Recipient Immunosuppression	Graft Outcome	References
1. **Direct UV-B Irradiation of Islet Grafts**	a) **Rat**			
	Lewis-to-ACI	–	Tolerance	8, 9
	WF-to-Lewis	CsA 30 mg/kg x3	Tolerance	9, 12
	Lewis-to-CD BB	CsA 30 mg/kg x3	Prolongation	9, 13, 14
	Lewis-to-AD BB	CsA 30 mg/kg x3	Prolongation	9, 13, 14
	WF-to-CD BB	CsA 30 mg/kg x3	Prolongation	9, 13, 14
	WF-to-AD BB	CsA 30 mg/kg x3	Rejection	9, 13, 14
	b) **Monkey**			
	ABO Compatible Cynomolgus Monkeys	CsA (Serum trough level of 150–400 ng/ml)	Modest Prolongation	15
	c) **Xenograft**			
	Lewis-to-B10/BR	–	Tolerance	9
	Lewis-to-BALB/C	–	Prolongation	9
2. **UV–B Irradiated DST**	**Rat**			
	Lewis-to-ACI	–	Tolerance	16
	WF-to-ACI	–	Prolongation	17
3. **UV–B Irradiated BMT**	**Rat**			
	WF-to-Lewis	–	Tolerance	24, 27
4. **Intrathymic UV–B Irradiated Donor Spleen Cells**	**Rat**			
	Lewis-to-ACI	Sublethal TBI	Tolerance	34, 35
	WF-to-Lewis	ALS	Tolerance	38

cells (APC) in the graft since UV-B irradiation of APC abolishes their ability to induce T-cell proliferation in a primary MLR.[7,8] We hypothesized that MHC-class II positive APC may not need to be eliminated from islets prior to transplantation, but rather be modulated by UV-B. Initially we showed that UV-B irradiation (dose range 600-900 J/m^2) is not detrimental to islet isograft function and leads to indefinite acceptance of Lewis islet allografts in streptozotocin (STZ)-induced diabetic ACI rats.[8] The animals remained permanently normoglycemic without recipient immunosuppression in this low responder combination of Lewis-to-ACI rats. In contrast, UV-B irradiated islets were promptly rejected in the high responder combination of WF-to-Lewis[9] where the recipient's MHC-class II positive APC can present the MHC-class I or minor antigens (Ag) on the UV-B irradiated islets through the alternate pathway of T cell activation.[10] However, transient immunosuppression of the recipient (Lewis) with peritransplant cyclosporine A (CsA), which blocks T-cell activation by inhibiting IL-2 production,[11] was found to be synergistic with UV-B irradiation of the donor islets (WF) in the induction of specific unresponsiveness; a brief course of peritransplant CsA (30mg/kg on days 0,1, and 2) led to permanent normoglycemia.[9,12] Transient recipient immunosuppression with CsA converted a metastable to a stable state of transplant unresponsiveness to UV-B-irradiated islets.

Studies of UV-B islet allografting were extended to the correction of diabetes mellitus in BB rats, one of the best animal models of IDDM. Transplantation of UV-B irradiated MHC disparate Lewis islets combined with a 3-day course of peritransplant CsA treatment led to permanent normoglycemia in chronically diabetic BB (CD-BB) rats while UV-B irradiated MHC matched WF islets were only moderately prolonged in CsA treated CD-BB rats.[9,13,14] In contrast, acutely diabetic BB rats (AD-BB) treated in a similar fashion accepted UV-B Lewis islets with only modest prolongation while WF islets were promptly rejected.[9,13] These observations suggest that destruction of the well-matched islet allografts is related to autoimmune disease and that the immune process may be much more active in the AD-BB rats than in the CD-BB rats where the specifically targeted autoimmune activity might have waned or be suppressed. Further work is needed to answer the questions raised regarding the timing of islet transplantation and the ideal source of donor islets for correction of spontaneous, autoimmune IDDM.

Monkey Allografts

Encouraged by the results in the rat islet allograft model, transplantation of UV-B irradiated islets were performed in the primate model using ABO-compatible cynomolgus monkeys in which ketoacidosis-prone IDDM was induced with STZ. Transplantation of UV-B irradiated (450-600 J/m^2) islets into recipients treated with CsA to maintain a serum trough level of 260-400ng/ml led to normoglycemia for 5 to 9 days without exogenous insulin in 3/9 animals.[15] The impairment of glucose tolerance observed in the control normal animals treated with CsA and the inadequate number of donor islets have made the interpretation of UV-B effect on primate islet allograft acceptance very difficult.

Islet Xenograft

Using UV-B irradiated Lewis islets in a xenograft model in which islets were transplanted into STZ diabetic mice, islets were accepted by STZ diabetic B10/BR recipients (low responder), while the high responder Balb/C showed modest prolongation of islet xenograft survival.[9] These findings demonstrate that UV-B irradiation may be useful in the manipulation of islet xenograft survival in the concordant xenograft model of rat-to-mouse in the absence of immunosuppression.

INDUCTION OF SPECIFIC UNRESPONSIVENESS TO ISLET ALLOGRAFTS BY UV-B IRRADIATED DST

The finding[7,8] that UV-B irradiation abolishes the allostimulatory capacity of APCs led us to hypothesize that MHC-class II expressing cells may not need to be eliminated from blood before its use for recipient pretreatment but may need to be modulated with UV-B. We reasoned that prevention of allorecognition and T-cell activation while leaving the MHC antigens intact may result in a state of anergy that leads to induction of donor-specific immunologic unresponsiveness. This concept was confirmed by the finding that all STZ-induced diabetic ACI rats that received UV-B irradiated donor-specific transfusions (UV-DST) at weekly intervals for 3 weeks prior to islet transplantation accepted permanently and specifically islet allografts and became normoglycemic.[16,17] In contrast, recipients of unmodified DSTs rejected their islet allografts in an accelerated fashion. In the high responder combination, when UV-DST from WF was given as pretransplant treatment, WF islet allografts were only moderately prolonged in ACI recipients.[17] The mechanism of acceptance of islet allografts in this model appears to be based primarily on the induction of suppressor immunoregulatory mechanism, as demonstrated by both in vitro co-culture experiments and more importantly by adoptive transfer experiments.

INDUCTION OF TOLERANCE TO ISLET ALLOGRAFTS BY RECIPIENT PRETREATMENT WITH UV-B BONE MARROW TRANSPLANTATION

Bone marrow transplantation (BMT) has been used recently for pretransplant conditioning of recipients in the induction of donor-specific transplantation tolerance to experimental organ allografts[18] and xenografts.[19] Unfortunately, the therapeutic use of BMT prior to clinical organ transplantation has remained very limited because BMT is associated with a high incidence of fatal graft-versus-host disease (GVHD).[20,21] Although ex vivo T-cell depletion (TCD) of bone marrow cells (BMC) prevents GVHD, it decreases the incidence of full BM engraftment.[21] We[22-24] and others[25,26] have employed UV-B irradiation of BMC before transplantation as a novel approach to the prevention of GVHD without compromising BM-engraftment. Such studies have been based on the finding that UV-B irradiated T-cells do not respond to or stimulate alloantigens in mixed lymphocyte reaction (MLR), while UV-B irradiation of APC prevents alloreactive responses.[7,8] This led us to hypothesize that ex vivo UV-B modulation of T cells in BM inoculum will prevent GVHD while UV-B modulation of the APCs contained in the BM inoculum will prevent BM rejection.

We have shown that reconstitution of lethally gamma irradiated recipients with UV-B irradiated admixture of allogeneic BMC and spleen cells (SC) induces a stable lymphohematopoietic chimerism without the development of GVHD in the rodent model.[22-24] Transplantation of UV-B irradiated BMC is associated with complete allogeneic chimerism with 94 to 98% of donor-type T-cells in long-term chimeras.[24,27,28] Such stable chimeras specifically and permanently accept donor-type and recipient-type isolated pancreatic islets,[24,27] cardiac,[23,24] and small intestinal[27] allografts. Lethally gamma irradiated Lewis rats that received UV-B irradiated (700 J/m^2) WF BMT demonstrate stable chimerism without any evidence of GVHD.[24,27] Streptozotocin induced diabetic Lewis chimeric recipients accept permanently (>300 days) BM donor (WF) and recipient type (Lewis) islets and become normo–glycemic. In contrast, they reject acutely (7-8 days) third-party (BN) islet cells. The animals that reject third-party (BN) islet allografts become normoglycemic permanently when retransplanted with BM donor (WF) islets. The results emphasize the specificity of the induction of tolerance in this model and the apparent lack of organ specific sensitization. It appears that the state of unresponsiveness to both donor and recipient Ag in the UV-B BMT model may be essential to the maintenance of self-tolerance. This new strategy of modulating T cells and accessory cells in BM inoculum offers a promising alternative approach to TCD of BMT in clinical BMT as well as an opportunity for pretransplant recipient conditioning with BMT in the induction of Ag-specific tolerance to organ allografts.

INDUCTION OF TOLERANCE TO ISLET ALLOGRAFTS BY RECIPIENT PRETREATMENT WITH INTRATHYMIC UV-B ALLOGENEIC SPLEEN CELLS, RESTING T-CELLS OR SOLUBLE PEPTIDES

The search for a new strategy for the induction of donor-specific immunologic unresponsiveness to transplantation antigens without the use of chronic immunosuppression has rekindled interest in the role of the thymus as an immunologic privileged site for the induction of tolerance. The surge of interest has resulted in the induction of donor-specific tolerance to cellular and vascularized organ allografts by intrathymic (IT) inoculation of donor cellular Ag.[29,30] This concept is based on the finding that intravenously administered radiolabeled resting mature T-cells and dendritic cells (DC) do not circulate through the thymus,[31] thus suggesting that lymphocyte traffic from the thymus is strictly unidirectional. It also relies on the well-known hypothesis that presentation of Ag not represented in the thymus to immature lymphocytes in the thymic micro-environment can induce self-tolerance.

We have employed IT-injection of donor UV-B irradiated (600 J/m^2) SC combined with recipient conditioning with 200 rads sublethal total body irradiation (TBI) to consistently induce donor-specific unresponsiveness to cardiac allografts[33,34] and islet allografts[34] in the Lewis-to-ACI rat combination.[35] The brief peritransplant immunosuppression with TBI more than likely modulates peripheral circulating T-cells that are capable of causing graft rejection prior to completion of "education" of putative antigen-tolerant T-cells and their migration to the periphery. Recently, we have further shown that IT-injection of donor resting T-cells (class I) but not resting B-cells or dendritic cells (class I and class II) combined with sublethal TBI or ALS led to permanent donor-type cardiac and islet allograft survival in the low responder Lewis-to-ACI[36,37] rat strain combination. IT inoculation of donor UV-B spleen cells, or T-cells combined with transient immunosuppression with ALS also induces specific unresponsiveness to islet allografts,[38] and to small intestinal allografts without clinical evidence of GVHD[39] in the high responder (WF-to-Lewis) rat strain combination. The finding that extrathymic inoculation of allogeneic cellular Ag via the intravenous route fails to prolong graft survival confirms the importance of the thymus in the induction of tolerance.[33,35,37] The inability of animals that were thymectomized at the time of heart transplantation, i.e. 7 days after IT inoculation of Ag, to maintain prolonged allograft survival suggests that the induction of tolerance is dependent on the continued transient presence of donor Ag in the thymus for at least about four weeks after Ag inoculation.[37] The observation that the long-term unresponsive recipients accepted a second-set, donor-type cardiac or islet allograft while rejecting a third-party allograft[35-39] reemphasizes the immunologic privileged position of the thymus in the development and maintenance of specific unresponsiveness of the immune system to self- or "pseudo-self" (modified alloantigens) antigens.

Our finding[40] that IT injection of purified resting allogeneic T-cells, but not DC induces specific tolerance led us to hypothesize that allopeptide presentation by thymic APCs may convey a tolerogenic signal to the recipient. We then examined if IT inoculation of allogeneic soluble Ag obtained from 3M KC1 extracts of purified resting T-cells can induce specific tolerance to cardiac allografts in transiently immunomodulated recipients. We have now shown that IT inoculation of donor soluble Ag combined with transient immunosuppression with ALS led to specific indefinite WF cardiac allograft survival (>200 days) in Lewis recipients.[41] This finding was not reproducible by intravenous injection of soluble Ag in ALS-treated animals. The unresponsive recipients accepted permanently donor-type but not third-party 2nd-set grafts. To define the role of recipient (self) APCs in Ag presentation, we have studied the presentation of soluble Ag in MLR. Our preliminary (unpublished) findings showed that primed T-cells obtained from Lewis rats sensitized to WF skin allografts responded to WF soluble Ag in MLR and that the proliferative response was enhanced by the addition of Lewis DC. Addition of anti-Lewis class II mab (0X3) blocked the alloresponse to soluble Ag, thus confirming the role of self APC in allorecognition. In contrast, WF primed Lewis T-cells failed to respond to ACI soluble Ag, thus demonstrating the specificity of allopeptide recognition. This observation emphasizes the importance of the alternate pathway of Ag presentation in the thymus. Extending this technique to islet allografts, in preliminary experiments we have now shown that IT inoculation of 1 mg 3M KC1 extracts of purified Lewis T-cells combined with 1 ml ALS pretransplant immunomodulation leads to 3/7 indefinite Lewis islet allografts survival (>200 days) in WF diabetic recipients. On the other hand, IT inoculation of 2.0 mg Lewis soluble Ag induces indefinite prolongation of islet allografts in unmodified (no ALS treatment) WF diabetic recipients. It therefore appears that induction of donor-specific unresponsiveness in this model depends on the dose of soluble Ag inoculated into the thymus. These findings strongly suggest that IT inoculation of donor soluble MHC peptides has potential therapeutic application in larger animals and eventually in clinical transplantation.

UNDERLYING MECHANISMS OF EFFECT OF UV-B IRRADIATION ON THE IMMUNE SYSTEM

UV-B Induced Anergy

We and others have shown that UV-B irradiated cells do not respond to or stimulate alloantigens in MLR.[7,8] The underlying mechanism of UV-B effect on APC function remains poorly defined; recent studies suggest that impairment of accessory cell function is due to defect(s) at the molecular level. It has been shown that suppression of DTH and GVHR by UV-B irradiation is associated with failure of production of accessory molecules (cytokines).[28,42,43] Lymphocytes obtained from UV-B treated and sensitized mice show a state of anergy in MLR due to suppression of IL-2 and IFNγ production associated with a concomitant increase in IL-4 secretion.[42,43] This raises the possibility that UV-B may selectively suppress Th1 T-cells, while augmenting or sparing the functional capacity of Th2 T-cells. We have studied the underlying mechanisms of the state of anergy produced by UV-B in vitro. Our results suggest that the inability of UV-B treated stimulators to induce T-cell activation is due to failure of production of IL-2 and IL-6.[28,44] These studies suggest that a UV-B induced defect in certain, as yet unidentified, accessory signals required for T-cell activation aborts the synthesis of IL-2 and other lymphokines. We speculate that these undefined accessory molecules modulated by UV-B may be adhesion molecules. This hypothesis receives support from our finding that UV-B irradiation abolishes the homing of T-cells and DCs to lymph nodes, and prevents their binding to frozen sections of lymph nodes.[31]. Our results suggest that UV-B modulates the expression or function of T-cell surface adhesion molecules (LFA-1 and VLA-4), which are necessary for HEV recognition through binding to ligands (ICAM-1, ICAM-2, and VCAM-1) present on the surface of endothelial cells.[45]

Molecular Defects Induced by UV-B

UV-B-radiation has been shown to alter the accessory function of a number of different cell types, including epidermal Langerhans cells,[46] dendritic cells,[47] and cells of macrophage/monocytic[48-50] origin. This effect has also been accepted to be applicable to other cell types that can acquire the function of antigen presenting cells, through the expression of MHC class II molecules, such as activated vascular endothelial cells[51] and islet β cells from prediabetic and diabetic pancreata.[52] Central to these observations is the identification of the defect that accompanies UV-B exposure. Loss of MHC class II determinants on lymphocytes, especially HLA-DP and HLA-DQ, following UV-B irradiation has been described,[53] as have alterations in IL-1 production and antigen processing.[54] However, the inability to completely restore the T cell proliferative response after binding to irradiated APCs by adding exogenous IL-1 or processed antigen suggested that additional accessory signals might be inhibited.

Intercellular adhesion molecule-1 (ICAM-1/CD54) and B cell activation antigen (B7/BB1), expressed by APCs, are necessary costimulatory signals for accessory cell function and T cell activation. The interaction of B7 and its ligand CD28 is known to stimulate T cell proliferation by directly affecting IL-2 gene transcription and expression,[55] while T cell activation is inhibited by mabs against ICAM-1.[56] Furthermore, mouse L cells co-transfected with ICAM-1 and HLA-DR can be rendered effective in presenting alloantigen to human lymphocytes.[57] Recent studies that focused on the effects of UV-B on ligand surface expression show that ICAM-1 and B7 surface expression is abrogated on irradiated prototype APCs. Human blood dendritic cells constitutively express high levels of these molecules, which are up-regulated after co-culture with allogeneic CD4+ T cells.[47] However, following alloreactive T cell binding, the de novo upregulated expression on UV-B-treated cells is abolished. Similarly, UV-B-exposure produces a dose-dependent decrease in ICAM-1 cell expression on human blood monocytes[48] and epidermal Langerhan cells,[46] associated with a corresponding decrease in cluster formation and primary alloreactive response.[48] T cell proliferation was severely abrogated without supplemental IL-2 while T cell alloreactivity was preserved in a secondary response.[47]

Based on these results, it has been proposed that UV-B might exert its immunomodulatory effects by altering costimulatory ligand expression on APCs, thereby inducing a state of T cell anergy. This hypothesis, however, is rooted on the assumption that alterations in ligand expression on irradiated APCs are not necessarily associated with the in vitro cytotoxicity caused by sublethal doses of UV-B. Evidence from two recent studies argues against this assumption: doses of UV-B that inhibit Langerhans cell function and ICAM-1 expression cause a delayed cytotoxic effect on these cells in vitro[58,59] and UV-B is a potent agent for the induction of programmed cell death, apoptosis, in human lymphocytic and monocytic cell lines.[60-65]

Following UV-B exposure, cell death can occur by two distinct mechanisms, those of necrosis and apoptosis. Mildly injurious doses cause the cell to trigger its endogenously programmed cell suicide, apoptosis, while necrosis is produced with higher, more directly damaging, doses.[60,61] The latter is a passive and degenerative process, characterized by swelling of mitochondria, immediate loss of membrane function, integrity, and cell lysis. In marked contrast, apoptosis is a gene directed process, which requires the active participation of the dying cell, either at the level of RNA and/or protein synthesis or protein kinase activity.[66,67] The cell mobilizes a cascade of highly ordered events, beginning with a reduction in cell volume and condensation of the cytoplasm (cell shrinkage) and ending with cell disintegration into intact vesicles, apoptotic bodies, which are subsequently phagocytosed. Although the onset of apoptosis is rapid, the membrane's structural integrity and transport function are maintained in the initial stages. Apoptotic cells exclude vital dyes, such as trypan blue and propidium iodide, and thus can be erroneously classified as viable.[68] They can be distinguished from both living and necrotic cells by a number of morphological, biochemical and molecular criteria. The major biochemical events of apoptosis are chromatin condensation and cleavage of chromosomal DNA, after activation of an endonuclease, into units of single or multiple nucleosome-sized fragments (approximately 180-200 bp), observable as a "DNA ladder" on gel electrophoresis. Since DNA from necrotic cells typically appears on electrophoresis as a smear of random-sized fragments, this highly characteristic pattern of DNA cleavage has come to be accepted as a molecular marker of apoptosis.[69,70] Nuclear DNA fragmentation and changes in the morphology of apoptotic cells affect their light scattering properties.[70] This makes possible the identification of cells undergoing apoptosis by flow cytometry light scatter measurements. An increase in orthogonal scatter and a decrease in forward scatter correspond to the reduction in cellular volume and increase in granularity typical of apoptotic cells. This simple assay has the advantage that it can be effectively combined with an immunofluorescent analysis of cell surface expression. Thus, it can both identify the particular phenotype of the apoptotic cell and correlate changes of the surface expression of specific molecules with DNA fragmentation.[68]

Lymphocytic and monocytic cell lines in response to sublethal doses of UV-B undergo apoptosis characterized by morphological changes and patterns of DNA fragmentation previously described. Furthermore, UV-B-induced apoptosis of HL60 cells and thymocytes requires extracellular Ca^{2+} and the process can be inhibited by the addition of Zn^{2+} to the culture medium in a dose dependent manner.[60,71] Such evidence raises the possibility that UV-B-induced alterations in cell surface expression of costimulatory signals might ultimately occur in cells undergoing apoptosis. We addressed this possibility by examining the effects of UV-B on DNA integrity and surface expression of MHC class I and class II antigens, ICAM-1 and B7 molecules on three model cell culture systems with relevance to transplantation: (1) the human monocytic cell line THP-1, established from a patient with monocytic leukemia which exhibits distinct monocytic markers that are maintained in tissue culture conditions.[72] The cytokine interferon-γ (IFNγ) up-regulates in this cell line cell surface expression of HLA and CD54 and the production of the cytokines IL-1b, TNF-α and IL-6[73]; (2) Human umbilical vein endothelial cells (HUVECs) established in primary culture in our laboratory from umbilical cord were used as monolayers following[2-4] passages for studies of adhesion molecule expression. The immunogenicity of these cells depends on expression of both MHC and costimulatory molecules.[74] Under standard culture conditions, they express class I but not class II. In our hands, HUVECs express basal levels of ICAM-1 while exogeneous IFNγ induces class II and upregulates the expression of both class I and ICAM-1 in these cells;[74] (3) the human islet β cell line HP62,[75,76] obtained by transfection of human pancreatic islet cells with SV40 viral DNA, maintains in vitro several of the characteristics of the parental cell. The maintenance of insulin secretion following early passages supports endocrine origin of these cells. Insulin production is, however, lost in subsequent passages. HLA and ICAM-1 expression is readily induced by IFN-γ and modulated with high doses of TNF-α;[76] (4) the rat insulinoma cell line RIN,[77] established from a rat cell tumor, is an insulin producing cell line that mimics the behaviour of β cells from the prediabetic and newly diabetic pancreas. Thus, these cells represent a valuable in vitro system for studying the induction pathways of HLA and costimulatory molecules. We used one sub-clone RINm5F which exhibits a class I response to IFN-γ. The pattern of constitutive and induced expression of the molecules under analysis on each cell type is illustrated in Figure 10.1. In summary, all cell types constitutively express high levels of MHC class I, whereas MHC class II and ligand B7 are constitutively expressed only by the monocytic cells. High levels of ICAM-1 can be detected on HUVEC and monocytes: ICAM-1 is expressed at low levels on the two islet cell lines. IFN-γ enhances the expression of these molecules de novo within 4-12 hours of treatment, both at a transcriptional and cell surface level in monocytes and HUVEC. However, a much longer period of treatment (5-7 days) is needed to induce class II expression of HP62 and RIN islet cells. Since we concentrated on the short-term effects of UV-B exposure immediately prior to incubation with IFN-γ, we did not study the upregulation of MHC class II in HP62 and RIN over this prolonged period of time. We also found that IFN-γ does not induce B7 ligand expression on islet cells or HUVECs.

To distinguish the effects of UV-B on constitutive and de novo induced expression, cells untreated and treated with IFNγ (500 to 1000 U/ml) were exposed to UV-B and 6-48h later were analyzed by FACS. Results obtained by such analysis are shown in Figures 10.1 and 10.2. Irradiation did influence the constitutive expression of these molecules. However, the expression of heat-shock proteins (HSP70) and the adhesion molecules Mac-1/CD11b and lymphocyte function an-

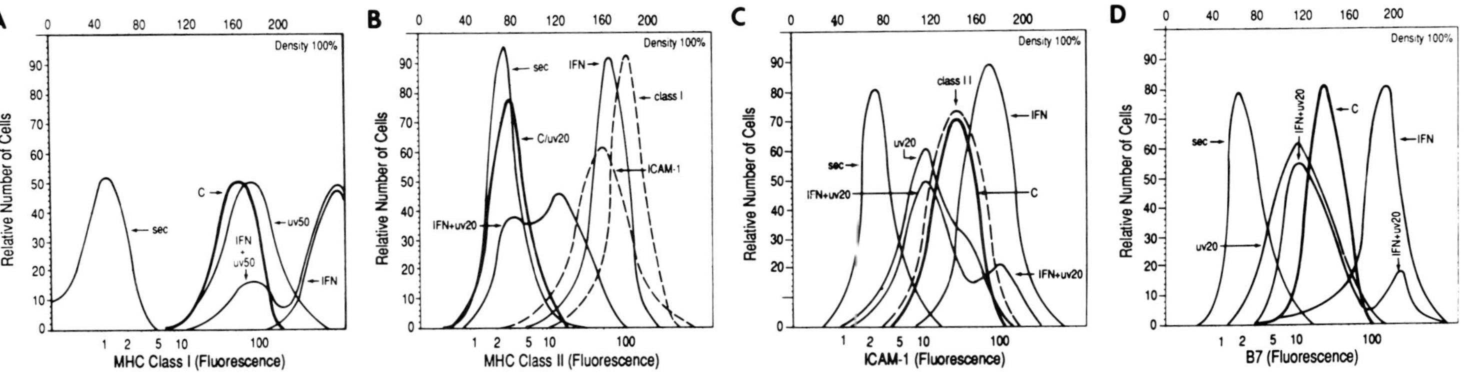

Fig. 10.1. Representative flow cytometric analysis of MHC class I (A) on RINm5F cells, MHC class II (B) on HUVEC, ICAM-1 (C) and B7 (D) on THP-1. C (control) in all histograms represents the constitutive expression of each of these molecules. IFN + UV-B; Cells were irradiated with UV-B at the various doses immediately prior to incubation with IFNγ at 500U/ml (HUVEC and THP-1) and 1000U/ml (RINm5F).

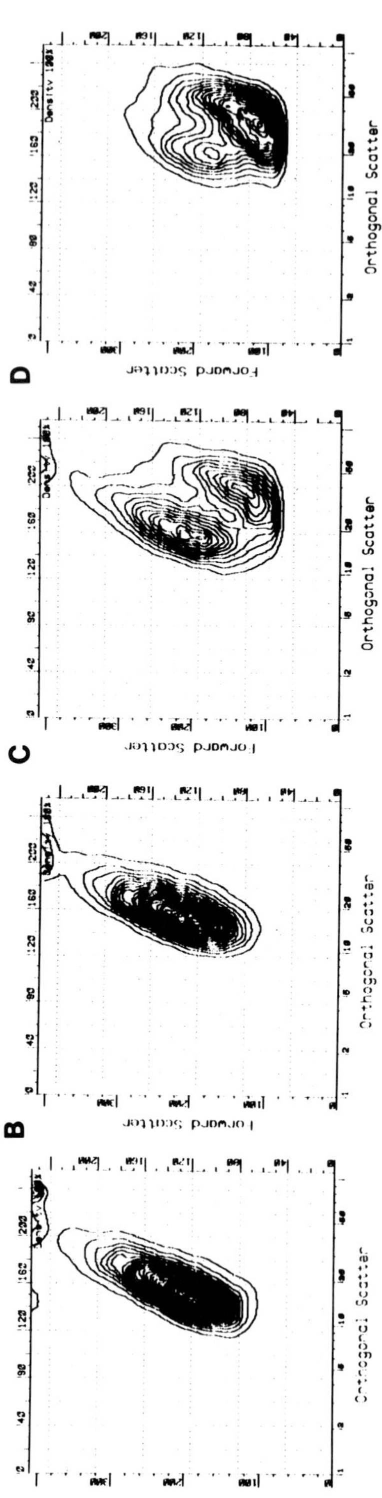

Fig. 10.2. Representative flow cytometric light scatter profiles of A: untreated THP-1 cells; B: IFNγ treated cells (500U/ml for 24h); C: IFN-γ + UV-B (20ml/cm^2); D: IFNγ+ UV-B (50ml/cm^2). UV-B irradiation was immediately prior to incubation with IFNγ.

tigen (LFA-1/CD11a) [used as controls, data not shown] was unaffected. The IFN-induced expression of MHC antigens (Figs. 10.1A and 10.1B), ICAM-1 (Fig. 10.1C) and B7 (Fig. 10.1D) when cells were harvested 6-24h after irradiation was inhibited in a portion of the cells. At a high dose (50 mJ/cm^2) of UV-B irradiation endothelial and monocytic cells uniformly exhibited down-regulation to basal levels (data not shown). Expression of these molecules could be detected up to 24h after exposure, when necrotic cell death began to occur. After electrophoresis in agarose gels and staining with ethidium bromide, DNA prepared from these cells was visualized and was found to be cleaved into nucleosomal-sized fragments (Fig. 10.3, Lanes 5 and 9). At lower doses (10-20mJ/cm^2), cells treated with IFN could be separated into two distinct subpopulations: one with high levels of molecule expression and a light scatter profile (High Forward/Low Orthogonal) characteristic of living cells (Fig. 10.2A and 10.2B) while the other exhibited only basal levels of expression and a light scatter profile (Low Forward/High Orthogonal) consistent with apoptosis (Fig. 10.2C and 10.D). Only the DNA prepared from the second cell population, after cell sorting, was found to be fragmented (Fig. 10.3, Lanes 3, 4, 7 and 8). Thus, UV-B at low doses injures the cells stochastically, with 20% cell survival after 24 hours. These cells and their progeny retain their ability to respond to IFNγ and to stimulate allogeneic T cells in a mixed lymphocyte reaction (data not shown). The induction of apoptosis by UV-B in transformed β cells suggests that freshly isolated islets (from both rat and human) might naturally have a system (genes, endogenous endonucleases, receptors) that initiates programmed cell death in response to UV-B. Despite being presently unable to isolate fresh islets with 100% purity, we attempted to analyze the effects of UV-B on fresh islets from human and rat pancreata. After digestion with collagenase and enrichment for islets by ficoll-gradient centrifugation (human) and hand-picking (rat), purity was judged to be 50-90% and 90% respectively. Cells were then irradiated in vitro at sublethal doses (15mJ/cm^2 and 60mJ/cm^2 respectively) and 6h, 12h and 24h later low molecular weight DNA was prepared and analyzed by electrophoresis. DNA fragmentation was detected in the 6h and 12h samples (data not shown), suggesting that fresh cells of endocrine origin might be sensitive to UV-B via apoptosis. In order to identify the phenotype of the cells undergoing apoptosis, we are currently performing flow cytometry analysis, staining digests of human pancreas of varying islet purity with a battery of mabs specific for islets (N-1),[78] acinar tissue (J-28),[79] reticuloendothelial and lymphoid cells. Apoptosis occurs in various cell types under normal and stressful physiological conditions. The mechanism of cell death under different circumstances is incompletely understood. Although the underlying biochemical processes might be unique for each cell type and each change in extracellular milieu, it is possible that all cells might share a common cell program.

In summary, our studies have shown: (1) UV-B-induced unresponsiveness to IFNγ-induction of MHC and costimulatory signal expression occurs in cells undergoing apoptosis, (2) cells which are spared the effects of UV-B continue to express both constitutive and up-regulated levels of these molecules and (3) cultured endothelial and β cells are sensitive to UV-B, some dying by apoptosis, a mode of cell death not previously described in these cells. Thus, in our models modulation of IFN-induced expression of MHC and adhesion molecules by UV-B is associated with apoptosis and is not a direct effect of UV-B light per se, as previous studies have suggested.

The most plausible implication of these new results is that islet interstitial APCs and lymphocytes might be selectively targeted by UV-B as they naturally possess an endogenous endonuclease which, following activation by UV-B, produces DNA fragmentation and are therefore hypersensitive to UV-B, as Arlett at al[65] have reported. Since they are important in islet recipient sensitization, their elimination by apoptosis might lead to a reduction in graft immunogenicity and prolongation of allograft survival. As described previously (vide supra) UV-B (70mJ/cm^2) is

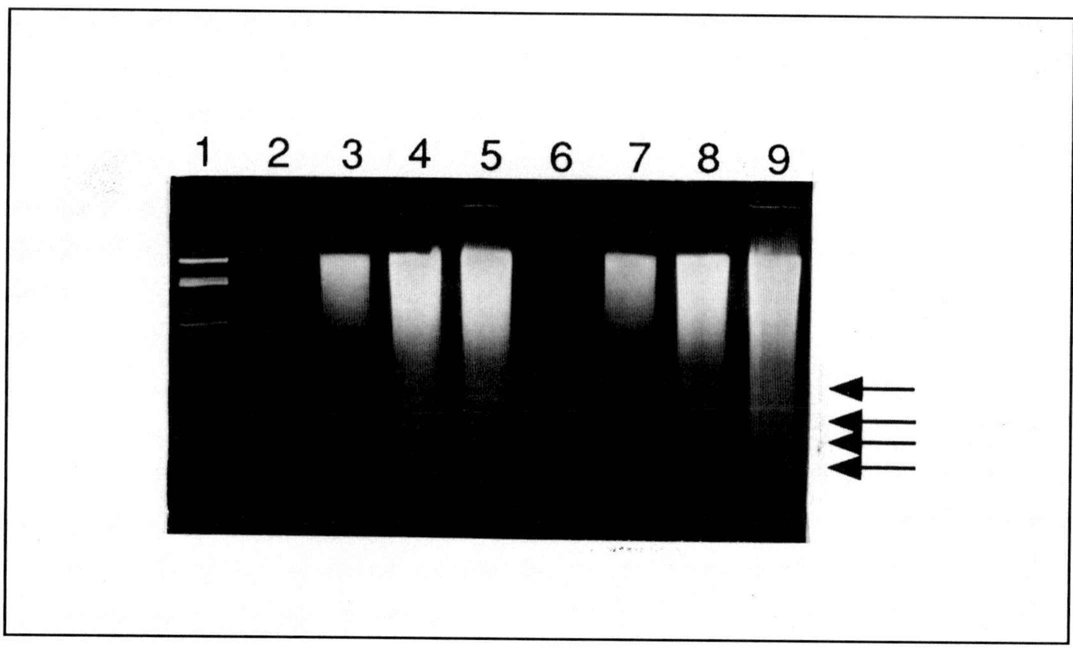

Fig. 10.3. Electrophoresis of DNA prepared from unirradiated, UV-B-irradiated and/or IFNγ treated THP-1 cells. Low molecular weight DNA was prepared from irradiated and/or IFNγ treated cells after 12h, electrophoresed on 1.5% agarose gels and stained with ethidium bromide. Cells were incubated with 500U/ml of IFNγ for 12 h immediately after exposure to UV-B at various doses.
DNA from:
Lane 1; Hind III digest of lamda-DNA and Hae III digest of -174-RF DNA respectively.
Lane 2; unirradiated cells.
Lane 3; UV-B, 10 mJ/cm²
Lane 4; 20 mJ/cm²
Lane 5; 50 mJ/cm²
Lane 6; IFNγ
Lane 7; IFNγ + UV-B, 10 mJ/cm²
Lane 8; IFNγ + UV-B, 20 mJ/cm²
Lane 9; IFNγ + UV-B, 50 mJ/cm²

not detrimental to the function of hand-picked Lewis rat islets, which successfully normalize blood glucose levels when transplanted into diabetic isogeneic, ACI, WF or BB recipients. Since rat islet β cells might also undergo apoptosis after exposure to UV-B (suggested by our preliminary data), UV-B at this dose might stochastically eliminate β cells, still leaving sufficient numbers, however, to reverse hyperglycemia. In the strongly responsive W/F-to-Lewis combination, a brief course of perioperative cyclosporine A, in addition to UV-B pretreatment of donor islets, results in indefinite islet graft survival. Cyclosporine A, by its ability to block the generation of IL-2,[80] might cause apoptotic cell death in certain mature alloreactive T cells: thus, we hypothesize that the synergy of UV-B and cyclosporine A is due to the induction of apoptosis both in donor APCs and sensitized recipient mature alloreactive T cells. Alternatively, apoptotic donor APCs might still anergize recipient alloreactive T cell clones induced in the absence of co-stimulatory signals. Although results from MLRs might give credence to this possibility, it remains to be shown which population of APCs, normal or apoptotic, induces T cell unresponsiveness. Finally, APCs dying by apoptosis, might retain their ability to activate suppressor T cells due to the persistence of an intact cell membrane and the expression of an as yet unidentified costimulatory signal.

ACKNOWLEDGEMENTS

This work was supported by NIH Grants CA52678 and HL14799, and The Kato Transplantation Fund.

REFERENCES

1. Pamphilon DH, Alnaqdy AA, Wallington TB. Immunomodulation by ultraviolet light:Clinical studies and biological effects. Immunol. Today 1991; 2:119-123.
2. Hardy MA, Oluwole SF. Effect of ultraviolet radiation on immunogenicity of tissues and organ allografts. Transplant. Rev. 1991; 5:46-62.
3. Snell GD. The homograft reaction. Ann. Rev. Microbiol. 1957; 2:439-458.
4. Lacy PE, Davie JM, Finke EH. Prolongation of islet allograft survival following in vitro culture (24°C) and a single injection of ALS. Science 1979; 204:312-313.
5. Lafferty KJ, Cooley MA, Woolnorgh S, Walker KZ. Thyroid allograft immunogenicity is reduced after a period in organ culture. Science 1975; 188:259-261.
6. Faustman D, Hauptfeld V, Lacy P, Davie J. Prolongation of murine islet allograft survival by pretreatment of islets with antibody directed to Ia determinants. Proc. Natl. Acad. sci. USA 1981; 78:5156-5159.
7. Lindahl-Kiessling K, Safwenberg J. Inability of UV-irradiated lymphocytes to stimulate allogeneic cells in mixed lymphocyte culture. Int. Arch. Allergy Appl. Immunol. 1971; 41:670-678.
8. Lau H, Reemtsma K, Hardy MA. Prolongation of rat islet allograft survival by direct ultraviolet irradiation of the graft. Science 1984; 223:607-609.
9. Hardy MA, Lau H, Weber C, Reemtsma K. Pancreatic islet transplantation:Induction of graft acceptance by ultraviolet irradiation of donor tissue. Ann. Surg. 1984; 200:441-450.
10. Sherwood RA, Brent L, Rayfield LS. Presentation of alloantigens by host cells. Eur. J. Immunol. 1986; 16:569-574.
11. Granelli-Piperno A, Inaba K, Steinman RM. Stimulation of lymphokine release from T-lymphoblasts. Requirement for mRNA synthesis and inhibition by cyclosporin A. J. Exp. Med. 1984; 100:1792-1802.
12. Lau H, Reemtsma K, Hardy MA. The use of direct ultraviolet irradiation and cyclosporine in facilitating indefinite pancreatic islet allograft acceptance. Transplantation 1984; 8:566-569.
13. Chabot JA, Lau H, Reemtsma K, Hardy MA. Long-term survival of islet allografts in spontaneously diabetic BB rats without chronic immunosuppression. Transplant. Proc. 1986; 18:1851-1853.
14. Chabot JA, Lau H, Reemtsma K, Hardy MA. Successful islet transplantation in BB rats without chronic immunosuppression. Transplant. Proc. 1987; 19:974-975.
15. Stegall MD, Chabot J, Weber C, Reemtsma K, Hardy MA. Pancreatic islet transplantation in cynomolgus monkeys. Transplantation 1989; 48:944-950.
16. Lau H, Reemtsma K, Hardy MA. Pancreatic islet allograft prolongation by donor-specific blood transfusions treated with ultra-violet irradiation. Science 1983; 221:754-756.
17. Hardy MA, Lau HT, Weber C, Reemtsma K. Pancreatic islet transplantation: Immunoalteration with ultraviolet irradiation. World J. Surg. 1984; 8:207-213.
18. Slavin S, Strober S, Fuks Z, Kaplan SJ. Induction of specific transplantation tolerance using mice:Long-term survival of allogeneic bone marrow and skin grafts. J. Exp. Med. 1977; 146:34-48.
19. Ildstat ST, Sachs DH. Reconstitution with syngeneic plus allogeneic or xenogeneic bone marrow leads to specific acceptance of skin allografts or xenografts. Nature 1984; 307:156-170.
20. Ferrara JLM, Deeg HJ. Graft-versus-host disease. N. Engl. J. Med. 1991; 324:667-674.
21. Martin PJ, Hansen JA, Storb B, Durnam D, Przepiorica D, O'Quigley J, Saunders J. Graft failure in the patients receiving T-cell depleted HLA-identical allogenic marrow transplants. Bone Marrow Transplant 1988; 3:445-456.
22. Pepino P, Hardy MA, Chabot J, Berger C, Marbow C, Wasfie T. UV-B irradiated allogeneic bone marrow transplantation in rats: Prevention of graft-versus-host disease without immunosuppression. Transplant. Proc. 1990; 49:886-889.

23. Chabot JA, Pepino P, Wasfie T, Stegall MD, Marboe C, Hardy MA. UV-B pretreatment of rat bone marrow allografts. Prevention of GVH and induction of allochimerism and donor-specific unresponsiveness. Transplantation 1990; 49:886-889.
24. Jin M, Engelstad K, Oluwole SF. Induction of stable chimerism and transplantation tolerance to rat islet and heart allografts by ultraviolet-B modulation of bone marrow cells. Transplantation 1992; 54:113-118.
25. Pamphilon DH, Alnaqdy AA, Godwin V, Preece AW, Wallington TB. Studies of allogeneic bone marrow and spleen cell transplantation in a murine model using ultraviolet-B light. Blood 1991; 77:2072-2078.
26. Cohn ML, Cahill RA, Deeg HJ. Hematopoietic reconstitution and prevention of graft-versus-host disease with UV-B irradiated haploidentical murine spleen and marrow cells. Blood 1991; 78:3317-3322.
27. Chowdhury NC, Jin MX, Oluwole SF. Prevention of graft-versus-host disease in rat small bowel transplantation by recipient pretreatment with UV-B modulated bone marrow cells. Transplantation 1993; 55:1229-1235.
28. Oluwole SF, Engelstad K, James T. Prevention of graft-versus-host disease and bone marrow rejection.Kinetics of induction of tolerance by UV-B modulation of accessory cells and T-cells in the bone marrow inoculum. Blood 1993; 81:1658-1665.
29. Posselt AM, Barker CF, Tomaszewski JE, Markman JF, Choh MA, Naji A. Induction of donor-specific unresponsiveness by intrathymic islet transplantation. Science 1990; 249:1293-1295.
30. Remuzzi g, Rossini M, Imberti O, Perico N. Kidney graft survival in rats without immunosuppressants after intrathymic glomeruli transplantation. Lancet 1991; 337:750-752.
31. Oluwole SF, Engelstad K, DeRosa C, Wang TST, Fawwaz RA, Reemtsma K, Hardy MA. Migration patterns of dendritic cells in the rat:Comparison of the effects of gamma and UV-B irradiation on the migration of dendritic cells and lymphocytes. Cell. Immunol. 1991; 133:390-407.
32. Oluwole SF, Chowdhury N, Fawwaz R, Hardy MA. Induction of tolerance to cardiac allografts by pretreatment with intrathymic UV-B donor spleen cells. Transplant. Proc. 1992; 24:2904-2905.
33. Oluwole SF, Chowdhury NC, Fawwaz RA. Induction of donor-specific unresponsiveness to rat cardiac allografts by intrathymic injection of UV-B irradiated donor spleen cells. Transplantation 1993; 55:1389-1395.
34. Jin MX, Chowdhury NC, James T, Engelstad K, Hardy MA, Oluwole SF. Prolongation of islet allografts by pretreatment with intrathymic UV-B donor spleen cells. Transplant. Proc. 1993; 25:291.
35. Oluwole SF, Jin MX, Chowdhury NC, James T, Fawwaz RA. Induction of specific unresponsiveness to rat islet allografts by intrathymic UV-B donor spleen cells. Transplantation 1993; 56:1142-1147.
36. Oluwole SF, Chowdhury NC, Fawwaz R, James T, Hardy MA. Induction of specific unresponsiveness to rat cardiac allografts by pretreatment with intrathymic donor major histocompatibility complex class I antigens. Transplant. Proc. 1993; 25:299-300.
37. Oluwole SF, Chowdhury NC, Fawwaz RA. Induction of donor-specific unresponsiveness to rat cardiac allografts by pretreatment with intrathymic donor MHC class I antigens. Transplantation 1993; 55:1396-1402.
38. James T, Jin MX, Chowdhury NC, Oluwole SF. Tolerance induction to rat islet allografts by intrathymic inoculation of donor spleen cells. Transplantation 1993; 56:1146-1152.
39. Chowdhury NC, Fawwaz RA, Oluwole SF. Induction of donor-specific tolerance to rat cardiac and small bowel allografts by intrathymic inoculation of donor T-cells. J. Surg. Res. 1993; 54:368-374.
40. Oluwole SF, Chowdhury NC, Jin MX. The relative contribution of intrathymic inoculation of donor leukocyte subpopulations in the induction of specific tolerance. Cell. Immunol. 1994 (in press).
41. Oluwole SF, Chowdhury NC, Jin M, Hardy MA. Induction of transplantation tolerance to rat cardiac allografts by intrathymic inoculation of allogeneic soluble peptides. Transplantation 1993; 56.

42. Ullrich SE. Suppression of the immune response to allogeneic histocompatibility antigens by a single exposure to ultraviolet radiation. Transplantation 1986; 42:287-291.
43. Araneo BA, Dowell T, Moon HB, Daynes RA. Regulation of murine lymphokine production in vivo:Ultraviolet radiation exposure depresses IL-2 and enhances IL-4 production in T-cells through an IL-1 dependent mechanism. J. Immunol. 1989; 143:1737-1744.
44. Oluwole SF, Stegall MD, Engelstad K, Reemtsma K, Hardy MA. Restoration of immunogenicity of UV-B-irradiated stimulator cells by the addition of lymphokines. Surg. Forum 1989; 40:378-381.
45. Shimizu Y, Newman W, Tanaka Y, Shaw S. Lymphocyte interactions with endothelial cells. Immunol. Today 1992; 13:106-112.
46. Simon JC, Krutmann J, Elmets CA, Bergstresser PR, Cruz PD. Ultraviolet B irradiated antigen-presenting cells display altered accessory signaling for T-cell activation: relevance to immune responses initiated in skin. J. Invest. Dermatol. 1992; 98:66S-69S.
47. Young JW, Baggers J, Soergel SA. High-dose UV-B radiation alters human dendritic cell costimulatory activity but does not allow dendritic cells to tolerize T lymphocytes to alloantigen in vitro. Blood 1993; 11:2987-2997.
48. Krutmann J, Kahn IU, Wallis RS, Zhang F, Rich EA, Ellner JJ, Elmets CA. Cell membrane is a major locus for ultraviolet B-induced alterations in accessory cells. J. Clin. Invest. 1990; 85:1529-1536.
49. Krutmann J, Kammer GM, Toossi Z, Waller RL, Ellner JJ, Elmets CA. UVB radiation and human monocyte accessory function: differential effects on pre-mitotic events in T-cell activation. J. Invest Dermatol. 1990; 94:204-209.
50. Hertl M, Kaplan DR, Fayen JD, Panuska JR, Ellner JJ, Elmets CA. The accessory function of B lymphocytes is resistant to the adverse effects of UV radiation. Eur. J. Immunol. 1991; 21:291-297.
51. Hughes CCW, Savage COS, Pober JS. The endothelial cell as a regulator of T-cell function. Immunol. Rev. 1990; 117:85-102.
52. Foulis AK, Farquharson MA. Aberrant expression of HLA-DR antigens by insulin-containing B-cells in recent-onset type I diabetes mellitus. Diabetes 1986; 35:1215-1224.
53. Deeg HJ, Sigaroudinia M. Ultraviolet B-induced loss of HLA class II antigen expression on lymphocytes is does, time, and locus dependent. Exp. Hematol. 1990; 18:916-919.
54. Rich EA, Elmets CA, Fujiwara H, Wallis RS, Ellner JJ. Deleterious effects of ultraviolet-B radiation on accessory function of human blood adherent mononuclear cells. Clin. Exp. Immunol. 1987; 70;116-126.
55. Fraser JD, Irving BA, Crabtree GR, Weiss A. Regulation of interleukin-2 gene enhancer activity by the T cell accessory molecule CD28. Science 1991; 251:313-316.
56. Makgoba MW, Sanders ME, Ginther Luce GE, Dustin ML, Springer TA, Clark EA, Mannoni P, Shaw S. ICAM-1 a ligand for LFA-1 dependent adhesion of B, T and myeloid cells. Nature 1988; 331:86-88.
57. Altmann DM, Hogg N, Trowsdale J, Wilkinson D. Cotransfection of ICAM-1 and HLA-DR reconstitutes human antigen-presenting cell function in mouse L Cells. Nature 1989; 338:512-514.
58. Tang A, Udey MC. Effects of ultraviolet radiation on murine epidermal langerhans cells: doses of ultraviolet radiation that modulate ICAM-1 (CD54) expression and inhibit langerhans cell function cause delayed cytotoxicity in vitro. J. Invest. Dermatol. 1992; 99:83-89.
59. Tang A, Udey MC. Doses of ultraviolet radiation that modulate accessory cell activity and ICAM-1 expression are ultimately cytotoxic for murine epidermal langerhans cells. J. Invest. Dermatol. 1992; 99:71S-73S.
60. Martin SJ, Cotter TG. Ultraviolet B irradiation of human leukaemia HL-60 cells in vitro induces apoptosis. Int. J. Radiat. Biol. 1991; 59:1001-1016.

61. Lennon SV, Martin SJ, Cotter TG. Dose-dependent induction of apoptosis in human tumour cell lines by widely diverging stimuli. Cell Prolif. 1991; 24:203-214.
62. Cotter TG, Lennon SV, Glynn JM, Green DR. Microfilament-disrupting agents prevent the formation of apoptotic bodies in tumor cells undergoing apoptosis. Cancer Research 1992; 52:997-1005.
63. Warters RL. Radiation-induced apoptosis in a murine T-cell hybridoma. Cancer Research 1992; 52:883-890.
64. Bazar LS, Deeg HJ. Ultraviolet B-induced DNA fragmentation (apoptosis) in activated T-lymphocytes and Jurkat cells is augmented by inhibition of RNA and protein synthesis. Exp. Hematol. 1992; 20:80-86.
65. Arlett CF, Lowe JE, Harcourt SA, Waugh APW, Cole J, Roza L, Diffey BL, Mori T, Nikaido O, Green MHL. Hypersensitivity of human lymphocytes to UV-B and solar irradiation. Cancer Research 1993; 53:609-614.
66. Wyllie AH, Kerr JFR, Currie AR. Cell death: the significance of apoptosis. Int. Rev. Cytol. 1980; 68:251-306.
67. Searle J, Kerr JFR, Bishop CJ. Necrosis and apoptosis: distinct modes of cell death with fundamentally different significance. Pathol. Ann. 1982; 17:229-259.
68. Darzynkiewicz Z, Bruno S, Del Bino G, Gorczyca W, Hotz MA, Lassota P, Traganos F. Features of apoptotic cells measured by flow cytometry. Cytometry 1992; 13:795-808.
69. Arends MJ, Morris RG, Wyllie AH. Apoptosis: the role of the endonuclease. Am. J. Pathol. 1990; 136:593-608.
70. Compton MM. A biochemical hallmark of apoptosis: internucleosomal degradation of the genome. Cancer Metast. Rev. 1992; 11:105-119.
71. Lennon SV, Kilfeather SA, Hallett MB, Campbell AK, Cotter TG. Elevations in cytosolic free Ca^{2+} are not required to trigger apoptosis in human leukaemia cells. Clin. Exp. Immunol. 1992; 87: 465-471.
72. Tsuchiya S, Yamabe M, Yamaguchi Y, Kobayashi Y, Konno T, Tada K. Establishment and characterization of a human acute monocytic leukemia cell line (THP-1). Int. J. Cancer 1980; 26:171-176.
73. Vey E, Zhang J-H, Dayer J-M. IFN-γ and $1,25(OH)_2D_3$ induce on THP-1 cells distinct patterns of cell surface antigen expression, cytokine production, and responsiveness to contact with activated T cells. J. Immunology 1992; 149:2040-2046.
74. Van Seventer GA, Newman W, Shimizu Y, Nutman TB, Tanaka Y, Horgan KJ, Gopal TV, Ennis E, O'Sullivan D, Grey H, Shaw S. Analysis of T cell stimulation by superantigen plus major histocompatibility complex class II molecules or by CD3 monoclonal antibody: costimulation by purified adhesion ligands VCAM-1, ICAM-1, but not ELAM-1. J. Exp. Med. 1991; 174:901-913.
75. Soldevila G, Buscema M, Marini V, Sutton R, James RFL, Bloom SR, Robertson RP, Mirakian R, Pujol-Borrell R, Bottazzo GF. Transfection with SV40 gene of human pancreatic endocrine cells. J. Autoimmunity 1991; 4:381-396.
76. Vives M, Soldevila G, Alcalde L, Lorenzo C, Somoza N, Pujol-Borrell R. Adhesion molecules in human islet B-cells: de novo induction of ICAM-1 but not LFA-3. Diabetes 1991; 40:1382-1390.
77. Ono SJ, Colle E, Guttmann RD, Fuks A. Interferon-γ induces transcription and differential expression of MHC genes in rat insulinoma cell line RINm5F. Diabetes 1989; 38:911-916.
78. De Krijger RR, Aanstoot HJ, Kranenburg G, Verkerk A, Jongkind JF, Van Strik R, Lafferty KJ, Bruining GJ. Enrichment of β cells from the human fetal pancreas by flourescence activated cell sorting with a new monoclonal antibody. Diabetologia 1991; 35:436-443.

79. Albers GHR, Escribano MJ, Daher N, Nap M. An immunohistologic study of the feto-acinar pancreatic protein (FAP) in the normal pancreas, chronic pancreatitis, pancreatic adenocarcinoma, and intraabdominal metastases of adenocarcinomas. Am. J. Clin. Pathol. 1990; 93:14-19.

80. Bunjes D, Hardt C, Rollinghoff M, Wagner H. Cyclosporin A mediates immunosuppression of primary cytotoxic T cell responses by impairing the release of interleukin 1 and interleukin 2. Eur. J. Immunol. 1981; 11:657-661.

CHAPTER 11

Antibodies Directed to MHC Determinants For Transplantation

Denise Faustman

This series on pancreatic islet transplantation covers many perspectives and topics from islet isolation, cryopreservation, proliferation, microencapsulation, immunomodulation to islet human clinical trials to reverse the hyperglycemia of diabetes.

The major theme of this chapter concerns the use of antibodies as a mode of therapy to prevent graft rejection of both allografts and xenografts. It is important to mention early in this review that although antibodies are the common topic of this chapter, the role of antibodies is probably broader and more significant because these immunologic reagents have allowed the research community to demonstrate important mechanisms of graft rejection as well as the development of specific strategies to interfere with rejection.

Table 11.1 demonstrates that antibody therapy has been used to prove the validity of three major targets of immune interference. This review of the literature demonstrated that although the transplantation field is broad and diverse, the transplantation of islets was often the first tissue or cells used to prove the validity of these concepts.

This chapter will discuss the use of antibodies from three perspectives. First, this chapter will discuss the administration of antibodies to the host to inactivate or destroy the host's T cells. These therapies are routinely used clinically and have demonstrated the validity of targeting host T cells in alleviating or slowing immune rejection. This will be followed by a discussion of the use of antibodies to specifically rid the donor tissue of passenger lymphocytes prior to transplantation. This was first demonstrated in the islet transplantation field and now this therapy has progressed to clinical trials in the renal transplantation field. Third, this chapter will discuss new data demonstrating the use of inactivated antibodies to disguise dominant donor antigens in all donor cells prior to transplantation. The use of antibodies in this case validated a new concept of direct donor antigen modification to prevent immune rejection. An important distinction between the three therapies discussed in Table 11.1 is the target, i.e., T cells versus

Pancreatic Islet Transplantation Volume II: Immunomodulation of Pancreatic Islets, edited by Robert P. Lanza, MD, William L. Chick, MD;

passenger lymphocytes versus donor tissue. Another important distinction of these three therapies is whether the therapy can be applied in vitro, prior to transplantation, to prevent host treatment. The advantages and disadvantages of these targets for immune interference will be discussed.

THEORY I: INACTIVATION OR DESTRUCTION OF HOST'S T CELLS WITH ANTIBODY

Conventional transplantation wisdom dictates that if donor organs or cells of identical genetic origin are not available for transplantation, then immunosuppressive drugs must be used to prevent immune rejection. This premise was formulated in 1944 by Sir Peter Medewar and has influenced transplantation research for many years.[1] The goal of modern transplantation research is to treat the immune system of the recipient to prevent graft rejection (Table 11.1, Theory 1).

The inactivation of the immune system of the transplant host has been achieved by traditional transplantation rejection drugs such as azathioprine (Imuran), prednisone (steroids), cyclophosphamide, cyclosporine A and FK506. Many of these drugs are targeted against T cells as well as all lymphoid cells thus effectively controlling rejection but leaving the host susceptible to infections.

To attempt to add specificity to the anti-rejection therapy regiment, antilymphocyte or antithymocyte serum has been widely used as anti-rejection drugs. Although considerable variation in antibody preparation exists, there is extensive human and animal data demonstrating the effectiveness of these immunosuppressants.[2]

With the advent of hybridoma technology, the ability to produce in vitro large amounts of homogenous monoclonal antibody for infusion, yielded pure and reproducable antibody preparations useful for transplantation. Furthermore, the production of antibodies directed against specific lymphoid cell lineages could be designed.

The most common monoclonal antibody used in transplantation research is OKT3, an antibody directed to the CD3 protein, a molecule linked to the T cell antigen receptor. In culture experiments, OKT3 blocks killing by cytotoxic human T cells and in vivo, OKT3 induces T cell removal from the circulation.[3-6]

Table 11.1. Contrasting immunologic targets to prevent rejection

Target	Route	Goal	Approaches	
I. Recipient T cells	In vivo	Destroy or Inactivate	Drugs:	Steroid, Aziothoprine, FK506, Cyclosporine A
			Antibodies:	Polyclonal Serum, CD3, CD4, ICAM, HLA Class II
II. Donor Passenger Lymphocytes	In vitro	Destroy or Inactivate	Culture:	24° C, 37° C, Hyperbaric Oxygen
			Antibodies:	HLA class II antibodies, CD45 antibodies
			Irradiate:	UV
III. Donor Tissue	In vitro	Camouflage, mask or	Antibodies:	Non-lytic masking antibodies to eliminate donor donor antigens transplantation antigens
			Genetic Engineering:	β_2-microglobulin gene ablation

Although many other monoclonal antibodies directed to other T cell epitopes have been tried, CD3 or OKT3 monoclonal antibody therapy has remained the most effective. But even with the specificity conferred by this highly antigen specific therapy, adverse reactions still exist as well as limitations in clinical effectiveness. OKT3 is a murine anti-human antibody, and host immune responses to the murine protein are common, especially with prolonged or repeat infusion. Other side effects include pulmonary edema, fever and ineffectiveness of repeat dosages. These side effects and dwindling clinical effectiveness with repeated use are presumably due to host antibodies to the murine hybridoma as well as possibly host anti-idiotype responses to the antigen binding regions of the antibody.

To date, clinical islet transplantation programs have relied on monoclonal and polyclonal antibody therapy of the recipient. This may have been driven by many causes but a realization in the islet transplant field of the apparent toxicity of drugs such as cyclosporine A or steroids directed against the islets has allowed the consideration of antilymphocyte antibody treatment of the host as a major mode of therapy.[7,8] In the case of cyclosporine A, direct islet toxicity from the drug may be possible. In addition, many islet transplants lie ectopically in the terminal portal vessels of the liver. Some studies have documented extraordinarily high portal vein levels of "first-pass" cyclosporine A prior to liver detoxification thus conferring higher islet drug exposure. Steroids, a common regimen of drugs of the transplant surgeon, have long been known to induce diabetes. Therefore two of the common pharmaceutical approaches to prevent transplant rejection, cyclosporine A and steroids, are particularly poorly suited for islets.

The infusion of polyclonal and monoclonal anti-T cell antibodies into the islet cell transplant host represent effective therapies for this type of cellular transplant. The most recent publication from Federlin and his colleagues of the International Islet Transplantation Registry, document the most successful human islet transplants, in the setting of underlying type I diabetes, used polyclonal antiserum or monoclonal OKT3 therapy without cyclosporine A.[9] Therefore, although islets were not the first tissue to be transplanted with in vivo antibody therapy directed towards host T cells, islets represent one of the longest lasting types of tissues to heavily rely on this form of immunosuppressive therapy.

Monoclonal antibody and polyclonal antiserum treatment of the host substantiated the validity of the host T cell as an integral part of the rejection circuit. This use of antibodies with restricted target specificity opened the doors for the design of a "specific" bullet. Although the antibody maintained high specificity, the toxicity of antibody infusions suggested further improvements could be identified with alternative strategies or targets.

THEORY II: ELIMINATE PASSENGER LYMPHOCYTES FROM THE DONOR CELLS PRIOR TO TRANSPLANTATION

In direct contrast to the past Medawar theory exists the passenger lymphocyte theory. This concept was proposed by George Snell in 1957 and suggests that the transplantation antigens on donor cells are not necessarily the primary barrier to rejection, but instead transplants contain donor passenger lymphocytes that are highly immunogenic. Endocrine tissues, especially islets of Langerhans, have been at the forefront of demonstrating the validity of this concept. Furthermore, this theory introduced the possibility that perhaps the graft could be modified prior to transplantation by donor passenger lymphocyte depletion; this was a dramatic conceptual departure from the belief that only treatment of the recipient would be successful. The use of antibodies was important in validating this concept. Antibody treatment of the donor tissue was a specific tool to definitely target and eliminate the passenger lymphocytes and prove these donor lymphoid cells were important triggers of graft rejection.

In the early 1970s several different groups investigated the effect of organ pretransplant culture on inducing passenger lymphocyte depleting the donor cells (Table 11.1, Theory II). For instance, Jacobs in 1967 demonstrated culture of ovaries prior to transplantation prolonged survival.[10] Lafferty and colleagues in 1976 demonstrated marked prolongation of thyroid allograft survival by a period of 95% oxygen culture for 3-5 weeks prior to transplantation.[11] In 1979, Lacy and colleagues successfully used in vitro 24° C culture of rat islets for 4 days combined with antilymphocyte treatment of the recipient to achieve 85% rat allograft survival beyond 100 days.[12] Naji and co-workers similarly demonstrated prolonged survival of parathyroid allografts with 95% O_2 survival.[13] Similar culture procedures were applied to other tissues as well as xenografts, and culture appeared to be beneficial in decreasing tissue immunogenecity.

Why did culture change the immunogenicity of the transplant? The overriding opinion at the time was the increased susceptibility of passenger lymphocytes to death or inactivation with cell culture compared to parenchymal cells. It was observed that organ culture caused rapid degeneration of the vascular bed and free floating blood elements and lymphocytes in culture demonstrated decreased immunogenicity after culture, especially at low temperature (25° C), a methodology highly effective for prolonging islet allografts.[14] In addition, Opelz and Terasaki demonstrated that lymphocytes lost their ability to stimulate allogeneic lymphocytes in vitro when cultured at 24° C for 4 days.[15] The most convincing data, at this time, of a pre-transplant change in passenger lymphocyte content altering immunogenecity as a primary mechanism came from two types of experiments. First, established thyroid allografts could be rejected when a second uncultured thyroid of donor origin was transplanted into the recipient[14] and established islet allografts could be rejected by the injection of donor passenger lymphocytes, i.e., donor cells were recognized by $CD8^+$ cytotoxic T lymphocytes if the host was given a proper trigger.[14,16] It appeared as if the donor graft antigens remained and were poorly immunogeneic. This, in total, suggested the successfully transplanted tissue maintained expression of donor antigens but these proteins were not the primary trigger of graft rejection. The primary triggers of graft rejection were HLA class II expressing donor lymphocytes.

During the late 1970s, it was unclear if islets expressed the classic transplantation antigens such as HLA class I and HLA class II. Although it was initially reported that islets lacked class I and class II antigens, this appears to be a technical artifact secondary to stripping off the antigens with improper fixation.[17] Later studies demonstrated in the mouse in 1980[18] and then in the human in 1981[19] that islets selectively express HLA class I but not HLA class II antigens.

This opened the door to try to specifically and selectively remove passenger lymphocytes and test the Snell hypothesis. Since all lymphoid cells bear HLA class II antigens, freshly isolated islets were briefly treated with HLA class II specific antibodies and complement prior to transplantation to specifically kill possible passenger lymphocytes without harming the class II negative donor parenchymal cells (Table 11.1, Theory II). Transplantation of such pretreated islets resulted in uniform allograft survival without any immune suppression of the recipient.[20] Similar to the previously discussed culture experiments, long-term fully allogeneic islet transplants briefly pretreated with HLA class II antibodies could be rejected by injecting the recipients with donor lymphocytes.[20] This again suggested that, at least in the case of allografts, the donor class I antigens by themselves, without accompanying passenger lymphocytes, were not necessarily immunogeneic triggers of rejection and passenger lymphocytes played a major role in triggering the rejection cascade.

Other experimental data accumulated and demonstrated the presumed role of donor passenger lymphocytes in the rejection cascade. In 1982, Batchelor's laboratory demonstrated that long-term surviving immunologically enhanced, rat kidney transplants when transplanted from a primary to a secondary host did not elicit rejection, (normal rejection-12 days).[21] This was again indirect evidence in favor of a loss of passenger lymphocytes. Sollinger, et al in 1983 used donor tissue passage in an athymic mouse as a way of eliminating short-lived donor passenger lymphocytes in vivo prior to transplantation into the allogeneic host.[22]

The direct visualization of HLA class II positive cells within the parenchymal tissues such as kidney was first demonstrated by Hart and Fabre.[23] The presence of HLA class II positive cells in islets was in 1984.[24] Furthermore, detailed characterizations of these scattered lymphoid cells with sub-set specific antibodies revealed the majority of these passenger lymphoid cells to be dendritic cells, a highly immunogeneic and excellent antigen presenting cells. As predicted, selective and specific removal of donor dendritic cells with dendritic cell specific serum prior to transplantation resulted in long-term islet allograft survival without any drug treatment of the murine recipients.[24] Therefore, passenger lymphocytes were visible in donor tissues with antibodies, could be specifically eliminated with lymphocyte specific antibodies and lymphocyte subset analysis revealed donor dendritic cells to be an important passenger lymphocytes in the rejection circuit.[25]

If passenger lymphocytes were important triggers of graft rejection, then other strategies to selectively inactivate these lymphoid cells would be tested (Table 11.1, Theory II). The immunologic literature in the early 1980s published extensively on ability of UV irradiation of inactivate antigen-presenting lymphocytes. In 1984, ultraviolet irradiation of donor rat allografts also abrogated rejection.[26]

If passenger lymphocytes could be selectively removed with lymphocyte specific antibodies in islet allografts, the strategy should work for other parenchymal tissue and cellular transplants. Lytic antibody pretreatment of donor rat cardiac transplants, donor pancreas transplants and even canine renal allografts demonstrated significantly prolonged survival with antibody directed to donor lymphocytes.[27-29] Most importantly, renal graft pretreatment with lymphocyte specific antibodies decreased the incidence of kidney allograft rejection episodes in humans.[30] Further clinical trials in the United States are being conducted to expand these results.

The successful and specific antibody mediated depletion of passenger lymphocytes prior to transplantation validated the role of passenger lymphocytes in allograft rejection. Furthermore, this experimental data demonstrated antibody treatment to delete passenger cells, was in and of itself, sufficient to achieve long-term transplant survival without the use of immunosuppressive drugs in the recipient.[20,24]

THEORY III: CAMOUFLAGE, MASK OR GENETICALLY ELIMINATE DONOR TRANSPLANT ANTIGENS PRIOR TO TRANSPLANTATION (TABLE 11.1)

Throughout the mid 1980s, a large body of literature defined the mechanisms of cytotoxic T lymphocyte (CTL) killing of targets. This literature defined CTL killing as three separate steps: CTL adhesion, CTL activation and CTL lysis of the target.[31] Each of these steps was possibly by a lock and key mechanism of reciprocal structures (proteins) between the CTL and target. In brief, adhesion, Step 1, was driven by reciprocal adhesion structures on both the target and CTL such as LFA-3, ICAM-1, LFA-1, etc. These steps were apparently reversible because separation of the two cells yielded no damage to the target, no T cell activation and no T cell memory. Step 2 involved the T cell receptor (TCR), CD3 protein and CD8 protein complex of the T cell binding to the HLA class I target molecule. These steps occurred after Step 1 and the CTL acquired immunologic memory of the event. Step 3 involved lytic events, i.e., the actual lethal hits to the target cell which would result in lysis.

This basic science definition of CTL and target interactions suggested that these concepts could be useful tools for averting transplant rejection. As defined earlier in this review, systemic injections of lytic CD3 antibodies (OKT3) were very effective in prolonging kidney transplants. Presumably this therapy interfered with Step 2 of CTL killing by eliminating the attacking T cell. In addition, our bias was again to develop strategies aimed at altering the donor cells in vitro prior to transplantation, not the attacking T lymphocytes located in the host.

In order to possibly accomplish this goal, we set out to define the dominant antigens on the surface of islets. Although adhesion structures were common on the vascular endothelium of whole organs, freshly isolated islets were virtually devoid of these determinants such as ICAM-1, LFA-3, LFA-1, etc.[32] As we had demonstrated 10 years previously, a prominent protein on the surface of islets was HLA class I itself.

The literature at this time suggested donor HLA class I would be a poor target to modify to prevent CTL killing. In fact, the literature contended that donor HLA class I was non-immunogeneic. For instance, donor islets or thyroid depleted of passenger lymphocytes were easily rejected by the recipient receiving injections of donor lymphocytes, evidence that HLA class I was present on the stably transplanted tissue and was available for attack. Injections of isolated donor class I antigens were either weakly immunogeneic or even beneficial in the growth of tumor transplant models. Furthermore, donor specific immunologic unresponsiveness could be induced by pretransplant injections of donor cells transfected with donor HLA class I genes[33] or pretransplant injections of class I enriched donor cells.[34]

We were not discouraged by this literature. Although the passenger lymphocyte was a very important cell for triggering graft rejection, possible interference with the actual donor target structures for averting activated CTL attack seemed an appropriate alternative target. Furthermore, just like CD3 antibodies inhibiting MLR (mixed-lymphocyte reactions) between host T cells and the tissue and target, Stock et al similarly demonstrated that HLA class I antibodies inhibition MLR between host T cells and islet tissue in vitro.[35]

Although there are many methods to possibly immunologically disguise or eliminate donor HLA class I antigens, we first chose antibodies to possibly demonstrate the validity of this concept. To maintain molecular specificity rendered by the antibody but remove antibody lytic function, the tail of the antibody (Fc region) was removed by enzymatic treatment with papain. This yielded specific antibody target binding $F(ab')_2$ fragments without Fc antibody region complement activating function.

"Masking" of freshly isolated donor human islets with these non-lytic HLA class I antibodies allowed long-term xenograft survival and function without immunosuppression of the murine recipients.[32] This methodology worked in a tough islet xenograft model as well as in a liver xenografts model. Most importantly, this strategy worked without immunosuppressive regimens against the recipients. Furthermore, the successfully transplanted xenograft recipients even developed graft specific tolerance.[32]

In the case of islets and liver cells, donor HLA class I masking was sufficient for long-term survival. In addition, in these tissues, although masking all donor surface molecules with non-lytic polyclonal serum similarly allowed survival, other less dense surface proteins such as LFA-3, ICAM-1, etc. played a less important role and allowed less extended xenograft survival when masked prior to transplantation.[32] Furthermore, masking only the passenger lymphocytes did not prolong xenograft survival. Although high affinity HLA class I masking antibodies were difficult to produce, the experiments demonstrated the ability to avert graft rejection by directly modifying donor parenchymal structures, such as HLA class I. The literature expanded to other tissues and other variations of class I masking (Table 11.2, Theory III).[36,37] For instance, Dr. Wu in 1992 demonstrated prolonged skin allograft survival with HLA class I associated β2-microglobulin antibody masking. For cardiac transplantation, using a non-lytic antibody to donor LFA-1 combined with a lytic ICAM-1 antibody to recipient T cells allowed impressive whole heart allograft survival.[37]

If HLA class I was a dominant protein, then permanent donor ablation of class I seemed like an attractive expansion of this theory. This "universal" donor animal was available due to the transgenic ablation of HLA class I associated β2-microglobulin by two research groups.[38,39] Without β2-microglobulin production, HLA class I has difficulties producing a correct 3-dimensional structure for endoplasmic reticulum exit to the cell surface. The transgenic mice therefore have tissue expressing extraordinarily low levels of MHC class I antigens.

Markmann and colleagues in 1992 demonstrated that islets isolated from donor class I deficient mice demonstrated indefinite survival in non-immunosuppressed fully allogeneic recipients.[40] This experimental approach confirmed the central importance of donor class I elimination or masking as an important strategy for promoting prolonged survival. Importantly, although the grafts were resistant to transplant rejection, the grafts were fully susceptible to recurrent autoimmunity when transplanted into the autoimmune NOD mouse.[40] The transgenic class I deficient donor mice also beautifully worked for whole kidney transplants as demonstrated by Coffman and colleagues in 1993.[41]

Most importantly, the β2-microglobulin deficient mice yielded some variability in transplant survival based on the tissue being transplanted (Table 11.3). Liver allogeneic cells from HLA class I deficient mice only demonstrated partial survival.[42] Skin allografts demonstrated no prolonged survival.[43] Liver xenografts from HLA class I deficient mice survived long-term into markedly disparate frog recipients.[42] The rules of transplantation generally in the past suggest that allografts are easier to perform than xenografts and cellular transplants are easier to perform than whole organ transplants. The transgeneic ablated class I transplant data yielded results not consistent with these beliefs.

A likely explanation for why different donor tissues from class I deficient transgenic mice survive for different times and xenografts are at times more successful in this model now appears to be evident. One of the most plentiful proteins in the serum of all species is β2-microglobulin. Could host β2-microglobulin rapidly reconstitute the HLA class I deficient graft after transplantation? Indeed this appeared to be the case. Culture experiments have confirmed the ability of serum containing β2-microglobulin or media specifically supplemented with β2-microglobulin to rapidly reconstitute formerly β2-microglobulin deficient tissues at varying rates; this correlates with varying transplant survival times, i.e., liver rapid, islets and kidney slow. This can be observed by observing the reappearance of class I in tissue culture experiments.[42] Furthermore, in vitro and in vivo transplantation evidence confirms that transplantation of β2-microglobulin deficient murine cells into discordant xenogeneic species with non-identical β2-microglobulin tracks with the ability of these discordant β2-microglobulins to reconstitute the transgeneic graft and restore donor class I.[42] Therefore in vitro and in vivo

Table 11.2. "Masking" approaches to transplantation*

Tissue	Methods	Journal
Islets/Liver	"Masking" Donor HLA class I	Science (91) 252:1700
Islets	Polyclonal serum "masking" all donor antigens	Science (91) 252:1700
Heart	"Masking" donor LFA-1 with lytic ICAM-1 to recipient	Science (92) 255:1125
Skin	"Masking" donor HLA class I associated β2-microglobulin	J. Immunol. Res. (92) 4:21

* Masking refers in this text to coating donor cells with non-lytic antibody or antibody fragments generated by $F(ab')_2$ production

β2-microglobulin reconstitution of donor class I negative transgenic tissues correlates with the species divergence of β2-microglobulin and possibly explains the enhanced survival of xenografts over allografts in this trangeneic donor model of class I ablation.

The results of the above transplant studies using "masking" of donor class I or genetic interference with class I expression suggest a new model for prolonging allografts and xenografts. The critical role of donor MHC class I antigens in stimulating the rejection cascade or more likely serving as a critical target for the host rejection response is substantiated by diverse methods. Matching of MHC class I antigens between donor and recipients is virtually impossible but concealment or genetic elimination of donor class I is feasible. Transgenic animals with permanent modifications of their donor antigens will play an important future role in organ and cellular transplantation. New ways to genetically eliminate class I such as Tap-1/2 ablation or direct genetic interruption of class I itself will be important in the coming years in the search to find a universal donor animal. Importantly, antibodies allowed the validity of a novel transplantation concept to be tested. Once again, islets were the first tissue to be transplanted using this new approach of donor antigen elimination prior to transplantation.

Although the ablation, camouflaging or genetic elimination of donor class I is a new concept introduced into the transplant field in 1991, perhaps mother nature has already encouraged this trickery of the immune system. A large body of literature exists in the tumor field documenting the frequent occurrence of class I deficiency on malignant tumor,[44-48] perhaps allowing tumors to escape CTL attack. Furthermore, there is some literature suggesting the possibility that tumor hosts protect their tumors with nonlytic antibodies, therefore averting cytotoxic T lymphocyte killing of the malignancy.[49] Perhaps we have even come more full circle in our beliefs. There is even now transplantation data that suggests tissue culture of donor cells prior to transplantation works by down-regulation of class I not by passenger lymphocyte ablation.[50,51]

SUMMARY

The results presented in the three sections above demonstrate the central role antibodies have played in the transplant community in validating three different pathways of immunologic rejection and the development of three targets for averting rejection. The central role of the host T cell in triggering target destruction is well substantiated by the ability of intravenous monoclonal and polyclonal anti-T cell antibodies against host T cells to avert rejection. The central role of the class II positive passenger lymphocyte is substantiated by the extensive experimental and clinical data using lytic antibodies against donor passenger lymphocytes. Third, the substantiation of the dominant role of donor class I as a target for immune manipulation is substantiated by concealment of donor antigens pre-transplantation with disguising antibodies. This strat-

Table 11.3. Use of HLA class I deficient mice as organ donors

Tissue	Method	Success/Failure	Journal
Islets	β2-microglobulin ablation	Success	Transplantation (92) 54:1085
Skin	β2-microglobulin ablation	Failure	J. Exp. Med. (92) 175:885
Liver	β2-microglobulin ablation	Partial	Transplantation (93) 55:311
Kidney	β2-microglobulin ablation	Success	J. Immunol. (93) 151:425
Islets	β2-microglobulin ablation	Success	Diabetes (93) 42:1520

egy prevented xenograft rejection. Whether antibodies in transplantation remain the central drug in the future is unknown but what is certain is the recognized role of antibodies as the critical immunologic reagent to prove the mechanism of rejection and the development of novel approaches of immunologic interference.

References

1. Medawar PB. The uniqueness of the individual. New York: Basic Books, 1957.
2. Russell PS. Antilymphocyte sera for immunosuppression. In: Haber E,Krause R, ed(s). Human Diagnosis and Therapy. New York: Raven Press, 1977: 303-355.
3. Ortho Multicenter Transplant Study Group. A randomized clinical trial of OKT3 monoclonal antibody for acute rejection of cadaveric renal transplants. N.E.J.M. 1985;313:337-342.
4. Thurlow PJ, Lovering E, d'Apice AJ et al. A monoclonal antipan-T cell antibody: in vitro and in vivo studies. Transplantation 1983;36:293-298.
5. Takahashi H, Okazaki H, Terasaki PI et al. Reversal of transplant rejection by monoclonal antiblast antibody. Lancet 1983;2:1155-1158.
6. Kirkman RL, Araujo JL, Busch GJ et al. Treatment of acute renal allograft rejection with monoclonal anti-T12 antibody. Transplantation 1983;36:620-626.
7. Kneteman NM, Marchetti P, Tordjman K et al. Effects of cyclosporine on insulin secretion and insulin sensitivity in dogs with intrasplenic islet autotransplants. Surgery 1992;111:430-437.
8. Metrakos P, Hornby L,Rosenberg L. Cyclosporine and islet mass—implications for islet transplantation. J. Surg. Res. 1993;54:375-380.
9. Hering BJ, Browatzki CC, Schultz A et al. Clinical islet transplantation-registry report, accomplishments in the past and future research needs. Cell Transplant. 1993;2: 269-282.
10. Jacobs BB. Ovarian allograft survival. Prolongation after passage in vitro. Transplantation 1974;18:454-457.
11. Lafferty KJ, Bootes A, Dart G et al. Effect of organ culture on the survival of thyroid allografts in mice. Transplantation 1976;22:138-149.
12. Lacy PE, Davie JM,Finke EH. Prolongation of islet allograft survival following in vitro culture (24° C) and a single injection of ALS. Science 1979;204:312-313.
13. Naji A, Silvers WK,Barker CF. Effect of culture in 95% O_2 on the survival of parathyroid allografts. Surgical Forum 1979;30:109-111.
14. Parr EL, Bowen KM,Lafferty KJ. Cellular changes in cultured mouse thyroid glands and islets of Langerhans. Transplantation 1980;30:135-141.
15. Opelz G,Terasaki PI. Lymphocyte antigenicity loss with retention of responsiveness. Science 1974;184:464-466.
16. Lacy PE, Davie JM,Finke EH. Induction of rejection of successful allografts of rat islets by donor peritoneal exudate cells. Transplantation 1979;28:415-420.
17. Parr EL. The absence of H-2 antigens from mouse pancreatic β cells demonstrated by immunoferritin labeling. J. Exp. Med. 1979;150:1-9.
18. Faustman D, Hauptfeld V, Davie J et al. Murine pancreatic β cells express H-2K and H-2D but not Ia antigens. J. Exp. Med. 1980;151:1563-1569.
19. Baekkeskov S, Kanatsuna T, Klareskog L et al. Expression of major histocompatibility antigens on pancreatic islet cells. Proc. Natl. Acad. Sci. USA 1981;78:6456-6460.
20. Faustman D, Hauptfeld V, Lacy P et al. Prolongation of murine islet allograft survival by pretreatment of islets with antibody directed to Ia determinants. Proc. Natl. Acad. Sci. USA 1981;78:5156-5159.
21. Lechler RI,Batchelor JR. Restoration of immunogenecity to passenger cell-depleted kidney allografts by the addition of donor strain dendritic cells. J. Exp. Med. 1982;155:31-41.
22. Sollinger HW, Burkholder PM, Kuperman OJ et al. Xenotransplantation. Prolonged survival of xenografts after organ culture. Transplant. Proc. 1977;9:359-362.

23. Hart DN,Fabre JW. Demonstration and characterization of Ia-positive dendritic cells in the interstitial connective tissue of rat heart and other tissues, but not brain. J. Exp. Med. 1981;154:347-361.
24. Faustman D, Steinman R, Gebel H et al. Prolongation of mouse islet allograft survival by pretreatment of islets with anti-dendritic cell antibody. Diabetes 1984;33:242-249.
25. Faustman D, Steinman R, Hauptfeld V et al. Localization of dendritic cells within freshly isolated islets. Transplantation Proc. 1984;12:153-156.
26. Lau H, Reemtsma K,Hardy MA. Prolongation of rat islet allograft survival by direct ultraviolet irradiation of the graft. Science 1984;223:607-609.
27. Sone Y, Sakagami K,Orita K. Effect of ex vivo perfusion with anti-IA monoclonal antibodies on rat cardiac allograft survival. Transplant. Proc. 1987;19:599-604.
28. Lloyd M, Buckingham M, Stuart F et al. Does depletion of donor dendritic cells an allograft lead to prolongation of graft survival in transplantation? Transplant. Proc. 1989;21:482-483.
29. Otsubo O, Sakai A, Watanabe T et al. Effect of anti-mouse Ia monoclonal antibody on canine renal allograft survival. Transplant. Proc. 1983;15:797-799.
30. Brewer Y, Palmer A, Taube D et al. Effect of graft perfusion with two CD45 monoclonal antibodies on incidence of kidney allograft rejection. Lancet 1989;2:935-937.
31. Spits H, van Schooten W, Keizer H et al. Alloantigen recognition is preceded by non-specific adhesion of cytotoxic T cells and target cells. Science 1986;232:403-405.
32. Faustman D,Coe C. Prevention of xenograft rejection by masking donor HLA class I antigens. Science 1991;252:1700-1702.
33. Madsen JC, Superina RA, Wood KJ et al. Immunological unresponsiveness induced by recipient cells transfected with donor MHC genes. Nature 1988;332:161-164.
34. Faustman D, Lacy P, Davie J et al. Prevention of allograft rejection by immunization with donor blood depleted of Ia-bearing cells. Science 1982;217:157-158.
35. Stock PG, Ascher NL, Chen S et al. Modulation of MHC class I antigen decreases pancreatic islet immunogenicity. J. Surg. Res. 1989;46:317-321.
36. Wu J, Menapace L, Barisoni D et al. An anti-beta-2-microglobulin monoclonal antibody prevents the reactive proliferation of lymphocytes elicited by allo-human epidermal cells. J. Immunol. Res. 1992;4:21.
37. Isobe M, Yagita H, Okumura K et al. Specific acceptance of cardiac allograft after treatment with antibodies to ICAM-1 and LFA-1. Science 1992;255:1125-1127.
38. Koller BH,Smithies O. Inactivating the beta-2 microglobulin locus in mouse embryonic stem cells by homologous recombination. Proc. Nat'l. Acad. Sci. USA 1989;86:8932-8935.
39. Zijlstra M, Bix M, Simister NE et al. Beta 2-microglobulin-deficient mice lack CD4-8+ cytolytic T cells. Nature 1990;344: 742-746.
40. Markmann JF, Bassiri H, Desai NM et al. Indefinite survival of MHC class I-deficient murine pancreatic islet allografts. Transplantation 1992;54:1085-1089.
41. Coffman T, Geier S, Ibrahim S et al. Improved renal function in mouse kidney allografts lacking MHC class I antigens. J. Immunol. 1993;151:425-435.
42. Li X,Faustman D. Use of donor β2-microglobulin-deficient transgenic mouse liver cells for isografts, allografts, and xenografts. Transplantation 1993;55:940-946.
43. Zijlstra M, Auchincloss H, Loring JM et al. Skin graft rejection by beta 2-microglobulin-deficient mice. J. Exp. Med. 1992;175: 885-893.
44. Doherty PC, Knowles BB,Wettstein PJ. Immunological surveillance of tumors in the context of major histocompatibility complex restriction of T-cell function. Adv. Cancer Res. 1984;42:1-65.
45. Hui K, Grosveld F,Festenstein H. Rejection of transplantable AKR leukaemia cells following MHC DNA-mediated cell transformation. Nature 1984;311:750-752.
46. Rees RC, Buckle AM, Gelsthorpe K et al. Loss of polymorphic A and B locus HLA antigens in colon carcinoma. Br. J. Cancer 1988;57:374-377.

47. Karre K, Ljunggren HG, Piontek G et al. Selective rejection of H-2-deficient lymphoma variants suggests alternative immune defense strategy. Nature 1986;319:675-678.
48. Smith ME, Marsh SG, Bodmer JG et al. Loss of HLA-A,B,C allele products and lymphocyte function-associated antigen 3 in colorectal neoplasia. Proc. Natl. Acad. Sci. USA 1989;86:5557-5561.
49. Manson LA. Does antibody-dependent epitope masking permit progressive tumour growth in the face of cell-mediated cytotoxicity? Immunol. Today 1991;12: 352-355.
50. Markmann JF, Jacobson JD, Kiumura H et al. Modulation of the major histocompatibility complex antigen and the immunogenicity of islet allografts. Transplantation 1989;48:478-486.
51. Barker CF, Markmann JF, Posselt AM et al. Studies of privileged sites and islet transplantation. Transplant. Proc. 1991;23: 2138-2142.

CHAPTER 12

Tolerance and the Costimulatory Pathway

David M. Harlan

Carl H. June

Two barriers stand in the way of the cure of insulinopenic diabetes by pancreatic islet transplantation: a ready supply of islets and a means of preventing the immune-mediated rejection of the islets once transplanted. The latter problem may be particularly difficult in patients with type 1 diabetes because of the underlying autoimmune pathogenesis of the disease such that the affected individuals' T lymphocytes are sensitized against pancreatic β cells even before any grafting is attempted.[1,2] Other chapters in this series document the myriad approaches being developed to address these two central problems facing the diabetologist. In this chapter, we will discuss the problems from an immunologist's perspective. We will first briefly review some basic immunology and definitions, then discuss our current understanding of T cell activation. With this background, we will turn to exciting new research that suggests it may be possible to induce antigen-specific T cell tolerance via manipulation of the T lymphocyte costimulatory pathway.

DEFINITIONS AND BACKGROUND

The vertebrate immune system has evolved with the capacity to recognize essentially any antigen, even those that might arise by a new mutation and therefore have never previously existed. This important and virtually unlimited capacity of the immune system is a function of the fact that the antigen specific T cell receptor (TCR) expressed on the surface of individual T lymphocytes is generated during T cell ontogeny via a stochastic process of TCR gene fragment recombination. There are problems however, with this random generation of TCRs. One, since TCRs are "restricted" to recognize antigens (Ag) presented by self major histocompatibility complex (MHC) molecules, the vast majority of T cells developing within the thymus will express TCRs that are incapable of the required self MHC recognition. Therefore these T cells are functionally useless and they die during the thymic developmental process, i.e. they are not "positively selected".[3] The other problem that results from the random generation of the TCR reper-

Pancreatic Islet Transplantation Volume II: Immunomodulation of Pancreatic Islets, edited by Robert P. Lanza, MD, William L. Chick, MD; ©1994 R.G. Landes Company.

toire is that a finite number of the antigen specific TCRs will recognize self Ag/MHC on the surface of the antigen presenting cell (APC). Viewed in this context, these potentially self-reactive T cells are a necessary price paid for the luxury of an immune system with almost unlimited recognition potential.

Fortunately, the immune system has also evolved a multilayered fail-safe system to protect against self-reactive T cell mediated disease. Collectively, this system is referred to as tolerance.[4,5] Over the past two decades, several specific mechanisms underlying tolerance have been elucidated. The only infallible means of incapacitating a potentially autoreactive T cell is to eliminate it. It is now well documented using a variety of experimental techniques that many T cells with potential autoreactivity are deleted, or "negatively selected", during the thymic maturation process.[6] This thymic clonal deletion, which occurs through the induction of thymocyte programmed cell death, occurs only when a thymocyte bearing a self-reactive TCR encounters that Ag/MHC within the thymus. Therefore, T cells bearing TCRs with specificity against other-than-thymic self-antigens will escape thymic deletion. Indeed, the presence in vivo of circulating self-reactive T cells is well documented experimentally, so non-deletional tolerance mechanisms must exist to prevent disease.[7,8] One of at least four, not mutually exclusive, forms of non-deletional T cell tolerance mechanisms (defined below) bridle these lymphocytes from causing disease.

The proposed non-deletional T cell tolerance mechanisms share the common characteristic of allowing the coexistence in vivo of both APCs bearing the Ag/MHC, and circulating autoreactive T cells. Immune ignorance is defined as tolerance due to the physical separation of these two cellular entities. It is known, for example, that circulating naive T cells migrate preferentially through lymphoid organs and therefore avoid many of the self antigens expressed via MHC class I molecules on non-lymphoid tissue cells.[9] What if a self-reactive T cell, and an APC bearing the self-Ag/MHC do come in contact? In this circumstance, immunologic civil war can still be averted if the potentially autoreactive T cell recognizes the self-Ag/MHC, and yet either does not achieve an activation threshold (indifference), or has somehow "learned" that the self-antigen is one to leave alone (anergy). Anergy is defined experimentally as the functional inactivation of a T cell such that when exposed to self-Ag/MHC under conditions that would otherwise have activated the T cell, it neither proliferates nor produces interleukin-2 (IL-2).[10,11] The important difference between the anergy and indifference tolerance mechanisms is that the former is an active "shutting off" of the T cell, while the latter is a neutral event for the T cell. The final general mechanism of tolerance, suppression, requires the presence of one or more other "suppressor" cells that function to prevent or blunt an immune response that would otherwise result when antigen-specific T cells and APCs bearing that self-Ag/MHC interact.[12,13] Each of these general tolerance mechanisms is now supported by sound experimental evidence, and each is almost certainly relevant in vivo as part of a redundant system to prevent autoimmune illness. Unfortunately, these redundant non-deletional tolerance mechanisms are not fool-proof and T cell mediated autoimmune diseases like type 1 diabetes result.

T CELL ACTIVATION

The two signal hypothesis of lymphocyte activation[14,15] first proposed by Bretscher and Cohn in 1970 to address the problem of self:non-self discrimination by B lymphocytes[16] was later generalized to explain the behavior of T lymphocytes.[14,17] Stated succinctly, the T cell was thought to express two general types of signalling receptors, the TCR which conferred antigen specificity to an immune response, and the costimulatory receptor which provided the on-off switch. Given the binary model of the two signal hypothesis, it was possible to predict three distinct potential outcomes consequent to APC:T cell cognate interactions (Fig. 12.1). If the T lymphocyte received both signal one via the TCR and a costimulatory signal, then the T cell produced sufficient IL-2 to drive autocrine clonal expansion and to develop effector functions. Alternatively, if the T lymphocyte received only the costimulatory signal, and no TCR driven antigen specific signal, the event would be a neutral one for the T cell. The final possibility, that of a T cell receiving only signal one via the TCR and not the costimulatory signal, would also fail to activate the T cell. In fact, work by Jenkins, Schwartz and others in the 1980s suggested that this latter type of APC:T cell interaction may not simply be a neutral event for the T cell. Collectively these and other investigators found that isolated delivery of signal one in vitro (whether it be by chemically fixed antigen presenting cells, immobilized anti-CD3 antibodies, or purified, immobilized then antigen-pulsed MHC class II molecules) all resulted in $CD4^+$ T cells unable to produce IL-2 when they were subsequently challenged with antigen/APC.[10] These anergic cells were able to proliferate normally to exogenous IL-2 however, demonstrating that the inactivation was antigen specific.

IDENTIFICATION OF CD28 AS A COSTIMULATORY RECEPTOR OF T CELLS

The T cell surface molecule CD28 (previously termed T44 or Tp44) is a T lymphocyte accessory receptor initially identified in humans as a T cell specific surface molecule by the monoclonal antibody (mab) 9.3.[18] The first indication that the T lymphocyte signal generated by the CD28 receptor was distinct from the TCR-mediated signal came following the observation that human peripheral lymphocytes stimulated in vitro with phorbol 12-myristate 13-acetate (PMA) to provide signal one and CD28 antibody induced vigorous and cyclosporine-independent T cell proliferation and IL-2 production.[19] Also, consistent with the two signal model of lymphocyte activation, treatment of cells with only the anti-CD28 antibody had no discernable effect on the cells. These and other characteristics of CD28 signalling fit well with the properties proposed by Schwartz and colleagues[10] for costimulatory signal transduction. Subsequently, experiments by Jenkins and colleagues demonstrated that the

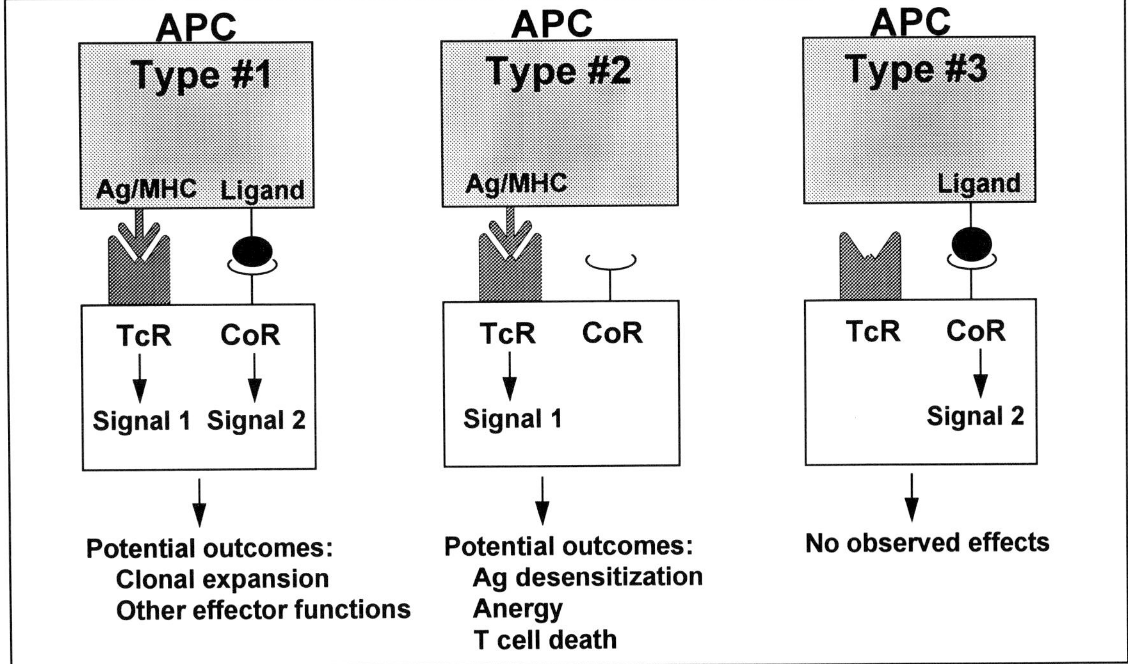

Fig. 12.1. Potential outcomes of T cell : antigen presenting cell (APC) interaction. APC independently expressing cognate Ag/MHC (↓) or costimulatory ligands encounter a resting T cell expressing an antigen specific T cell receptor (TcR) and an antigen non-specific costimulatory receptor (CoR).

signal generated by CD28 was necessary for both antigen specific proliferation and IL-2 production by human T cell clones.[20] In related work, Allison and colleagues showed the response of a mouse T cell clone to an antigenic challenge by stimulated APCs could be blocked by Fab fragments of an anti-CD28 antibody.[21] These studies thus demonstrated that the CD28 receptor was both necessary and sufficient for the antigen-driven activation of T cell clones in vitro. Damle and colleagues extended these observations by studying allogeneic mixed lymphocyte reactions (MLR) and found that anti-CD28 Fab fragments could inhibit the proliferative response of primary resting human T cells as well.[22]

EFFECTS OF CD28 ON T LYMPHOCYTES IN VITRO

Activation of human T cells through the CD28 pathway produces two distinct effects in T cells.[23] One, in thymocytes and peripheral blood T cells that have received an initial activation signal (signal one), is engagement of CD28 provides a second signal that allows the cells to proliferate. Two, CD28 activation enhances the effector function of activated T cells. CD28 costimulation markedly augments the mRNA expression and secretion of specific lymphokines, including IL-1 α,[24] IL-2,[25] IL-3,[26] IL-4,[27] IL-5,[25] IL-6,[28] IL-13,[29] colony stimulating factor-1 (CSF-1),[30] tumor necrosis factor (TNF)-α,[25] interferon-γ (IFNγ),[25] and GM-CSF.[25] The mechanisms of this augmentation include specific inhibition of lymphokine mRNA degradation[31] and enhanced lymphokine gene transcription, possibly through an NFkB-like element.[32-34] Moreover a CD28-mediated costimulatory signal is required for the demonstration of cytolytic T cell (CTL) function in vitro.[35] The mechanism of CD28 signalling in T cells has recently been reviewed.[36]

IDENTIFICATION OF B7 AS A STIMULATORY LIGAND FOR THE CD28 ACTIVATION PATHWAY

Linsley and colleagues first demonstrated that a natural ligand for CD28 was the B7 cell surface molecule (see reference 37 for a review). Their initial supporting evidence was that the adhesion of activated B lymphocytes to CHO cells transfected to express CD28 could be specifically blocked with an anti-B7 antibody. They and others have subsequently shown that cells transfected to express B7 could provide the necessary costimulatory signal to activate T cells receiving signal one via Ag/MHC or mitogen stimulation of the TCR.[38,39] In addition, Jenkins and coworkers showed that a T lymphocyte MLR triggered by Epstein-Barr virus (EBV) transformed B cells could be blocked by anti-B7 antibody treatment.[20] These studies thus established that the B7 molecule was a natural ligand for the CD28 costimulatory pathway of T cells.

BOTH CD28 AND B7 BELONG TO FAMILIES OF RELATED RECEPTORS

Analysis of the human CD28 gene[40,41] and of the B7 gene[42] suggested that both are members of the immunoglobulin superfamily. To complicate matters, other immunoglobulin superfamily members that bear either a structural and/or functional relationship to CD28 or B7 have been identified. For example, in 1987 Golstein and colleagues reported the cloning of an immunoglobulin superfamily member they named CTLA-4 because it was the fourth cDNA they identified from a cytolytic T lymphocyte associated library.[43] Subsequent work from the same group documented that CTLA-4 and CD28 shared significant (31%) amino acid sequence identity (Table 12.1). Moreover, both CTLA-4 and CD28 consisted of single IgV-like extracellular domains, a single membrane spanning domain, and a short intracellular domain.[44,45] These similarities, plus the facts that the two genes shared a similar exon/intron structure and co-localized on band q33 of human chromosome 2, and on band c of mouse chromosome 1, strongly suggested that the two receptors arose by gene duplication. In contrast to CD28 which is expressed on the majority of T lymphocytes at rest however, CTLA-4 expression appeared to be limited to activated T cells.[46-48] The exact function of CTLA-4 has remained obscure, and only

Table 12.1. Conservation amongst members of the B7 and CD28 receptor families

Receptor	Conservation (% identity)					
	Overall	Signal	Ig-V	Ig-C	Tm	Cytoplasmic
hCD28						
mCD28	69	72	66		67	80
hCTLA4						
mCTLA4	74	65	67		83	100
hCD28	31	16	30		42	34
mCD28	27	16	27		42	26
hB7-1						
mB7-1	45	24	46	59	20	23
hB7-2	25	17	24	34	23	6
mB7-2	23	9	30	24	21	8
hB7-2						
mB7-2	50	56	66		17	10

limited information is available on the surface expression of CTLA-4.[47]

The importance of CTLA-4 to this discussion is not limited to the point that CD28 has close gene family members. In 1991, Linsley and colleagues produced a chimeric CTLA-4 immunoglobulin (CTLA4Ig) fusion protein that combined the extracellular domain of CTLA-4 with the Fc domain of human immunoglobulin of the IgG1 isotype.[49] This CTLA4Ig reagent was found to bind B7 with 20-fold higher affinity than a similar construct containing the extracellular domain of CD28,[49] and CTLA4Ig therefore could effectively compete with CD28 for B7 engagement. This characteristic of CTLA4Ig allowed its use as a tool to study the role of the CD28:B7 interaction in vivo (discussed below), and to identify other members of the B7 family of receptors.

In an effort to further delineate the functional relevance of the CD28:B7 interaction in vivo, B7 knockout mice were created.[50] Surprisingly, these mice were not found to have any profound immune defects. Further study disclosed that immune responses of these mice could be suppressed by CTLA4Ig, strongly suggesting that redundant B7-like ligands were subserving the costimulatory ligand function in these animals. This suspicion was quickly confirmed when two groups recently and independently cloned a cDNA for a new B7 family member named B7-2 by one group[51] and B70 by the other.[52] Comparison of the nucleotide sequence of B7-2 and B70 has confirmed that they were indeed from the same gene. The cloning of this new B7 family member had been presaged for some time by the presence of additional CTLA4Ig-binding molecules on the surface of activated mouse B cells[53,54], and by reports of discordant staining of human cells with two different anti-B7 antibodies.[55-57] In fact, evidence already exists for the presence of yet another B7 family member, tentatively identified as B7-3, based on differential binding of various anti-B7 mabs and CTLA4Ig to activated B cells.[58]

IN VIVO EVIDENCE SUPPORTING THE ROLE OF THE COSTIMULATORY MOLECULE IN IMMUNE RESPONSES

The importance of the B7:CD28 costimulatory pathway in vivo has recently been demonstrated using three general experimental approaches. In the first, tissue cells have been genetically engineered to express the B7-1 costimulatory ligand and the effect of this induced B7 expression on immune function has been observed. The second experimental approach has been to utilize homologous recombination to create mice in which either the CD28 or the B7-1 genes have been inactivated or "knocked out". The final approach has been to use CTLA4Ig to block the interaction of B7 family of receptors with the CD28 family of receptors.

Townsend and colleagues[59] as well as Linsley and coworkers[60] for example have studied rejection of tumor cells transfected to express B7-1 compared with untransfected cells. Both groups found that the tumors expressing B7 underwent immune rejection, while untransfected tumors were not rejected. In both studies, treatment with monoclonal antibodies to deplete the host's $CD8^+$ T cells prevented immune rejection of the tumor, while anti-$CD4^+$ antibodies had little or no effect. Thus, these studies demonstrated that the CD28-B7 interaction may play a crucial role in an immune response to cancer and that $CD8^+$ T lymphocytes are essential for the effector arm of the immune mediated killing.

We have recently created trangenic mice that express B7-1 on pancreatic β cells under the control of the insulin promoter as another test of the role of the costimulatory pathway in vivo.[61] These mice never spontaneously developed either insulitis or diabetes. When these mice were bred with mice expressing both a viral glycoprotein (GP) via MHC class 1 on their β cells and a transgene encoded TCR specific for that viral glycoprotein on their T cells,[62] all the resulting "triple transgenic" mice spontaneously developed immune mediated β cell destruction and diabetes. Other mice expressing any two of the transgenes never spontaneously developed either insulitis or diabetes. We have interpreted these data as reflecting the redundant levels of tolerance discussed earlier. That is mice with β cell expression of B7 with or without the coexpression of GP never developed spontaneous diabetes because of immune ignorance: their β cell antigen-specific T cells did not circulate to the islets, and were thus never activated. To test this model further, we have demonstrated that induction of low grade insulitis using multiple low dose streptozotocin[63,64] resulted in diabetes in all the B7 transgenic mice, but in none of their non-transgenic littermates (manuscript in preparation). On the other hand, mice expressing both β cell GP and the GP-specific TCR on their T cells never developed diabetes because of indifference or anergy. In other words, when a rare encounter of a T cell with a β cell occurred, the absence of a coincident costimulatory signal prevented the T cell from becoming activated.

The second general approach employed to study the CD28:B7 costimulatory pathway in vivo has been the disruption of both the CD28 and B7 genes to create "knockout" mice. The B7-1 knockout mouse with apparently normal immune function has already been discussed. In contrast, the CD28 deficient mouse has been found to have several rather profound defects in immune function.[65] While thymic T cell development was evidently normal in these mice, their peripheral T cells had impaired lymphokine secretion after stimulation with the lectin concanavalin A (which polyclonally activates T cells by crosslinking their surface receptors). Further, the mice were found to have only about one-fifth the basal immunoglobulin concentrations of their wild-type littermate controls. This result suggested a CD28 role in either the T:B lymphocyte interaction required for efficient antibody function or in the function of plasma cells, as the expression of CD28 has been found on both mouse and human plasma cells.[66] Interestingly, cytotoxic T lymphocyte activity was normal in the CD28 knockout mice; a result inconsistent with in vitro data which has suggested that CD28 activity is required for CTL generation.[35,67]

The final general approach used to study the importance of the CD28:B7 interaction in vivo has been to administer CTLA4Ig to mice. Using this approach, Linsley and coworkers have demonstrated the importance of the CD28:B7 interaction for normal T cell dependent antibody responses.[68] Even more impressive have been several recent studies documenting the effect of CTLA4Ig on graft rejection.

BLOCKING THE COSTIMULATORY PATHWAY TO INDUCE GRAFT TOLERANCE

In 1992 Lenschow and colleagues reported the exciting finding that CTLA4Ig was able to permit the long-term survival of human pancreatic islets transplanted into diabetic mice in the absence of immune suppression.[69] For these studies, mice were rendered insulin dependent using streptozotocin prior to the grafting of human pancreatic islets under the renal capsule. Control mice had a mean graft survival of only 6 days while animals treated for 2 weeks with intraperitoneal CTLA4Ig all maintained graft function for the duration of the study. The mechanism of the apparent state of tolerance was further evaluated by surgically excising the kidney containing the grafted islets, and injecting other human islets under the remaining renal capsule. If the newly transplanted islets were from a human donor unrelated to the first, the graft was promptly rejected. On the other hand, if the islets were from the original human donor the animals maintained the grafts even without any immunosuppressive therapy at the time of the second grafting procedure. These data suggested that CTLA4Ig had induced in the treated mice a prolonged state of antigen specific immune unresponsiveness. The investigators asked whether the CTLA4Ig they had administered was blocking mouse B7 receptors, or human B7 receptors present on cells within the grafted human islets. Anti-human B7 antibody treatment was also found to produce prolonged graft survival suggesting that costimulatory ligands on the grafted tissue were playing an important role in the T cell activation that resulted in graft rejection.

This initial sanguine report has been followed by other less optimistic studies of the effect of CTLA4Ig on allograft survival. Turka and colleagues performed cardiac allografts in rats and found that graft survival was prolonged by CTLA4Ig, but that the grafts were all eventually rejected.[70] These investigators subsequently used their cardiac allograft model to determine whether graft survival could be improved. By administering a donor specific transfusion at the time of the cardiac allografting, followed by a single dose of CTLA4Ig 2 days later, long-term graft survival was achieved in all animals studied.[71] The rationale for these manipulations was not simply empiric. The administration of the donor specific transfusion was performed to insure that all the hosts circulating T cells would be exposed to alloantigen at the time of the CTLA4Ig mediated CD28:B7 interaction blockade. The immunology underlying the rejection of allografts is complex. Two potential routes of graft antigen presentation to the recipient immune system are possible and their relative contribution toward graft rejection is still debated. The indirect route in which graft antigens are presented by recipient APCs in regional lymph nodes, and the direct route in which graft cells act as the APCs to stimulate host T cells. Lin and colleagues[71] planned the timing of CTLA4Ig administration to coincide with the peak migration of graft dendritic cells into the recipients lymphoid organs, identified by others as occurring 2 days after graft transplantation.[72] The success of this strategy certainly does not resolve the conflict over direct versus indirect alloantigen presentation, but taken together these studies further support the concept that the costimulatory pathway can be manipulated to achieve long-term graft survival.

DISCORDANT XENOGRAFTS

While the rejection mediated by the activated T cell is an important obstacle in the way of practical xenotransplantation, it is not the only one. The phenomena of hyperacute rejection is known to occur when grafts are transplanted across species barriers, especially in cases of so called "discordant combinations" where preformed anti-graft cytotoxic antibodies exist in the host.[73-75] Hyperacute rejection appears to be mediated by host IgM binding to the graft endothelium with resultant activation of the alternative complement pathway and the formation of platelet and fibrin thrombi. While these discordant combinations have created problems for researchers interested in xenotransplantation, solutions to the problem of hyperacute rejection may be on the horizon.[73,76]

CONCLUDING REMARKS

We began this chapter by identifying the two problems, islet availability and host rejection of the islets, that stand in the way of a using islet transplants to cure insulinopenic diabetes in man. The dramatic ability of CTLA4Ig to induce in diabetic mice an apparent state of human islet cell specific tolerance could solve both problems if a similar therapy can be found for xenogeneic islets transplanted into man. The more recent studies using CTLA4Ig to block allograft rejection in rats, while still quite promising, point out that inducing graft tolerance to cure human disease will require more elaborate intervention. The induction of tolerance may be further facilitated by the use of immunoprivileged sites, by tissue transplantation into the thymus to allow clonal deletion and/or tolerization of islet antigen specific T cells, and by modulation of islets to decrease their antigenicity by culture or masking their MHC determinants with antibodies. Manipulation of the costimulatory pathway in conjunction with other transplantation strategies may well permit the long sought after cure for diabetes to be realized.

ACKNOWLEDGEMENTS

Supported in part by Naval Medical Research and Development Command grant #63706N M0095.004.1412. The views expressed in this article are those of the authors and do not reflect the official policy or position of the Department of the Navy, Department of Defense, nor the United States Government.

REFERENCES

1. Rossini AA, Greiner DL, Friedman HP, Mordes JP. Immunopathogenesis of diabetes mellitus. Diabetes Reviews. 1993;1:43-75.
2. Birk OS, Cohen IR. T-cell autoimmunity in type 1 diabetes mellitus. Curr Opin Immunol. 1993;5:903-9.
3. Blackman M, Kappler J, Marrack P. The role of the T cell receptor in positive and negative selection of developing T cells. Science. 1990;248:1335-41.
4. Reich E-P, Janeway CA, Visintin I, Sherwin RS. Role of T-lymphocytes in murine IDDM. Diabetes Reviews. 1993;1:174-90.
5. Fowlkes BJ, Ramsdell F. T-cell tolerance. Curr Opin Immunol. 1993;5:873-9.
6. Kappler JW, Roehm N, Marrack P. T cell tolerance by clonal elimination in the thymus. Cell. 1987;49:273-80.
7. Burtles SS, Trembleau S, Drexler K, Hurtenbach U. Absence of T cell tolerance to pancreatic islet cells. J Immunol. 1992;149:2185-93.
8. Fowell D, Mason D. Evidence that the T-cell repertoire of normal rats contains cells with the potential to cause diabetes-characterization of the CD4+ T-cell subset that inhibits this autoimmune potential. J Exp Med. 1993;177:627-36.
9. Mackay CR. Homing of naive, memory and effector lymphocytes. Curr Opin Immunol. 1993;5:423-7.
10. Schwartz RH. A cell culture model for T lymphocyte clonal anergy. Science. 1990;248:1349-56.
11. Lake RA, O'Hehir RE, Verhoef A, Lamb JR. CD28 mRNA rapidly decays when activated T cells are functionally anergized with specific peptide. Int Immunol. 1993;5:461-6.
12. Dorf ME, Kuchroo VK, Collins M. Suppressor T cells: some answers but more questions. Immunol Today. 1992;13:241-3.
13. Qin S, Cobbold SP, Pope H, et al. "Infectious" transplantation tolerance. Science. 1993;259:974-7.
14. Liu Y, Linsley PS. Costimulation of T-cell growth. Curr Opin Immunol. 1992;4:265-70.
15. June CH. Signal transduction in T cells. Curr Opin Immunol. 1991;3:287-93.
16. Bretscher PA, Cohn M. A theory of self discrimination. Science. 1970;169:1042-9.
17. Jenkins MK. The role of cell division in the induction of clonal anergy. Immunol Today. 1992;13:69-73.
18. Hansen JA, Martin PJ, Nowinski RC. Monoclonal antibodies identifying a novel T-cell antigen and Ia antigens of human lymphocytes. Immunogenetics. 1980;10:247-60.

19. June CH, Ledbetter JA, Gillespie MM, Lindsten T, Thompson CB. T-cell proliferation involving the CD28 pathway is associated with cyclosporine-resistant interleukin 2 gene expression. Mol Cell Biol. 1987;7:4472-81.
20. Jenkins MK, Taylor PS, Norton SD, Urdahl KB. CD28 delivers a costimulatory signal involved in antigen-specific IL-2 production by human T cells. J Immunol. 1991;147:2461-6.
21. Harding FA, McArthur JG, Gross JA, Raulet DH, Allison JP. CD28-mediated signalling co-stimulates murine T cells and prevents induction of anergy in T-cell clones. Nature. 1992;356:607-9.
22. Damle NK, Doyle LV, Grosmaire LS, Ledbetter JA. Differential regulatory signals delivered by antibody binding to the CD28 (Tp44) molecule during the activation of human T lymphocytes. J Immunol. 1988;140:1753-61.
23. Lee KP, June CH, Thompson CB. The CD28 signal transduction pathway in T cell activation. In: Mond JJ, Cambier J, Weiss A, eds. Advances in Regulation of Cell Growth. New York: Raven Press Ltd.; 1991:141-60.
24. Cerdan C, Martin Y, Brailly H, et al. IL-1 alpha is produced by T lymphocytes activated via the CD2 plus CD28 pathways. J Immunol. 1991;146:560-4.
25. Thompson CB, Lindsten T, Ledbetter JA, et al. CD28 activation pathway regulates the production of multiple T- cell-derived lymphokines/cytokines. Proc Natl Acad Sci U S A. 1989;86:1333-7.
26. Guba SC, Stella G, Turka LA, June CH, Thompson CB, Emerson SG. Regulation of interleukin 3 gene induction in normal human T cells. J Clin Invest. 1989;84:1701-6.
27. Holter W, Majdic O, Kalthoff FS, Knapp W. Regulation of interleukin-4 production in human mononuclear cells. Eur J Immunol. 1992;22:2765-7.
28. Lorre K, Kasran A, Van Vaeck F, de Boer M, Ceuppens JL. Interleukin-1 and B7/CD28 interaction regulate interleukin-6 production by human T cells. Clin Immunol Immunopathol. 1994; 70:81-90.
29. Minty A, Chalon P, Derocq JM, et al. Interleukin-13 is a new human lymphokine regulating inflammatory and immune responses. Nature. 1993;362:248-50.
30. Cerdan C, Razanajaona D, Martin Y, Courcoul M, Pavon C. Contributions of the CD2 and CD28 T lymphocyte activation pathways to the regulation of the expression of the colony-stimulating factor (CSF-1) gene. J Immunol. 1992;149:373-9.
31. Lindsten T, June CH, Ledbetter JA, Stella G, Thompson CB. Regulation of lymphokine messenger RNA stability by a surface-mediated T cell activation pathway. Science. 1989;244:339-43.
32. Verweij CL, Geerts M, Aarden LA. Activation of interleukin-2 gene transcription via the T-cell surface moleculue CD28 is mediated through an NF-kB-like response element. J Biol Chem. 1991;266:14179-82.
33. Civil A, Geerts M, Aarden LA, Verweij CL. Evidence for a role of CD28RE as a response element for distinct mitogenic T cell activation signals. Eur J Immuno 1992;22:3041-3.
34. Ghosh P, Tan TH, Rice NR, Sica A, Young HA. The interleukin 2 CD28-responsive complex contains at least three members of the NF kappa B family: c-Rel, p50, and p65. Proc Natl Acad Sci U S A. 1993;90:1696-700.
35. Azuma M, Cayabyab M, Phillips JH, Lanier LL. Requirements for CD28-dependent T cell-mediated cytotoxicity. J Immunol. 1993;150:2091-101.
36. June CH, Bluestone JA, Nadler LM, Thompson CB. The B7 and CD28 receptor families. Immunol Today. 1994; July.
37. Linsley PS, Ledbetter JA. The role of the CD28 receptor during T cell responses to antigen. Annu Rev Immunol. 1993;11:191-212.
38. Linsley PS, Brady W, Grosmaire L, Aruffo A, Damle NK, Ledbetter JA. Binding of the B cell activation antigen B7 to CD28 costimulates T cell proliferation and interleukin 2 mRNA accumulation. J Exp Med. 1991;173:721-30.

39. Gimmi CD, Freeman GJ, Gribben JG, et al. B-cell surface antigen B7 provides a costimulatory signal that induces T cells to proliferate and secrete interleukin 2. Proc Natl Acad Sci U S A. 1991;88:6575-9.
40. Aruffo A, Seed B. Molecular cloning of a CD28 cDNA by a high-efficiency COS cell expression system. Proc Natl Acad Sci U S A. 1987;84:8573-7.
41. Lee KP, Taylor C, Petryniak B, Turka LA, June CH, Thompson CB. The genomic organization of the CD28 gene. Implications for the regulation of CD28 mRNA expression and heterogeneity. J Immunol. 1990;145:344-52.
42. Freeman GJ, Freedman AS, Segil JM, Lee G, Whitman JF, Nadler LM. B7, a new member of the Ig superfamily with unique expression on activated and neoplastic B cells. J Immunol. 1989;143:2714-22.
43. Brunet JF, Denizot F, Luciani MF, et al. A new member of the immunoglobulin superfamily--CTLA-4. Nature. 1987;328:267-70.
44. Buonavista N, Balzano C, Pontarotti P, Le Paslier D, Golstein P. Molecular linkage of the human CTLA4 and CD28 Ig-superfamily genes in yeast artificial chromosomes. Genomics. 1992;13:856-61.
45. Harper K, Balzano C, Rouvier E, Mattëi MG, Luciani MF, Golstein P. CTLA-4 and CD28 activated lymphocyte molecules are closely related in both mouse and human as to sequence, message expression, gene structure, and chromosomal location. J Immunol. 1991;147:1037-44.
46. Lindsten T, Lee KP, Harris ES, et al. Characterization of CTLA-4 structure and expression on human T-cells. J Immunol. 1993;151:3489-99.
47. Linsley PS, Greene JL, Tan P, et al. Coexpression and functional cooperation of CTLA-4 and CD28 on activated T lymphocytes. J Exp Med. 1992;176:1595-604.
48. Freeman GJ, Lombard DB, Gimmi CD, et al. CTLA-4 and CD28 mRNA are coexpressed in most T cells after activation. Expression of CTLA-4 and CD28 mRNA does not correlate with the pattern of lymphokine production. J Immunol. 1992;149:3795-801.
49. Linsley PS, Brady W, Urnes M, Grosmaire LS, Damle NK, Ledbetter JA. CTLA-4 is a second receptor for the B cell activation antigen B7. J Exp Med. 1991;174:561-9.
50. Freeman GJ, Borriello F, Hodes RJ, et al. Uncovering of functional alternative CTLA-4 counter-receptor in B7-deficient mice. Science. 1993;262:907-9.
51. Freeman GJ, Gribben JG, Boussiotis VA, et al. Cloning of B7-2: A CTLA-4 counter-receptor that costimulates human T cell proliferation. Science. 1993;262:909-11.
52. Azuma M, Ito D, Yagita H, et al. B70 antigen is a second ligand for CTLA-4 and CD28. Nature. 1993;366:76-9.
53. Lenschow DJ, Huei-Ting Su G, Zuckerman LA, et al. Expression and functional significance of an additional ligand for CTLA-4. Proc Natl Acad Sci U S A. 1993;90:11054-8.
54. Wu Y, Guo Y, Liu Y. A major costimulatory molecule on antigen-presenting cells, CTLA4 Ligand-A, is distinct from B7. J Exp Med. 1993;178:1789-93.
55. Nickoloff BJ, Mitra RS, Lee K, et al. Discordant expression of CD28 ligands, BB-1, and B7 on keratinocytes in vitro and psoriatic cells in vivo. Am J Pathol. 1993;142:1029-40.
56. Turka LA, Linsley PS, Paine R, Schieven GL, Thompson CB, Ledbetter JA. Signal transduction via CD4, CD8, and CD28 in mature and immature thymocytes. Implications for thymic selection. J Immunol. 1991;146:1428-36.
57. Augustin M, Dietrich A, Niedner R, et al. Phorbol-12-myristate-13-acetate-treated human keratinocytes express B7-like molecules that serve a costimulatory role in T-cell activation. J Invest Dermatol. 1993;100:275-81.
58. Boussiotis VA, Freeman GJ, Gribben JG, Daley J, Gray G, Nadler LM. Activated human B lymphocytes express three CTLA4 counterreceptors that costimulate T-cell activation. Proc Natl Acad Sci U S A. 1993;90:11059-63.
59. Townsend SE, Allison JP. Tumor rejection after direct costimulation of $CD8^+$ T cells by B7- transfected melanoma cells. Science. 1993;259:368-70.

60. Chen L, Ashe S, Brady WA, et al. Costimulation of antitumor immunity by the B7 counterreceptor for the T lymphocyte molecules CD28 and CTLA-4. Cell. 1992;71:1093-102.
61. Harlan DM, Hengartner H, Huang ML, et al. Transgenic mice expressing both B7 and viral glycoprotein on pancreatic β cells along with glycoprotein-specific transgenic T cells develop diabetes due to a breakdown of T lymphocyte unresponsiveness. Proc Natl Acad Sci U S A. 1994; 91:3137-3141.
62. Ohashi PS, Oehen S, Buerki K, et al. Ablation of "tolerance" and induction of diabetes by virus infection in viral antigen transgenic mice. Cell. 1991;65:305-17.
63. Like AA, Rossini AA. Streptozotocin-induced pancreatic insulitis: new model of diabetes mellitus. Science. 1976;193:415-7.
64. Rossini AA, Like AA, Chick WL, Appel MC, Cahill GFJ. Studies of streptozotocin-induced insulitis and diabetes. Proc Natl Acad Sci U S A. 1977;74:2485-9.
65. Shahinian A, Pfeffer K, Lee KP, et al. Differential T cell costimulatory requirements in CD28-deficient mice. Science. 993;261:609-12.
66. Kozbor D, Moretta A, Messner HA, Moretta L, Croce CM. Tp44 molecules involved in antigen-independent T cell activation are expressed on human plasma cells. J Immunol. 1987;138:4128-32.
67. Harding FA, Allison JP. CD28-B7 interactions allow the induction of CD8+ cytotoxic T lymphocytes in the absence of exogenous help. J Exp Med. 1993;177:1791-6.
68. Linsley PS, Wallace PM, Johnson J, et al. Immunosuppression in vivo by a soluble form of the CTLA-4 T cell activation molecule. Science. 1992;257:792-5.
69. Lenschow DJ, Zeng Y, Thistlethwaite JR, et al. Long-term survival of xenogeneic pancreatic islet grafts induced by CTLA4Ig. Science. 1992;257:789-92.
70. Turka LA, Linsley PS, Lin H, et al. T-cell activation by the CD28 ligand B7 is required for cardiac allograft rejection in vivo. Proc Natl Acad Sci U S A. 1992;89:11102-5.
71. Lin H, Bolling SF, Linsley PS, et al. Long-term acceptance of major histocompatibility complex mismatched cardiac allografts induced by CTLA4Ig plus donor-specific transfusion. J Exp Med. 1993;178:1801-6.
72. Larsen CP, Morris PJ, Austyn JM. Migration of dendritic leukocytes from cardiac allografts in host spleens. J Exp Med. 1990;171:307-13.
73. Fischel RJ, Matas AJ, Platt JL, et al. Cardiac xenografting in the pig-to-rhesus monkey model: manipulation of antiendothelial antibody prolongs survival. J Heart Lung Transplant. 1992;11:965-73; discussion 973-4.
74. Dalmasso AP, Vercellotti GM, Fischel RJ, Bolman RM, Bach FH, Platt JL. Mechanism of complement activation in the hyperacute rejection of porcine organs transplanted into primate recipients. Am J Pathol. 1992;140:1157-66.
75. Platt JL, Fischel RJ, Matas AJ, Reif SA, Bolman RM, Bach FH. Immunopathology of hyperacute xenograft rejection in a swine-to-primate model. Transplantation. 1991;52:214-20.
76. Auchincloss H, Jr. Xenogeneic transplantation. A review. Transplantation.1988;46:1-20.

CHAPTER 13

ORAL TOLERANCE

Mohamed H. Sayegh

Howard L. Weiner

Charles B. Carpenter

Oral tolerance is a state of specific immunologic unresponsiveness induced by oral administration of antigens. The observation that orally administered antigens could suppress immune responses was recognized long before the era of modern immunology. It was first described by Wells in 1911 where systemic anaphylaxis in guinea pigs was prevented by previous feeding of hen egg proteins.[1] In 1946, Chase demonstrated suppression of contact sensitivity responses by feeding the hapten DNFB to guinea pigs.[2] Over the past two decades studies have been focused on studying the mechanisms of oral tolerance, and the potential clinical applications in autoimmune diseases as well as in allograft rejection.[3,4]

ANIMAL MODELS

Oral administration of antigens suppresses the immune response in several experimental models. Thompson and Staines[5] and Nagler-Anderson et al,[6] initially described suppression of collagen-induced arthritis by feeding type II collagen in the rat. Studies by our group[7-9] and others[10-11] demonstrated suppression of experimental autoimmune encephalomyelitis (EAE) by orally administered myelin antigens. Subsequently, we investigated oral tolerance in experimental models of autoimmune uveitis,[12] diabetes in the NOD mouse,[13] adjuvant arthritis,[14] and transplantation.[15-16] Other investigators have also demonstrated suppression of other autoimmune models, such as myasthenia gravis[17] and immune complex disease,[18] by orally administered antigen.

The "effector" mechanisms of oral tolerance appear to be determined primarily by the the dose of antigen fed. Low doses of antigen favor the generation of regulatory cells which suppress the specific immune response in the target organ, whereas high doses of antigen induce an antigen-specific anergic state in the peripheral immune system, although these mechanisms need not be mutually exclusive.[19] The exact cellular interactions in the gut immune system which lead to the "induction" of oral tolerance are not well understood. As shown in Figure 13.1, low doses of orally administered antigen is taken up by gut associated antigen presenting cells. These cells,

Pancreatic Islet Transplantation Volume II: Immunomodulation of Pancreatic Islets, edited by Robert P. Lanza, MD, William L. Chick, MD;

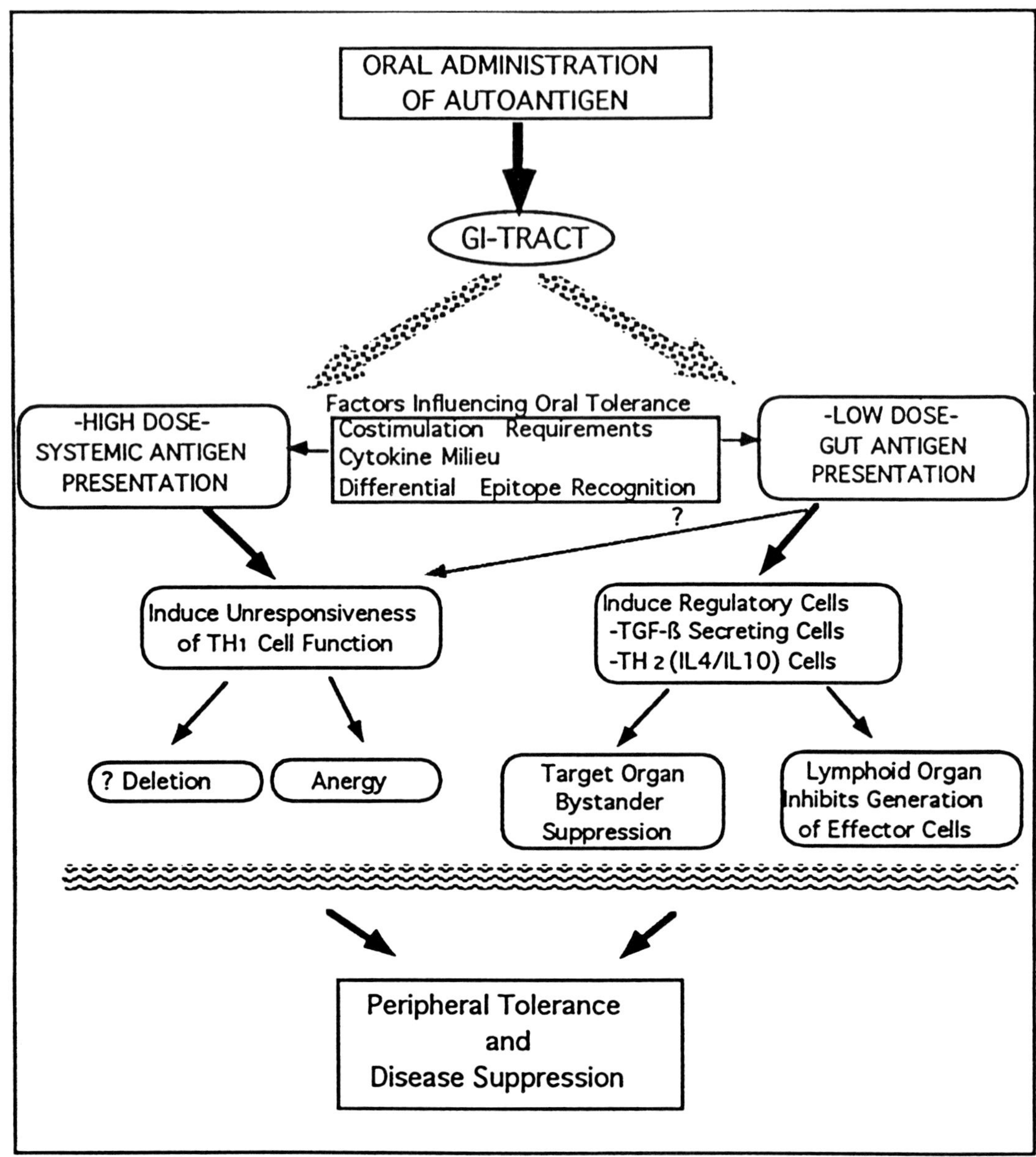

Fig. 13.1. Effector mechanisms of oral tolerance. An antigen is fed and leads to the generation of regulatory cells (with "low dose" antigen) and/or anergy (with "high dose" antigen) leading to a state of systemic unresponsiveness. The regulatory cells act by secreting inhibitory cytokines such as TGFβ, IL-4, and/or IL-10.[4] The exact cellular interactions in the gut mileau leading to the induction of oral tolerance have not been established.

through complex cellular interactions, preferentially induce regulatory T cells which upon recognition of antigen in the target organ, secrete suppressive cytokines such as TGFβ, IL-4, and IL-10.[20-22] One of the most interesting findings related to the generation of regulatory cells is that it is not necessary to feed the exact antigen which ultimately is responsible for the induction of the immune response and the disease process. This phenomenon is known as antigen-driven bystander suppression,[23] i.e. any antigen which is expressed in the target organ could potentially be used to induce specific oral tolerance. High doses of orally administered antigen, on the other hand, appear to pass through the gut and enters the systemic circulation either as intact or processed protein. High doses of antigen induces unresponsiveness of T cell function primarily via clonal anergy, and is specific for the fed antigen.[4]

NOD diabetic mice spontaneously develop an autoimmune form of diabetes associated with insulitis. This is a naturally occurring disease and its autoimmune nature is suggested by lymphocytic infiltration of the islets of Langerhans which precedes the destruction of insulin producing β cells. In addition, immunosuppressive therapy targeted at T lymphocyte function has been successful in preventing the disease. Oral administration of porcine insulin at a dose of 1 mg orally twice a week for 5 weeks and then weekly until 1 year of age resulted in delay in the onset of diabetes as well as decreased severity of the lymphocytic infiltration of pancreatic islets. Furthermore, a decreased incidence of diabetes was seen in animals followed for one year. Splenic T cells from animals orally treated with insulin adoptively transferred protection against diabetes in unmodified NOD mice, demonstrating that oral insulin generates active regulatory mechanisms which suppress the autoimmune response. As expected, orally administered insulin had no metabolic effect on blood glucose levels.[13] Additional studies have demonstrated the ability to suppress insulitis by administering insulin peptides or the B chain of insulin.[4]

In an initial series of experiments, we studied the effects of oral administration of major histocompatibility (MHC) antigens on the alloimmune response in the rat. Lymphocytes from inbred LEW ($RT1^l$) rats that were pre-fed allogeneic WF ($RT1^u$) splenocytes or their lysates exhibited significant antigen-specific reduction of the mixed lymphocyte response (MLR) in vitro and delayed type hypersensitivity (DTH) response in vivo, when compared to unfed controls. In an accelerated allograft rejection model, LEW rats were presensitized with BN ($RT1^n$) skin allografts 7 days before challenging them with (LEWxBN)F1 or BN vascularized cardiac allografts. While sensitized control animals hyperacutely reject their cardiac allografts within 2 days, animals pre-fed with BN splenocytes maintained cardiac allograft survival to 7 days, a time similar to that observed in unsensitized control recipients. This phenomenon was antigen-specific, as third party WF grafts were rejected within 2 days. Immunohistologic examination of cardiac allografts harvested on day 2 from the fed animals had markedly reduced deposition of IgG, IgM, C3, and fibrin, in addition to significantly less cellular infiltrates of total white blood cells, neutrophils, macrophages, T cells, IL-2 receptor positive T cells, and mononuclear cells with positive staining for the activation cytokines IL-2 and IFNγ. Interestingly, there was marked upregulation of intragraft IL-4. Therefore, oral administration of allogeneic splenocytes down-regulates the systemic cell-mediated alloimmune response in vitro and in vivo, and prevents sensitization by skin allografts and transforms accelerated rejection of vascularized cardiac allografts to an acute form.[15] These phenomena appear to be mediated by selective inhibition of Th1 cell and sparing of Th2 cell function.[16] Similar findings were reported in the pig, where islet allograft survival was prolonged by oral administration of islet tissue.[24]

Since oral administration of allogeneic splenocytes or their lysates was effective in down-regulating the systemic alloimmune response, we studied the tolerogenicity of orally administered synthetic class II MHC allopeptides in the same rat strain combination. Inbred LEW ($RT1^l$) rats, used as responders, were immunized in the foot pad with a mixture of 8 class II synthetic MHC allopeptides emulsified in complete Freund's adjuvant (CFA). These sequences represent the full length hypervariable domain of $RT1.B^u$ and $RT1.D^u$ (DR or I-E like) β chains of the WF rat. In vitro, responder lymphocytes harvested from popliteal and inguinal lymph nodes of immunized animals exhibited significant proliferation to the MHC allopeptide mixture. In addition, these responder lymphocytes had significantly increased proliferation to allogeneic WF ($RT1^u$) stimulator cells, when compared to naive controls in the standard MLR. In vivo, peptide immunized LEW animals were challenged in the ear 2 weeks after immunization with either the allopeptide mixture, the individual allopeptide sequences, or allogeneic WF splenocytes. When compared to controls, these animals had significant DTH responses to the allopeptide mixture, and to allogeneic WF splenocytes, but not to syngeneic LEW splenocytes, or to third party allogeneic BN splenocytes. Oral administration of the allopeptide mixture to LEW responder rats daily for 5 days before immunization effected significant reduction of DTH responses both to the allopeptide mixture and to allogeneic splenocytes. This reduction was antigen specific, since there was no reduction of DTH responses to mycobacterium tuberculosis, the antigen present in CFA. Only the immunogenic peptides (2 from RT1.B and from 2 RT1.D) were tolerogenic, when administered orally.[25] Immunohistological studies of DTH skin lesions of orally tolerized rats showed marked reduction in mononuclear cell infiltration, fibrin deposition, IL-2 and IFNγ expression, but increased expression of IL-4 and preservation of TGFβ expression. These data confirm that oral tolerance is associated with immune deviation to a predominance of Th2 cell function.[22] Studies are underway to determine the effects of oral administration of synthetic MHC allopeptides on vascularized allograft survival. Perhaps the best evidence to indicate that processed allo-MHC in the form of polymorphic peptide fragments can be a potentially viable approach for induction of transplantation tolerance comes from recent studies where we demonstrated that intrathymic injection of the polymorphic class II MHC allopeptides mixture leads to antigen-specific systemic unresponsiveness and prolongs renal allograft survival.[26] Similar to oral tolerance the unresponsive state could be induced by intrathymic injection of the immunogenic peptides, although the mechanisms of intrathymic unresponsiveness appear to involve a state of peripheral T cell anergy and/or deletion.[27]

ORAL TOLERANCE IN HUMANS

In order to determine whether orally ingested autoantigens could affect the clinical course and immune responses in patients with an autoimmune disease, 15 patients with relapsing remitting multiple sclerosis were fed a capsule containing 300 mg of bovine myelin or placebo daily for one year.[28] Results demonstrated a decrease in the precursor frequency of circulating MBP reactive cells of myelin fed patients, as compared to placebo fed controls. Clinical scores demonstrated that 12 of 15 placebo-fed patients had major MS attacks whereas only 6 of 15 in the control group had attacks ($p = 0.06$). It appeared that a subgroup of patients that were either males or negative for HLA-DR2 preferentially responded to the oral tolerization. Based on the results of this small phase I-II trial, a 500-patient multi-center double blind placebo controlled trial of oral bovine myelin in relapsing remitting MS patients prospectively randomized is underway.

In a separate study a double-blind trial of oral collagen administration to patients with rheumatoid arthritis was conducted.[29] Patients who were previously on immunosuppressant drugs, such as methotrexate, were taken off these medications and fed collagen for a 3 month period. In the first month they received 100 μg of collagen per day, and in the second and third months 500 μg per day. These doses were extrapolated from studies in the adjuvant arthritis model in the rat. There were no toxicities or evidence of sensitization to type II collagen in fed patients. Analysis of the data demonstrated a significant decrease in joint swelling and disease index in patients fed chicken collagen, as compared to placebo fed controls. Four patients in the collagen-treated group apparently had complete remission of their rheumatoid arthritis. There was no linkage to either DR type or sex in the patients who responded. Given the biologic effects seen, a multi-center 230-patient phase II double blind dosing study is planned, and will involve a washout period and 6 months therapy.

Finally, based on preliminary open label studies in patients with uveitis using the retinal S-antigen, a double-blind trial of 45 patients is currently underway.[4] In addition, studies are currently planned in type I diabetes both for new onset diabetics and for the prevention of diabetes in high risk populations by oral tolerization with insulin or other islet specific antigens.[4]

FUTURE DIRECTIONS

The results in animal models of autoimmunity and in transplantation, together with initial studies in humans suggest that oral administration of antigen provides a novel strategy for the treatment of human organ-specific autoimmune diseases, as well as a novel approach to induce transplantation tolerance. Such an approach would have the advantages of being orally-administered, non-toxic, and antigen-specific. Because of the potential diversity of the immune response to polymorphic MHC molecules, the principal targets of the immune response to allografts, oral tolerance to transplantation antigens may not be as straightforward as in autoimmune diseases, where autoreactivity to a particular antigen is the main defect. Therefore, extensive experimentation using synthetic MHC peptides or recombinant proteins to define potentially all polymorphic and immunogenic epitopes are required. Optimal dosing, timing, and the concomitant administration of immunomodulatory drugs may be required to obtain the desired specific tolerogenic effects.

REFERENCES

1. Wells, H. 1911. Studies on the chemistry of anaphylaxis. III. Experiments with isolated proteins, especially those of hen's egg. J. Infect. Dis. 9:147-51.
2. Chase, M.W. 1946. Inhibition of experimental durg allergy by prior feeding of the sensitizing agent. Proc. Soc. Exp. Biol. Med. 61:257-59.
3. Mowat, A.M. 1987. The regulation of immune responses to dietary protein antigens. Immunol. Today 8:93-8.
4. Weiner, H.L., Friedman, A., Miller, A., Khoury, S.J., Al-Sabbagh, A., Santos, L., Sayegh, M.H., Nussenblatt, R.B., Trentham, D.E., Hafler, D.A. 1994. Oral Tolerance: Immunologic mechanisms and treatment of murine and human organ specific autoimmune diseases by oral administration of autoantigens. Ann. Rev. Immunol. in press.
5. Thompson, H.S.G., Staines, N.A. 1986. Gastric administration of type II collagen delays the onset and severity of collagen-induced arthritis in rats. Clin. Exp. Immunol. 64: 581-86.
6. Nagler-Anderson, C., Bober, L. A., Robinson, M.E., Siskind , G.W., Thorbecke , F.J. 1986. Suppression of type II collagen-induced arthritis by intragastric administration of soluble type II collagen. Proc. Natl. Acad. Sci. USA 83: 7443-46.
7. Higgins, P., Weiner, H.L. 1988. Suppression of experimental autoimmune encephalomyelitis by oral administration of myelin basic protein and its fragments. J. Immunol. 140:440-45.
8. Khoury, S.J., Lider, O., Al-Sabbagh, A., Weiner, H. L. 1990. Suppression of experimental autoimmune encephalomyelitis by oral administration of myelin basic protein. III. Synergistic effect of lipopolysaccharide. Cell. Imunol. 131:302-10.
9. Brod, S.A., Al-Sabbgh, A., Sobel, R.A., Hafler, D.A., Weiner, H.L. 1992. Suppression of experimental autoimmune encephalomyelitis by oral administration of myelin antigens. IV. Suppression of chronic relapsing disease in the Lewis rat and strain 13 guinea pig. Ann. Neurol. 29: 615-622.
10. Bitar D.M., Whitacre, C.C. 1988. Suppression of experimental autoimmune encephalomyelitis by the oral administraiton of myelin basic protein. Cellular Immunol. 112:364-370.
11. Fuller, K.A., Pearl, D., Whitacre, C.C. 1990. Oral tolerance in experimental autoimmune encephalomyelitis: Serum and salivary antibody responses. J. Neuroimmunol. 28:15-26.

12. Nussenblatt, R.B., Caspi, R.R., Mahdi, R., Chan, C.C., Roberge, F., Lider, O., Weiner, H. L. 1990. Inhibition of S-antigen induced experimental autoimmune uveoretinitis by oral induction of tolerance with S-antigen. J. Immunol. 144: 1689-95.
13. Zhang, J.A., Davidson, L., Eisenbarth, G., Weiner, H.L. 1991. Suppression of diabetes in NOD mice by oral administration of porcine insulin. Proc. Natl. Acad. Sci. USA 88: 10252-56.
14. Zhang, J.Z., Lee, C.S.Y., Lider, O., Weiner, H.L. 1990. Suppression of adjuvant arthritis in Lewis rats by oral administration of type II collagen. J. Immunol. 145: 2489-93.
15. Sayegh, M.H., Zhang, Z.J., Hancock, W.W., Kwok, C.A., Carpenter, C.B., Weiner, H. L. 1992. Down-regulation of the immune response to histocompatibility antigen and prevention of sensitization by skin allografts by orally administered alloantigen. Transplantation 53:163-66.
16. Hancock, W.W., Sayegh, M.H., Kwok, C.A., Weiner, H.L., Carpenter, C.B. 1993. Oral but not intravenous alloantigen prevents accelerated allograft rejection by selective intragraft Th2 cell activation. Transplantation 55:1112-1118.
17. Wang, Z-Y., Qiao, J., Link, H. 1993. Suppression of experimental, autoimmune myasthenia gravis by oral administration of acetylcholine receptor. J. Neuroimmunol. 44:209-14.
18. Devey, M.E., Bleasdale, K. 1984. Antigen feeding modifies the course of antigen-induced immune complex disease. Clin. Exp. Immunol. 56: 637-44.
19. Friedman, A., Weiner, H.L. Induction of anergy or active suppression following oral tolerance is determined by frequency of feeding and antigen dosage. 1994. Proc. Natl. Acad. Sci. USA, in press.
20. Miller, A., Lider, O., Roberts, A.B., Sporn, M., Weiner, H.L. 1992. Suppressor T cells generated by oral tolerization to myelin basic protein suppress both in vitro and in vivo immune responses by the release of TGFβ following antigen specific triggering. Proc. Natl. Acad. Sci. USA 89: 421-25.
21. Khoury, S.J., Hancock, W.W., Weiner, H.L. 1992. Oral tolerance to myelin basic protein and natural recovery from experimental autoimmune encephalomyelitis are associated with downregulation of inflammatory cytokines and differential upregulation of transforming growth factor β, interleukin 4, and prostaglandin E expression in the brain. J. Exp. Med. 176:1355-64.
22. Hancock, W.W., Khoury, S.J., Carpenter, C.B., Sayegh, M.H. 1994. Differential effects of oral versus intrathymic administration of polymorphic MHC class II peptides on mononuclear and endothelial cell activation and cytokine expression during a delayed-type hypersensitivity response. Am. J. Pathol. in press.
23. Miller, A., Lider, O., Weiner, H.L. 1991. Antigen-driven bystander suppression following oral administration of antigens. J. Exp. Med. 174: 791-98.
24. Hrstka, J., Hesse, U.J., Hrstka, V., Danis, J., Schmitz-Rode, M., Tunggal, B., Hordegen, P., Peters, S. 1992. Prolongation of islet allograft survival following immunologic conditioning by antigen feeding in the pig. Transplant. Proc. 24:663-64.
25. Sayegh, M. H., Khoury, S.J., Hancock, W.H., Weiner, H.L., Carpenter, C. B. 1992. Induction of immunity and oral tolerance with polymorphic class II major histocompatability complex allopeptides in the rat. Proc. Natl. Acad. Sci. USA 89:7762-66.
26. Sayegh, M.H., Perico, N., Imberti, O., Hancock, W.W., Carpenter, C.B., Remuzzi, G. 1993. Thymic recognition of class II MHC allopeptides induces donor specific unresponsiveness to renal allografts. Transplantation 56:461-465.
27. Sayegh, M.H., Perico, N., Gallon, L., Imberti, O., Hancock, W.W., Remuzzi, G., Carpenter, C.B. 1994. Mechanisms of aquired thymic unresponsiveness to renal allografts: Thymic recognition of immunodominant allo-MHC peptides induces peripheral T cell anergy. Transplantation, in press.

28. Weiner, H.L., Mackin, G.A., Matsui, M., Orav, E.J., Khoury, S.J., Dawson, D.M., Hafler, D.A. 1993. Double-blind pilot trial of oral tolerization with myelin antigens in multiple sclerosis. Science. 259:1321-24.

29. Trentham, D.E., Dynesius-Trentham, R.A., Orav, E.J., Combitchi, D., Lorenzo, C., Sewell, K.L., Hafler, D.A., Weiner, H.L. 1993. Effects of oral administration of collagen on rheumatoid arthritis. Science. 261:1727-1730.

CHAPTER 14

Immunomodulation of Islet Transplantation: Future Prospects

Francis T. Thomas

An overview of immunomodulation for islet transplantation is necessarily complex with the current availability of multiple chemical immunosuppressants as well as the so-called biological response modifiers which can achieve potent immunosuppression.[1,2] In addition, during the last few years immunomodulation protocols have clearly shifted to techniques for generation of tolerogenicity or tolerance in transplantation which has now been achieved in higher animals and has undergone clinical trials in the human.[3,4] These trials continue to expand and attract more attention as the limitation of current non-specific immunosuppression become more evident. For a host of reasons discussed later in this paper, chronic immunosuppression appears to be an unacceptable option for the diabetic receiving an islet transplant if the full potential of this procedure is to be achieved. In addition, current clinical transplantation seems poised towards potential application of xenografting and strong evidence has now accumulated that the islet xenograft reaction is quite different and requires entirely new concepts and techniques of immunomodulation.[1,5] Perhaps most significantly, a small but verifiable data base now suggests that immune tolerance to disparate xenografts is possible without drastic life-threatening suppressive protocols.[6] Immunomodulation of pancreas islets is a uniquely exciting area because it permits protocols which have not been achieved to date in transplantation. Some new areas of immunomodulation available in islet transplantation include donor pretreatment of islets in culture with a variety of techniques to decrease immunogenicity,[7] the transgenic modification by germ cell or somatic transgenes of donor islets to decrease immunogenicity,[8] unique techniques of transplantation including the use of multiple donors, multiple sequential transplants, subimmunogenic transplants done in sequence, as well as, unique sites of placement of the grafts.[1,2,9,10] Finally, the newer concepts of islet encapsulation to achieve immunoisolation represent a powerful form of immunomodulation which is treated separately in these volumes on islet transplantation. Thus, the field of islet transplantation and as

Pancreatic Islet Transplantation Volume II: Immunomodulation of Pancreatic Islets, edited by Robert P. Lanza, MD, William L. Chick, MD; ©1994 R.G. Landes Company.

Ricordi has previously noted, perhaps cellular transplantation in general opens a "Pandora's box" of new techniques which challenge the innovativeness of the transplant immunologist.[11]

In this chapter, I will deal with techniques of donor graft modulation to achieve successful islet transplantation as well as techniques of immunomodulation with particular focus on the "Holy Grail" of transplantation, the creation of donor-specific tolerance which has the potential to release the recipient from the oppression of chronic suppressive drug therapy and perhaps even make islet xenotransplantation without chronic immunuosuppression possible. Although I will focus on these areas, I confess to a bias that the final common goal of islet transplant—to create a long-term successful islet transplantation without requirement of chronic immunosuppression and with a potential for complete patient rehabilitation and excellent glycemic control may well be best achieved by either techniques of immunoisolation which are discussed in another volume in this series or by induction of immune tolerance. Furthermore, my final bias is that the technique with the highest potential for immediate success may well be the induction of donor-specific tolerance by transfer of donor stem cells probably in the form of fractionated donor bone marrow cells given along with the islets to achieve microchimerism.[12]

Islet transplantation was made possible by the classic work of Lacy's group developing techniques for isolation of viable islets from the whole pancreas.[13] Progress in this field has been slow however, and isolation techniques were inefficient and cumbersome until the late 1980s. The description by Ricordi, first in the human islets and later with pig islets of techniques using collagenase digestion with perfusion and recirculation in a chamber followed by density gradient separations to achieve efficient isolation of islets[14,15] revolutionized this field and increased the islet yield 2-4 times or more. More recently a number of groups have achieved the desirable level of achieving enough islets from a single pancreas for complete reversal of hypoglycemia in a diabetic animal or patient.[1,2]

It is important for the person studying or treating islets with immunomodulatory techniques to understand some basic non-immune factors in islet isolation and transplantation which can cause considerable variability in islet success independent of immunological factors. Many of the early problems in transplantation involving incomplete reversal of diabetes, late failure of the islets, etc. seem related to some of the variables in isolation and transplantation of the islets[1] Indeed one of the key factors in achieving successful immunomodulation of islet transplants is to separate the immune from non-immune factors in early and late islet failure. Another set of factors is poised on a middle ground between these two areas and involves such things as primary nonfunction of the islets where islet isolation variables may be contributory as well as unique immune reactions, such as the primary nonfunction inflammatory reaction apparently mediated by macrophage type pro-inflammatory activity in the peri-transplant period.[16] The whole organ graft has posed a similar dilemma in the quest to differentiate cyclosporine islet toxicity which can be quite severe from the immunological damage to incompatible islets which is often the primary mechanism suspected in any transplant system. Overseeing this complex maze of transplant interactions juxtaposed against the basic drama of an incompatible graft placed in a hostile, immune environment is confusing to say the least. It is this final interplay with which we concern ourselves in this chapter recognizing that much of the stage for the final result has been set prior to the time the players came onto the field. Perhaps most importantly, much of the action and final outcome may depend upon non-immune variables poorly understood and thus immunomodulation must be viewed in a somewhat limited perspective of the overall transplant panorama.

Since chemical immunosuppression has formed the mainstay of immunomodulation for transplantation to date, it is a good place to begin. Current pancreas islet transplants have utilized the traditional immunomodulatory protocols devised by whole organ transplanters including immunosuppression with steroids, cyclosporine A, Imuran and a whole new set of drugs coming on the horizon with some such as FK506 nearly ready for widespread clinical application and others such as Deoxyspergualin (DSG) approved for human use but not widely accepted for specific application to transplantation. RS16443 is another drug which is in an advanced phase of clinical evaluation and has shown promise in experimental islet transplantation.[17] An important perspective in this area is the appreciation of the inherent limitations of chronic immunosuppression for islet transplantation in diabetics who do not tolerate the rigors of immunosuppression well. In addition, the islet transplanter has his work made more difficult by the known islet toxicity of virtually all of the conventional drugs including prednisone, cyclosporine A, Imuran and FK506. RS16443 acting in many respects much like Imuran would be highly suspect as having a inherent islet toxicity since it has been considered a type of "super Imuran". However, DSG, has been shown by our group and others, to be nontoxic to islets in culture[1,2] and this may be a factor in some of it's early clinical success.[18]

The inherent toxicity of these conventional drugs coupled with the general inadvisability of chronic immunosuppression in islet transplantation clearly dampens our enthusiasm for reliance on these drugs in future islet immunomodulation protocols. There seems little doubt that the immediate future of islet transplantation will be dependent on some of these drugs but highly doubtful that they will form the mainstay of the immunomodulatory techniques in the long run.

Previous techniques of incompatible transplantation without steroids have been essentially unsuccessful. One of the best examples was the use of cyclosporine initially as monotherapy in whole organ grafting. Starzl's description of the early requirement for steroids which appears to continue in most patients with this drug, represented a major advance leading to the success of CsA modulation. Unfortunately, steroids seem to be about the most toxic of the suppressive drugs for the islets. On the other hand, islet transplantation has recently been demonstrated to be feasible experimentally without steroid immunosuppression, a happy situation, which is only rarely seen in other organ transplants. Thus, future efforts at immunomodulation will most certainly involve minimal use or complete discontinuance of steroid therapy. Imuran or RS16443 are acceptible and effective immunosuppressants for islet transplantation. Experimentally deoxyspergualin (DSG) has been shown to effect strikingly prolonged islet graft survival with adjunctive steroids and using a short (14-28 day) course which results in induction of functional tolerance with islet xenografts.[6,19] This impressive work needs to be reproduced and further studied. Cyclosporine A has been the major drug contributing to the recent improvements in allograft survival and it is a likely candidate as a primary drug for early islet transplantation. However, a number of investigators have reported clear-cut in vitro and in vivo evidence for cyclosporine islet toxicity and thus, the drug has major limitation for immunomodulation of islet transplants in the future. FK506 has produced some of the most impressive islet survivals, but it too, has toxic effects on islets with some species variability. The drug does appear to have a special utility in xenografts however.[20]

Deoxyspergualin was first reported to be immunosuppressive in pancreas islet grafts by Nakiyama and Dickneite[18] although the drug was poorly effective in these studies. Hsu and Thomas reported the drug to be more effective than FK506 and cyclosporine in xenografts in 1988.[20] Ochiai confirmed that the drug was more effective than FK506 in 1989.[21] DSG effects were summarized for clinical and experimental results which demonstrated a particular utility of this drug in pancreatic islet grafts in 1991 and 1992.[18] This summary is the most comprehensive review of this drug to date and summarizes the potential of the drug to induce tolerance in islet transplantation as well as its overall efficacy in islet xenografting.[18] In 1993, Gores and Sutherland reported the use of the drug in two diabetics without steroids, one of whom became insulin independent.[22]

The efficacy of DSG in pancreas islet grafting and especially in xenotransplantation have not been explained to date. The overall effectiveness of the drug may be a result of a combination of factors. It has been suggested but not proven, that the drug acts on macrophages to decrease antigen presentation and other deleterious proinflammatory responses of macrophages. The drug is unique in that it does not appear to have toxic effects on transplanted islets unlike virtually all other suppressive agents used at present, including steroids, cyclosporine A, FK506 and Imuran. A combination of effectiveness in blocking early efferent rejection arc, as well as a lack of toxicity of the agent on islets are apparently major factors in the effectiveness of this agent in islet transplantation. It should be pointed out, however, that the agent is also effective in islet allotransplatation and indeed in allotransplantation of most organs. In a study in our laboratory, fully allogeneic cardiac grafts were prolonged more effectively by this agent than by cyclosporine.[18] The agent has been used in clinical transplantation with good results although its use has been largely confined to Japan, where the major source of donors is the living related donor and thus the agent needs further testing in cadaveric transplantation. The action of this agent is characterized by a strong antihumoral activity which blocks the development of humoral antibodies more effectively than any other suppressive agent available.[18] This may give the agent a special utility in transplantation of highly presensitized patients and may also go far towards explaining its special utility in xenografting where humoral antibody is known to be central to the xenograft rejection. Kaufman et al have implicated the macrophage as the major mediator or primary nonfunction in islet grafts and have attributed the beneficial effects of DSG to the blocking of macrophage activity in islet grafts.[16] In our own studies, the addition of anti-macrophage agents such as silica were unable to reduce the rate of PNF beyond that seen with DSG alone.[24] PNF was also favorably influenced by splenectomy and thus we have concluded that humoral antibody may be a major mediator of primary nonfunction of pancreas islets similar to the effect it has in primary nonfunction of other transplanted organs. The most striking effect of DSG in islet grafting is its ability to produce functional tolerance of the islet grafts and the survival of the grafts 100-200 days beyond the administration of the last dose of ATG. This effect was first reported by Thomas et al in 1993.[19] These authors grafted adult pig xenogeneic islets into the difficult NOD mouse and found survival of the islets to over 200 days beyond the last dose of immunosuppressive drug given (DSG on day 14). These results would appear to be most exciting since the goal of permitting long-term islet graft survival without chronic immunosuppressive drugs has been a major aim of islet immunosuppression. A number of authors have noted that the islet transplants will only have a large success in diabetics if they are able to replace islet function satisfactorily without requiring the administration of chronic immunosuppressive drugs, since the drugs have morbidity and mortality that rivals that of the type I diabetic condition itself and thus one is only trading one disease, diabetes, for another of chronic immunosuppression.[1,2,9]

In summary, the ability of DSG to induce this tolerance of such a striking nature in long-term grafts of highly disparate tissue from adult pigs is of great interest. A similar effect is seen with grafting of disparate xenograft hearts in other models. The result is unexplained, but is most likely due to the early blockade of humoral antibody since DSG is effective in blocking early rejection of xenografts in the nude rat where T cell function is ablated. Under these conditions, rejection occurs by a B cell mechanism but can be strikingly prolonged from 3 days to over 100 days by administration of DSG and splenectomy to block the humoral antibody response.[18]

In summary, DSG is one of the most effective and promising agents for future immunosuppression and islet grafting, especially islet xenograft-ing. The agent appears to act primarily by blockage of humoral antibody, although an effect on the macrophage has not been ruled out. The agent is effective in blocking primary nonfunction in early graft rejection of islets and has produced the most striking and prolonged function of discordant xenograft islets in both the STZ and NOD mouse model. Of potentially great importance is the ability of DSG to induce a functional tolerance of discordant xenograft such that the grafts survive up to 200 days or more beyond the administration of DSG. This is recognized to be one of the most laudible aspects of this drug.

Monoclonal and polyclonal anti-T cell reagents have been used to prolong islet graft survival. Unfortunately, most of the work with monoclonal agents use the mouse recipient where graft acceptance between weak and strong barriers is strikingly easy to obtain in contrast to higher animals and even other forms of rodents.[25,26] In early experiments in our laboratory, marked prolongation to over 100 days was achieved with some of the most disparate xeno-combinations available such as human islets into mouse. When we attempted to repeat this phenomena in the Lewis rat, however, early graft rejection occurred despite strong immunosuppression. Major questions as to the validity of the mouse recipient model for islet testing have recently been raised by at least two laboratories.[27,28] In the studies of Brayman et al, mouse recipients clearly tolerated islet grafts with high degrees of antigenic disparity that evoked strong rejection in other rodent recipients. The subject of the validity of the mouse model was the focus of a presentation and publication from the 2nd International Xenograft Conference in which mouse survival was noted to be easy to obtain and a variety of different xenografts is contrasted to rat recipient survival. At present, it seems incumbent for all investigators to attempt to apply findings that are promising in the mouse to other animal models, at least other rodent species although extension to higher animals would be even more desirable. Unfortunately, attempts to induce tolerance in higher animals with single monoclonal antibodies have been uniformly unsuccessful,[26] although Bromberg et al did induce tolerance in rodent vascularized grafts with a cocktail of anti-CD2 and anti-CD3 monoclonal antibodies.[29] Finally, it needs to be noted that the enthusiastic results of transplants with anti-CD4 monoclonal antibodies have not been reproduced by some groups even in the mouse.[25] In the case of xenotransplantation of islets, the anti-CD4 antibody does not appear to be effective with only temporarily prolongation of xenograft survival of less than 4 weeks seen in most animals tested.[30]

The polyclonal antilymphocyte and antithymocyte globulins, especially rabbbit ATG, are markedly effective in prolonging islet allografts in mice and rats.[2] Potential explanations for this immunosuppresive effect which appears to be far stronger than the effects seen with most monoclonal antibodies was developed recently by Rebellato et al who reported high titers of multiple monoclonal antibodies specificities in a polyclonal ATG preparation.[31] These included antibodies to the adhesion molecules, macrophages, T and B cells, and other specificities which are only beginning to be understood in allograft rejection. These agents may be important in synergizing with drugs such as DSG in the future immunosuppressive protocols and are also notable for their lack of systemic toxicity in a variety of animals. The agents, as could be expected, have no known toxic effects on islets which tends to place them in the non-toxic category of DSG making them especially useful for islet grafting.

A number of authors have reported recently on the ability of new monoclonal antibodies, such as the CTL4 fusion protein, to induce long-term tolerance of grafts. This effect is postulated to be related to the blocking of the second (costimulatory) signal for T cell activation. While these results are exciting, both from a conceptual and a practical point of view, recent studies have suggested that additional cell epitopes maybe involved in costimulation and B7 (now designated B7-1 vs. B7-2) blockade may not be sufficent to block costimulation.[32,33]

Perhaps the most exciting potential development in islet immunomodulation today is the possibility of development of techniques of donor specific tolerance in higher animals. Tolerance has long been considered the "Holy Grail" of transplantation and was pointed out by Medawar as the long-term goal of transplantation immunomodulation many years ago. Unfortunately, little solid progress was made in this field until the last few years. However, in the last few years a number of exciting new reports have indicated that increased knowledge in this area may well permit satisfactory techniques of donor-specific tolerance in the future.[3,4,12,34]

Most importantly, donor-specific tolerance has been developed in larger animals in non-islet grafting, specifically the dog and Rhesus primates.[35,36] These results were important in indicating the development of tolerance in animal models was not limited to rodent models with their associated vexaciousness but rather could be applied to models such as the Rhesus primate which represents a preclinical model and provides a scientific and ethical justification for application of this technique to the human. Barber et al did a randomized prospective study in kidney recipient transplants with donor kidneys procured from the same cadaver donor, one transplanted in the control group and one kidney placed into a experimental group treated with donor bone marrow to induce donor specific tolerance. Despite the number of problems with logistics and scientific rationale for the use of various donor bone marrow elements related to the need for better knowledge of the mechanism involved in this effect, Barber was able to achieve a significant improvement in graft survival to a level of 90% cadaver graft survival in a longstanding unit for survival in a control group as well as a historical control group had been in the range of 70% for many years.[4]

In addition to the clear empirical development of donor specific tolerance in these higher animal models including man, results have been noted recently indicating that a type of microchimerism occurs in the recipients which gives rise to the exciting possibility that long-term stable tolerance may be generated by a known mechanism which can be quantitated and further developed. Studies in our laboratory have demonstrated that DR depleted donor bone marrow is more effective than fractionated marrow in generating donor specific tolerance and that adjuvant protocol such as posttransplant TLI may be more effective than the polyclonoal ATG used previously.[37,38] Long-term survival without any chronic immunosuppression up to 3 and 4 years posttransplant has recently been achieved in primates. Present studies are in progress looking at development of donor specific tolerance in islets in primates and other higher animals. If these studies show effectiveness of the donor specific transplant protocol using donor bone marrow then a clear scientific and ethical rationale will be available for application of this technique to the human diabetic. A system of donor specific tolerance coupled with techniques for islet transplantation which could be achieved with minimal morbidity and mortality such as outpatient injection of islets into the portal vein for example would represent a potentially satisfactory technique for trials of islet transplantation early in the development of diabetes in younger people. This would permit a more reasonable test of the ability of islet transplantation to reverse secondary complications of diabetes since the transplantation could then be applied to patients before the development of severe and irreversable disease such as that seen in diabetic with renal failure or other irreversible severe complications present in the bulk of patients referred for pancreas transplantation at the present time.

Immunomodulation of donor islets has been a subject of great interest for many years. The donor islets are an unusual graft which can be cultured and modulated over a period of 14-21 days. Indeed, the islets can even be frozen away for prolonged periods of time and biopreservation per se appears to produce a decrease in immunogenicity of the islets in many of these studies reported. Early studies of endocrine tissue in culture developed the concept that the culturing of these tissues could produce a decreased immunogenecity although the precise mechanism by which this occurred was not clear. Lafferty et al were one of the first groups to demonstrate the decreased immunogenecity of islets in culture and attributed this to a loss of the so-called passenger leukocyte compartment of the islets which is responsible for a strong stimulatory response of donor tissue.[7] Some authors have noted the ability of islets cultured at 24° C, islets cultured with UV treatment, islets treated with gamma irradiation and culture, and a variety of other islet treatments to be subimmunogeneic when transplanted.[1,2] More recently it has been suggested that a modification of the class I immunogenicity of islets in culture may be responsible for the long-term graft survival of cultured islets. Hardy's group has done elegant work in demonstrating that ultraviolet light treatment of islets acts to reduce immunogenicity of the donor graft.[39] A most exciting paper was reported recently by Markmann et al in which islets from transgenic mice in which homologous recombination was used to develop a mouse lacking class I antigens on all germ line cells had an indefinite survival in an incompatible recipient.[8] These results suggest that matching for class I disparities in islet grafting may be of importance although this was not seen with whole organ graft pancreas grafting.[1,2,9] Our laboratory has independently obtained the same results reported by Markmann et al in a different recipient species, thus adding to the validity of this finding. However, Markmann's studies additionally demonstrated that class I depletion did not result in prolonged survival of islet xenografts. Desai et al have also reported deficiencies in islet allograft rejection in class I deficient recipients, thus providing an elegant model for further studies of T cell subpopulations in islet rejection and immunomodulation.[40] Much more work needs to be done in this field which offers the exciting potential for transgenic modification of donor tissue to achieve prolonged graft survival.

Empirically it seems quite clear that islets cultured for a minimal period of 5 days will produce better graft survival than is seen with fresh islets unless the islets can be isolated by hand picking with the use of minimal collagenase digestion enzymes which disrupts exocrine tissue and produces a strong proinflammatory response. Markedly prolonged times of islet preservation using cryotechniques has also given evidence that further culturing may be useful in decreasing the immunogenecity of islets. It may be important to note that few clinical studies to date have utilized prolonged islet culture and that this may be a technique which should be used more extensively in islet transplantation in the future.

The transplantation of islets to naturally immunologically privileged sites (in contrast to artifical techniques of immunoisolation using bioexclusion membrane) is an area of great interest. In some systems such as transplantation of islets into brain tissue or the testes the evidence for immune privilege seems clear cut.[41] The value of immune privileged sites in prolonging allografts has been shown repeatedly in animal models involving the hamster cheek pouch, the anterior chamber of the eye and numerous other models. Recently a potentially useful new area of transplantation was developed using the intrathymic islet transplants by Naji's group.[42] The precise technique by which this intrathymic islet transplantation works is not known. The immunologically privileged nature of the thymic stroma may be one factor but Naji's work suggests that a generalized tolerance is produced which may relate to the positive and negative selection of cells in the thymus which are reactive to donor islet cells. This technique needs to be applied to higher animals in the future. Early attempts to apply the technique to larger animals have apparently been unsuccessful to date. The system is also plagued by the severe involution of thymic tissue which occurs in the late juvenile and adult period of life. Thus, it is difficult on autopsy dissection to identify pancreas tissue and would undoubtedly be quite difficult to inject islets into the fibrostroma which represents the remnants of a earlier and more identifiable mass of thymus tissue. The technique might be useful however in young adults if it could be made innocuous by techniques of minimally invasive implantation of the islets coupled with the use of low doses of immunosuppression or perhaps no immunosuppression at all with one of the donor specific tolerance protocols.

An important need for future studies is improvement in the models available for testing techniques of immunomodulation in islets. As mentioned, the use of the mouse in islet transplantation is a questionably valid technique of potentially low relevance to higher animals. Most authorities agree that future techniques need to be carried in testing to the primate prior to their application to islet transplantation in the human. Another thorny issue is the use of animals made diabetic by streptozotocin (STZ) or other chemical toxins. Animals treated by STZ clearly retain the capacity to regenerate islets in the native pancreas. The use of the subcapsular kidney injection of islets permits testing of this vexacious variable by nephrectomy which produces prompt diabetes if euglycemia is being maintained by the transplanted islets alone. In addition, these animals do not have the high degree of propensity to autoimmune disease recurrence that is seen in the NOD mouse and the BB rat. In this respect it should be mentioned that newer developments in transgenic technology have permitted the creation of a NOD scid mouse which can be reconstituted selectively with immune elements to assay the potential contribution of these immune element to the immune reactivity associated with both islet rejection as well as autoimmune graft recurrence. These transgenic techniques including techniques for modification of class I and class II antigens on the surface of islets offer great potential for studying mechanisms of islet rejection and immunomodulation which no doubt will lead to a better understanding and better treatment for future islet transplantations.[8,40] It is difficult to overestimate the importance of these elegant techniques in future studies. It is important to point out also that the transgenic techniques are especially applicable to xenograft studies where modulation of donor tissue can be achieved and indeed donor tissue can be used as a vector so to speak for the transplantation of insulin producing transgenic tissue to a recipient with deficient action of his insulin producing tissue mass.[1,2]

A number of authors have worked with systems of so-called nesidioblastosis attempting to generate mature functioning insulin producing tissue from primative pluripotent cells as seen in embryos or other sources of undifferentiated pancreatic tissue. While this tissue may have logistic advantages in terms of the availability of large amounts of islet tissue, the best immunological evidence to date suggests that there is little if any immune advantage conferred upon these cells by their immaturity.[43] On the positive side, the use of fetal tissue could certainly go as a long way towards bridging the gap in donor tissue shortage especially in countries where abortion is widely practiced and ethical constraints on abortion and the use of fetal tissue are minimal. Apparently, fetal tissue is a major source of the islets transplanted to date in countries such as China.[44] Current ethical controversies over abortion in the Western World will likely produce severe constraints on fetal tissue transplantation in the near future. Overall, fetal tissue seems useful primarily to ease donor shortages while no clear-cut advantage in immunogenecity or immunomodulation can be seen with use of fetal tissue.

Finally the ultimate form of immunomodulation of pancreas islets would be immunomodulation to prevent the development of IDDM in islets prior to their irreversable destruction by this inexorable disease process. Progress along these lines awaits the development of techniques for blocking autoimmunity which has a striking resemblance to the rejection reactions seen with pancreas islets.[9] The best knowledge of mechanisms of rejection of these pancreas islets may in turn permit the development of better knowledge of the immune processes which create the islet immune destruction in the first place. Following the development of techniques to treat autoimmune islet disease the expansion of systems for early diagnosis of this disease in susceptible individuals such as the use of the GAD (glutamic acid decarboxylase) enzymes or islet cell antibody measurements to detect early prediabetic state would permit application of drugs at an early time in hopes of evading the autoimmune process given rise to IDDM. Early clinical studies using such drugs as cyclosporine have been instituted but the efficacy of these techniques to date has not been established. From the point of view of islet transplantation such techniques would not necessarily sound a death knell for islet transplantation in the immediate future since there remains a large number of juvenile diabetics with irreversable damage to their islets. In addition recent studies have suggested that islet transplantation may be applicable to type II diabetics who suffer from a disease (NIDDM) which is not apparently an autoimmune disease process and would not therefore yield to immunomodulation to abort an immune process destroying the islets.[45] Although amyloid peptide has been linked to this disease, the amyloid process is probably a late and secondary immune process and could not be halted by early immune treatment. Reversal of the NIDDM process has been achieved in four animal models.[1,2,45] In these studies four animal models of NIDDM given islet transplants had essentially all glycemic parameters return to normal but the precise role of transplantation treatment of this disease has not been established to date although early experimental results are promising.

CONCLUSION

This chapter has attempted to provide a broad overview of the prospects for future treatment of diabetes by pancreas islets with focus on immunomodulation to achieve long-term pancreas graft survival. The incredible complexity of this field has been noted, a situation which provides both many problems as well as many opportunities to the islet transplanter of the future. The ability to modify donor islet tissue in culture is currently a technique of extraordinary potential. The history of transplantation to date has not recorded such a large potential for donor tissue modification, a technique which represents a highly desirable form of immunomodulation since it does not compromise the immune system of the recipient. It is difficult to underestimate the potential for transgenic techniques to improve future islet transplantation in the future. Transgenic techniques could permit a number of major immunomodulatory steps to reduce the immunogenecity of islets including the down regulation or complete removal of the class I, II or both antigens of the allogeneic cells in culture or by manipulation of xenogeneic islets. In many of these systems, the largest potential can clearly be found in the xenograft islets. It should be noted that it is not at all clear that the immune barrier to xenotransplantation is refractory to current immunomodulatory therapy in the case of cellular transplants such as islets which are not rejected hyperacutely. Our own experience to date suggests that xenografts are strikingly easy to prolong and, indeed, even induce tolerogenicity to using DSG and polyclonal ATG.[1,2,6,18,19,24] The xenogeneic rejection reaction with respect to the central cell in rejection to date (the T cell) is a remarkably weak one. The bulk of immune reactivity in the xenograft occurs apparently in the endothelial antigen reaction[47] which is minimal to absent in islets. The islet cell antibody response is not clearly strong enough to destroy islets in most cases and it may be possible in the future with the use of drugs which better control the immune response to xenografts such as DSG to achieve long lasting graft survival. Of perhaps greatest excitement in immunomodulation is the recent progress in the field of tolerance of a donor specific nature to disparate tissues both allogeneic and xenogeneic. Such donor specific tolerance would permit the long-term graft survival without chronic immunosuppression which is necessary for the successful treatment of diabetics at an early stage in their disease. Techniques to modulate the immune system with immunosuppressants such as RS16443 or Rapamycin may well prove fruitful also and other techniques for donor tissue modulation in culture may be rewarding and some may, as yet, be undiscovered. It is the personal bias of this reviewer that future techniques for immunomodulation of islets will carefully examine the potential for immunomodulation by immuno exclusion techniques using bioreactors of types which have already shown potential in higher animals.

There is a rational need at the present time to apply many of these systems, especially immune tolerance and techniques of immunoexclusion, which appear to be useful to the human in preliminary studies. In some cases, the ethical and medical basis for these studies will reside in preclinical primate testing which has been shown to be feasible and available. Clearly, the future goals of these techniques is to permit the use of transplantation in the early course of diabetes before irreversible complications have occurred and without the use of chronic immunosuppression. It is only by achieving this goal that islet transplantation will be perceived as a reasonable alternative to the chronic and morbid diseases of conventionally treated Type I diabetes.

References

1. Thomas, F. Isolated Pancreas Islet Xenografting. in Xenotransplantation. DKC Cooper, DJG White and E Kemp (eds.). Springer-Verlag, New York, pp. 275-296, 1991.
2. Thomas, FT. Panreas islet transplantation. Current Surgery 1991; 343-353.
3. Thomas, JM, Carver, FM, Cunningham, PR, Olson, LC, Thomas, FT. Kidney Allograft Tolerance in Primates Without Chronic Immunosuppression—The Role of Veto Cells. Transplantation. 1991; 51(1):198-207.
4. Barber, WH. Induction of Tolerance to Human Renal Allografts with Bone Marrow and Antilymphocyte Globulin. Transplantation Reviews. July 1990; 4(1):68-78.
5. Thomas, FT, Demasi, RJ, Araneda, D, Marchman, W, Alqaisi, M, Larkin, EW, Condie, RM, Carobbi, A, Thomas, JM. Comparative Efficacy of Immunosuppressive Drugs in Xenografting. Transplant Proceed. 1990; 22(3):1083-5.
6. Henretta J, Pittman K, Thomas J, and Thomas F. Deoxyspergualin and rabbit antithymocyte globulin markedly prolong discordant pig pancreatic islet xenografts. Transplant Proceed 1993; 25(1): 412-413.
7. Simeonvic, CJ, Bowen, KM, Kotlarski, I, Lafferty, KJ. Modulation of Tissue Immunogenicity by Organ Culture. Transplantation. 1980; 30:174.
8. Markmann JF, Bassiri H, Desai NM, Odorico JS, Kim JI, Kollmer BH, Smithies O, and Barker CF. Indefinite survival of MHC Class I-deficient murine pancreatic islet allografts. Transplantation 1992; 54(6): 1085-1089.
9. McClaren, N, and Lafferty, K. Perspectives in Diabetes: The 12th International Immunology and Diabetes Workshop. Diabetes. 1993; 42:1099.
10. Gotoh, M, Maki, T, Porter, J, and Monaco, AP. Augmented Survival of Pancreatic Islets Transplantation Using H-2 Incompatible Multiple Donors . Transplant Proceed. 1987; 19(2):957-959.
11. Ricordi, C, Starzl, TE. Cellular Transplants. Transplant Proceed. 1991; 23(1):73.
12. Thomas, JM, Verbanac, KM, Thomas, FT. The Veto Mechanism in Transplant Tolerance. Transplantation Reviews. 1991; 5(4):209-229.
13. Lacy, PE, Kostianovsky, MA. A Method for the Isolation of Intact Islets of Langerhans From the Rat Pancreas. Diabetes. 1967; 16:35.
14. Ricordi, C, Lacy, PE, Finke, EH, Olack, BJ, Scharp, DW. Automated Method for Isolation of Human Pancreatic Islets. Diabetes. 1988; 37:413.
15. Ricordi, C, Socci, C, Davalli, AM, Staudacher, C, Baro, P, Vertova, A, Sassi, I, Gavazzi, F, Pozza, G, DiCarlo, V. Isolation of the Elusive Pig Islet. Surgery. 1990; 107:688.
16. Kaufman, DB, Platt, JL, Rabe, FL, Dunn, DL, Bach, FH, Sutherland, DER. Differential Roles of MAC-1+ Cells, and CD4+ and CD8+ T Lymphocytes in Primary Non Function and Classic Rejection of Islet Allografts. J Exp Med. 1990; 172:291-302.

17. Coulombe, M, Hao, L, Calcinaro, F, Gill, RG, Eugui, EM, Allison, AC, Lafferty, KJ. Tolerance Induction in Adult Animals: Comparison of RS61443 and Anti-CD4 Treatment. Transplant Proceed. 1991; 23 (2/2):31-2.
18. Thomas FT, Tepper MA, Thomas JM, and Haisch CE. 15-Deoxyspergualin: A novel immunosuppressive drug with clinical potential. Annals of New York Academy of Sciences. 685:175-192, June 1993.
19. Thomas FT, Pittman K, Henretta J, Haisch CE, and Thomas, J. Induction of tolerance to discordant pancreas islet xenografts by a short course of deoxyspergualin (DSG) and rabbit antithymocyte globulin (RATG). Transplant Science. 1994; 3(1):41-43.
20. Hsu, S, Thomas, J, Thomas, F. Synergism of FK-506 and Rabbit Antithymocyte Globulin in Prolongation of Xenografts. Surg Forum. 1988; 18:374-376.
21. Ochiai, T, Nakajima, K, Sakamoto, K, Ochiai, T, Asano, T, Isono, K. Effects of 15-Deoxyspergualin and FK506 on the Histology and Survival of Hamster-to-Rat Cardiac Xenotransplantation. 1989; 21(1): 546-548.
22. Gores, PF, Najarian, J, Stephanian, E, Kelly, S, Sutherland, DE. Insulin Independence in Type I Diabetes After Transplantation of Unpurified Islets From a Single Donor With 15-Deoxyspergualin. Lancet. January 1993.
23. Marchman, W, Araneda, D, DeMasi, R, Taylor, D, Larkin, E, Alqaisi, M, Thomas, F. Prolongation of Xenograft Survival After Combination Therapy with 15-Deoxyspergualin and Total Lymphoid Irradiation in the Hamster-to-Rat Xenograft Model.Transplantation 1992; 53(1):30-34.
24. Pittman, K, Thomas, F, McFadden, T, Haisch, C, Thomas, J. Reduction in Primary Nonfunction of Pancreas Islet Transplants With Antithymocyte Globulin Agents, Deoxyspergualin, and Splenectomy. Transplant Proceed. 1993; 25(1):986-987.
25. Kawai, M, Gotoh, M, Monden, M, Yamamoto, H, Ichikawa, T, Valdivia, LA, Mori, T, Uenaka, A, Nakayama, E. Effect of L3T4 and Lyt-2 Monoclonal Antibodies on Islet Xenograft (Rat to Mouse) Rejection. 1989; 21(1):2709-2710.
26. Wood KJ, Pearson TC, Darby C, and Morris. CD4: A potential target molecule for immunosuppressive therapy and tolerance induction. Transplant Reviews 1991; 5(3): 150-164.
27. Brayman, KL, Morel, P, Field, J, Lloveras, JJ, Leventhal, J, Nakhleh, R, Jessurun, J, Platt, J, Matas, AJ, Najarian, JS, et al. A Comparison of Mice and Rats as Recipients for Canine Islet Xenografts. Transplant Proceed. 1992; 24(2):651-2.
28. Araneda, D, Moon, S, Pittman, K, Thomas, F. Consideration of the Validity of Mouse-Rat Xenograft Combinations in Xenograft Testing. Transplant Proceed. 1994. In press.
29. Chavin, KD, Qin, L, Lin, J, Yagita, H, Bromberg, JS. Combined Anti-CD2 and Anti-CD3 Receptor Monoclonal Antibodies induce Donor Specific Tolerance in a Cardiac Transplant Model. J Immunol 1993; 151(12:7249-59.
30. Simeonovich, CJ, Ceredig, R, and Wilson, JD. Effect of GK1.5 Monoclonal Antibody Dosage On Survival of Pig Proislet Xenografts in CD4+ T Cell-Depleted Mice. Transplantation. 1990; 49(5):849-856.
31. Rebellato, LM, Gross, U, Verbanac, KM, Thomas, JM. A Comprehensive Definition of the Major Antibody Specificities in Polyclonal Rabbit Antithymocyte Globulin. Transplant. 1994; 57:84-88.
32. Lombard, LA, Gray, GS, Lee, MN. Cloning of B7-2: A CTLA-4 Counter Receptor That Costimulates Human T Cell Proliferation. Science. 1993; 262:909.
33. Freeman, GJ, Borriello, F, Hodes, RJ, Reiser, H, Hathcock, KS, Laszlo, G, McKnight, AJ, Kim, J, Du, L, Lombard, DB, Gray, GS, Nadler, LM, Sharpe, AH. Uncovering of Functional Alternative CTLA-4 Counter-Receptor in B-7 Deficient Mice. Science. 1993; 262:907-909.
34. Thomas, JM, Carver, FM, Cunningham, PR, Gross, U, Verbanac, KM, Rebellato, LM, Riley, R, Thomas, FT. Donor Bone Marrow Infusion Suppresses Alloantibody Response In RATG-Treated Recipients: A Correlate of Long Survival. Transplant Proceed. 1993; 25(1):342-343.

35. Hartner, WC, DeFazio, SR, Markees, TG, Maki, T, Monaco, AP, Gozzo, JJ. Specific Tolerance to Canine Renal Allografts Following Treatment with Fractured Bone Marrow and Antitlymphocyte Serum. Transplant Proceed. 1987;19(1):476-477.
36. Thomas, JM, Carver, FM, Kasten-Jolly, J, Haisch, CE, Rebellato, LM, Gross, U, Vore, SJ, Thomas, FT. Further Studies of Veto Activity in Rhesus Monkey Bone Marrow in Relation to allograft Tolerance and Chimerism. Transplantation. 1994; 57(1): 101-115.
37. Thomas, J, Carver, M, Cunningham, P, Park, K, Gonder, J. Promotion of Incompatible Allograft Acceptance in Rhesus Monkeys Given Posttransplant Antithymocyte Globulin and Donor Bone Marrow: I. In Vivo Parameters and Immunohistologic Evidence Suggesting Microchimerism. Transplantation.1987; 43(3):332.
38. Thomas, JM, Alqaisi, M, Cunningham, P, Carver, M, Rebellato, L, Gross, U, Patselas, T, Araneda, D, Thomas, F. The Development of a Posttransplant TLI Treatment Strategy That Promotes Organ Allograft Acceptance Without Chronic Immunosuppression. Transplantation. 1992; 53(2): 247-58.
39. Hardy, MA, and Oluwole, SF. Effect of Ultraviolet Radiation on Immunogenecity of Tissues and Organ Allografts. Transplantation Reviews. January 1991; 5(1):46-62.
40. Desai, NM, Bassiri, H, Kim, J, Koller, BH, Smithies, O, Barker, CF, Naji, A, Markmann, JF. Islet Allograft, Islet Xenograft, and Skin Allograft Survival in CD8+ T Lymphocyte-Deficient Mice. Transplantation. 1993; 55(4):718-722.
41. Selawry, HP, Whittington, KB, Bellgrau, D. Abdominal Intratesticular Islet-Xenograft Survival in Rats. Diabetes. 1989; 38 Suppl 1:220-3.
42. Posselt, AM, Campos, L, Mayo, GL, O'Connor, TP, Odorico, JS, Markmann, JF, Barker, CF, Naji, A. Selective Modulation of T Cell Immunity by Intrathymic Cellular Transplantation. Transplantation Reviews. 1993; 7(4):200.
43. Andersson, A, and Sandler, S. Fetal Pancreatic Transplantation. Transplantation Reviews. 1992; 6(1):20-38.
44. Hu, YF, Gu, ZF, Zhang, HD, Ye, RS. Fetal Islet Cell Transplantation in China. Transplant Proceed. 1989; 21:2605-607.
45. Thomas F, Pittman K, McFadden T, Haisch C, Peterson R, and Thomas J. Reversal of Type II diabetes by pancreas islet transplant in four separate animal models of Type II diabetes. Transplant Proceed 1993; 25(1): 992-993.
46. Auchincloss, H, Jr. Xenografting: A Review. Transplantation Reviews. 1990; 4(1):14-27.
47. Haisch, CE, Lodge, PA, Huber, SA, Thomas, FT. The Vascular Endothelial Cell is Central to Xenogeneic Immune Reactivity. Surgery. 1990; 108(2):306-11.

INDEX

Page numbers in italics denote figures (f) and tables (t).

D

E

F

G

H

I

J

K

L

M

N

O

P

R

S